T0276122

Ethics in Everyday Places

Basic Bioethics
Arthur Caplan, editor

A complete list of the books in the Basic Bioethics series appears at the back of this book.

Ethics in Everyday Places

Mapping Moral Stress, Distress, and Injury

Tom Koch

Esri Press
Redlands, CA

The MIT Press
Cambridge, Massachusetts
London, England

Copublished by the MIT Press and Esri Press.

This book was set in Stone Serif and Stone Sans by Toppan Best-set Premedia Limited.

Library of Congress Cataloging-in-Publication Data

Names: Koch, Tom, 1949– author.
Title: Ethics in everyday places : mapping moral stress, distress, and injury / Tom Koch.
Description: Cambridge, MA : MIT Press, 2017. | Series: Basic bioethics | Includes bibliographical references and index.
Identifiers: LCCN 2017016888 | ISBN 9780262037211 (hardcover : alk. paper), ISBN 9780262546621 (paperback)
Subjects: LCSH: Ethics. | Cartography—Miscellanea.
Classification: LCC BJ1012 .K55 2017 | DDC 170—dc23 LC record available at https://lccn.loc.gov/2017016888

For Margaret Cottle, Ken Hirsh, Harvey Pasternak, and Nancy Withers:
Friends, physicians, and teachers all.

Contents

Series Foreword

Glenn McGee and I developed the Basic Bioethics series and collaborated as series coeditors from 1998 to 2008. In fall 2008 and spring 2009 the series was reconstituted, with a new Editorial Board, under my sole editorship. I am pleased to present the forty-ninth book in the series.

The Basic Bioethics series makes innovative works in bioethics available to a broad audience and introduces seminal scholarly manuscripts, state-of-the-art reference works, and textbooks. Topics engaged include the philosophy of medicine, advancing genetics and biotechnology, end-of-life care, health and social policy, and the empirical study of biomedical life. Interdisciplinary work is encouraged.

Arthur Caplan

Preface

This is about that sinking feeling that comes when you've done everything right, played by the rules, and yet know you've done something wrong. It attempts to understand the dilemma that occurs when you seek to do good but find your best intentions stymied. It isn't about simple "moral intuitions" or making the best possible choice. Rather, it is about those situations in which moral intuitions do not serve because every alternative is bad.

Moral distress is a hot topic these days in moral philosophy and psychology. My work differs from that of most writers in those areas in several immediately obvious ways. First, I reject the assumption that moral stress, distress, and injury are limited largely to members of this or that particular profession. Rather, I argue they are a chronic and pervasive reality in modern Western society. Second, I refuse allegiance to one or another school of moral philosophy and remain constitutionally suspicious of theoretical propositions not grounded in the concrete realities of everyday life. Thus while I do discuss the insights of moral philosophers and ethicists, I build my argument from the ground up, on the experiential basis of normal folk in daily life.

Perhaps most significantly, this investigation relies on maps, which I present as cultural artifacts in which issues of ethics and morality are embedded. Professional cartographers and the works they produce provide an evidentiary backbone in this work not because mapmakers face unique problems but because they do not. The ethical dilemmas they confront, and the questions that maps may raise, are little different in kind from those I have heard from doctors, nurses, and social workers in medicine; graphic artists and reporters; demographers and statisticians; research librarians and others I have sometimes counseled and who, for this project, I have consulted.

The idea of "mapping morals" is an old one, born in the "moral statistics" developed in the nineteenth century to analyze public data in the early days of what we today call social science. Almost from the start, those statistics were mapped to present a comprehensible visual argument that focused reams of data bearing on social realities. The first great work in this field was André-Michel Guerry's *Essay on Moral Statistics* (*Essai sur la statistique morale de la France*, 1833), in which maps distilled and then presented data on a variety of subjects of social concern: charity, illiteracy, illegitimacy, criminal activity, health, poverty, and so on. Maps of incidence in this or that place and at one or another scale powered the search to understand clinical and social phenomena in a manner that might promote specific and what in the day were enlightened responses to them.

I employ that conjunction of morals and social circumstance here in an attempt to image what we mean by ethics, morals, and their traces in our daily lives. As chapter 2 explains, I began with questions raised by professional mapmakers about moral and ethical issues arising in their daily work lives. I quickly realized that their concerns were not specific to mapping but offered general examples of a greater problem. Thus mapping became not the subject but the medium for ethical exploration.

It is in part the sheer ubiquity of the map that recommends it to this kind of study. Maps are everywhere, from the morning newspaper to the evening newscast, embedded in academic journals and lofty tomes on a bewildering range of subjects. Maps proliferate across the World Wide Web. And, as I hope to demonstrate, all come bundled with a series of assumptions and presumptions that make of them not simple, factual presentations but ones whose construction is ethically grounded. As Mary Midgley put it in another context, "Facts are not gathered in a vacuum, but to fill gaps in a world-picture which already exists."[1] Mapping pictures a preconceived world within which a set of facts is chosen, organized, analyzed, and then argued.

In the main, "historians and philosophers struggle sternly to conceal their own interests and personalities behind a screen of graphs and statistics, vainly hoping that this will make them look as impersonal as physicists."[2] Let me state without apology that this work draws on my personal experiences. It began with questions that I couldn't answer at a meeting of cartographers in 2005. It continues with problems I considered but could not easily resolve. Chapter by chapter, it reviews subjects that have been the focus of my work for more than twenty years. It thus draws on my varying areas of expertise in ethics and bioethics, on the one hand, and on cartography, mapping, journalism and public health, on the other. Since I cannot pretend to Olympian objectivity, let me instead use this foreword to introduce myself, as well as the chapter-by-chapter program that resulted. There is nothing wrong with honest bias as long as it is clearly stated.

I am a US citizen by birth and a Canadian citizen by choice. My worldview, and that of this work, is therefore fundamentally North American. I make no general claims for the universality of its conclusions, although I believe that the materials presented, chapter by chapter, reflect more than a parochial perspective. Although I have studied, translated, and worked in other languages (Chinese, Spanish, and Japanese), English remains my primary working language. Thus the references at the back of the book are primarily to English-language works.

I have served for several decades as a gerontologist and as a medical ethicist specializing in chronic and palliative care. In those roles, I have struggled with the ethical conflicts and moral dilemmas expressed by patients who find the world they knew disappearing and, separately, the doctors, nurses, and social workers professionally enjoined to attend to those patients' needs. I have listened as some described how the vocational hopes they once entertained had been dimmed if not wholly extinguished by the realities of professional regulations and strictures.

The book's organization is more circular than linear in its attempt to bridge experience and theory, ethics, morals, and their practice. That is, as the book advances, it sometimes circles back to ideas earlier introduced. Chapter 1 reviews the idea of moral stress, distress, and injury as historical subjects and philosophical concerns. It briefly reviews that voluminous literature and places it firmly within a context of lived experience. The general theoretical grounding will be critical to some, but certainly not all, readers. Readers suspicious of philosophy and theory are invited to begin their reading with chapter 2. They can return to the first chapter's comments at need and at their leisure.

Chapters 2 through 4 are more ethnographic than philosophical, presenting what some might call a Foucauldian archaeology or at least anthropology. Chapter 2 describes the meeting of working cartographers where I was first challenged to transpose the broad strokes of ethical discourse into something relevant to the mundane working world of professional mapmakers. If the attendees had ever taken an undergraduate course in applied ethics or philosophy, the lessons half learned in those classes seemed, they said, to offer little guidance in their daily lives and their resulting dilemmas. The question for me was how to create a space—both figural and literal—in which they might better consider the ethical issues that seemed to them problematic.

Chapter 3 presents the program I developed to explore the unease those cartographers described and, by extension, that members of other trades and professions—graphic artists, journalists, and social scientists—similarly experience. The goal was to create a scenario that raised issues but did not dictate solutions. From the start, what I called "the Tobacco Problem" was fashioned in a manner permitting me to investigate the troubling questions raised by classroom students and working professionals participating in seminar settings. It was in the teaching that what began as a question of ethics became an exercise in moral anthropology.

Over time the context of questions about ethical problems and moral foundations expanded. This was, again, as much a reflection of my own history as it was of the lessons learned in the evolving project or the lectures I was asked to give. I spent many years as a daily journalist writing for newspapers, magazines, the Canadian Broadcasting Corporation, and a wire service. So it is no surprise that journalistic examples appear across these pages. Because public media are voracious consumers of maps (and charts, graphs, and tables), expanding from the map to its published context seemed logical and, in retrospect, perhaps inevitable. And, too, it was clear early on that journalists and mapmakers are in a similar ethical bind. Chapter 3 therefore expands its focus from the cartographic specific to mapped arguments in popular media and finally in scientific journals.

Chapter 4, "The Morals in the Map," describes what happened when I took the problem of cartographic ethics into the classroom. In presenting audiences—undergraduate, graduate, and professional—with an ethical question for which there is no clear answer. I was able to draw from participants their views, encouraging them to perceive the manner in which ethics and their moral underpinnings informed their work. Their responses taught me a great deal about how issues of ethics and morals are perceived and then understood by average citizens. Those lessons prompted me to review things I had, in other contexts, considered earlier.

There the book stalled until Alexandria Enders, a geographer at the University of Montana, kindly sent me a map of governmentally defined poverty in US counties. What was this poverty, and why should I care about it? How did the map describe itself, and what was hiding in its presentation? In its facticity, I wondered, where *were* its ethics, and why was I not immediately outraged by the map's bald statement that more than one in eight Americans, citizens of my birth country, were living in poverty? Answering those questions, or at least raising them, is the subject of chapter 5 and the beginning of the "evidentiary" section of this book.

Because poverty and public education are intimately related, chapter 6 focuses on poverty's effects on the education of the US urban poor, and thus on society at large. At the University of British Columbia, my friend Ken Denike and I had explored and written about a seminal US court case that focused on the systemic links between education and poverty. Here that earlier work is reviewed and expanded as a way of locating the real effects (short- and long-term) of the poverty mapped in the previous chapter. The focus becomes not simply poverty, or the fact of poverty's effect on student education, but also the moral violation that results.

In the late 1980s, I spent a year at Ohio State University, studying transportation analytics with geographer Howard Gauthier. Chapter 7 draws on that experience in a case study of the means by which transit mapping (and thus planning) may hide the effect of travel barriers on persons who have mobility limits. Here was a way to build from my experiences as an arthritic with low vision to fashion a detailed study of the means by which people with physical or other differences are excluded from participation in our shared world. In this chapter, I focus on London's famous transit system and its iconic map. In the gulf between my map of mobility-restricted opportunities and the "official" map of London transit, I found a wide gulf between the ethical promise of inclusion and the realities of systemic exclusion.

Chapter 8 takes as its focus the US graft organ transplant system that I first studied in the 1990s. Here was a perfect subject for issues of not simply mapping but also statistics, as well as the way in which the force of our moral declarations is diminished (and sometimes denied) in the name of utilitarian practicality. Like its predecessor, this chapter finds the traces of poverty's effects in an area that, by law, is supposed to be egalitarian and noneconomic. Again, my earlier work was reviewed, revised, and extended with newly available data.

In the book's final part, chapters 9 and 10 attempt to bring these individual case studies together, to map (if you will) a coherent argument across the various insights their predecessors advanced. Readers who are looking for an easy fix, a straightforward, uncomplicated ethical rule, or an inflexible moral standard will be disappointed. It is simply not that easy, not ever. There is no one thing that makes the "right" always crystal clear and the "good" blindingly obvious. It's a messy world, as John Law says,[3] one in which complexity rather than simplicity rules.[4]

But because it is messy does not mean it is incomprehensible. A close analysis of mapped arguments does provide a kind of nested hierarchy that is prescriptive, rejecting both the anarchy of individual eccentricities ("I believe … no matter what you think or say") and the bludgeon of social imperatives ("You'll believe what we tell you to accept … no matter what"). We can understand conflicts by attending to the ethical propositions they present, and to the sometimes conflicting moral declarations an ethical proposition may invoke. The result is an experiment in ethics that seeks to join a consequential consideration of thick realities to the overriding presence of thinly principled value declarations. It is not the answer but *an* answer, a beginning but hopefully not the last word in assessing the moral queasiness of modern professional and social realities.

If the effort is successful, those of us who have known moments of uncertainty and distress will at the least be able to identify the source of our moral queasiness. Once ethics in places are seen as real (again, I want to say "mapped"), we can look for the linkages that will identify their associations in a manner permitting not only a better understanding of our dilemmas but, perhaps, at least a partial resolution.

This is a book about ethics and morals as understood through maps and what they say. That said, it is also about the arguments we make and the rationales on which they are based in societies that promise but do not always deliver on their best ideals. In thinking about those things, it also is about the distance between truth as a simple thing and truth as something shifting, uncertain, and dependent on the experiences we have and the perspectives we accept in the societies where we live.

It is hard to talk about ethics and morality without thinking about truths, because our judgments about good and bad, right and wrong, are bound up in the assumption that truth is an objective thing. It isn't. Instead the things we call truths are grounded in the values we hold as citizens, members of social groups, and professionals. That doesn't mean all truth is relative and can thus be dismissed as a chimera. Rather, it is to say that the truths we proclaim evolve over time as our societies evolve and change. Think of them as tectonic plates that support the world while shifting, slowly, beneath its surface.

There are no simple solutions to the complex questions of ethics, no litmus test that firmly establishes moral verities. There is no road map that ensures you or I can live easily and conscience free in a society where what we believe is right is so often a question of what is practical. What I can offer, perhaps, is some insight into what makes ethics and morality difficult things. I can point out the alternatives we face as persons in society and the result of those alternatives for society at large. I can offer some direction to the dilemmas we face in a world composed of coworkers, family members, neighbors, fellow citizens, and species members with whom we share the world.

That's not everything, of course. It may not even be much. But it's a beginning.

Acknowledgments

Writing may be a solitary craft, but it would be impossible without the assistance of a range of persons whose active support first informed its thinking and then enabled its production. This work, the culmination of almost three decades of work in cartography-geography, ethics and bioethics, and public health, has incurred more debts than most.

I am grateful indeed to four anonymous peer reviewers who evaluated the original manuscript and offered a series of critical suggestions that were incorporated into what is now the final text. The reviewers came from several disciplines, including, I deduced from their comments, ethics, geography, medical anthropology, and philosophy. Their insights were critically informative, approving of the general idea and its approach in a text that was vastly improved by their suggestions. Peer review, especially of book-length manuscripts, is a tiresome and unremunerative task. Those who undertake it are rarely acknowledged. It is therefore a pleasure to thank those who in this case undertook the responsibility and did so with care and attention.

In the same vein, this book owes its existence to the acquisitions editors at both Esri Press, which published my earlier *Cartographies of Disease*, and the MIT Press, which published my book *Thieves of Virtue: When Bioethics Stole Medicine*. Kathleen Morgan of Esri worked with MIT Press's Phil Laughlin to structure a copublishing arrangement in which Esri supported MIT's production of the book. This was an unusual and perhaps unique collaboration between a focused technical press dedicated to mapping and an academic press willing to take a chance on a major interdisciplinary work. Esri's support permitted the use of the myriad graphics that might otherwise have been excluded on the basis of production costs. I was then gifted with talented designers and editors, including Judith Feldmann and Bill Henry, who are the personnel critical for the myriad details that transform a manuscript into a completed work.

In the same vein, this book is presented as part of an MIT Press series in basic ethics whose independent editorial board is headed by Arthur Caplan. While I am sure my views may differ from his and from those of other board members, they have supported this and other works that offer what hopefully are challenging and new perspectives. For that generosity of mind and the resulting support I am very much obliged.

I am also obliged to members of the North American Cartographic Information Society (NACIS), whose annual meeting in 2005 was the origin of this work. As chapter 2 makes clear, it was in their questions and my attempts to answer them, first in person and then in their journal, *Cartographic Perspectives*, that the basic focus of *Ethics in Everyday Places* came into being. Then, as chapters 3 and 4 demonstrate, I was fortunate in having participants willing to explore the book's issues in classes at the University of British Columbia, the University of Regina, and Clark University. This book attempts to address questions they asked, which, *in medias res*, I sometimes found myself unable to answer adequately.

My early work on the issues of morality, education, and poverty is indebted to my friend, onetime collaborator, and former teacher Ken Denike. Now an emeritus professor at the University of British Columbia, he was for many years a local school trustee. It was in association with him that I first explored the legal issues and the spatial grounding of educational funding. Only later did I link that earlier work to the issues of ethics and morality that are my focus here.

I am obliged as well to other geographers for their assistance and support in the chapter on transportation. The late Warren Gill, Simon Fraser University geography professor and vice president, as well as then geography transportation professor Ray Torchinsky, contributed to my analysis of the means by which supposedly universal public transit systems may be systematically exclusive.

My thinking about moral stress, distress, and injury was informed by discussions with Dr. Kenneth Hirsh (Capt. MC, USN), an expert in the treatment of post-traumatic distress at Tripler Army Medical Center in Hawaii. His experience with military patients and more generally as a physician-psychiatrist was invaluable in helping me to frame these issues. And, too, it was Dr. Hirsh who awakened me to the early twentieth-century history of "moral injury" as a social rather than individual disorder.

Across the many years of research, study, and writing, this book would have been impossible without the assistance of the research librarians who time and again helped find answers in various literatures to my unending array of technical and general questions. They are the unsung heroes and heroines of many books, and we are all indebted to them.

As an adjunct professor of geography at the University of British Columbia under three chairs—David Ley, Graeme Wynn, and most recently Marwan Hassan—I have had access to a superb university library collection of digital documents and databases without which much of this work could not have been realized. Thanks to them, I also have had ready access to computer GIS programs and expert advice on their use. Acknowledging their support is not simply a pro forma thank you but a true pleasure.

Personally, over the years I have been gifted by the intellectual insights and personal support of various friends. These include, in a very partial list, Clark University philosopher Walter Wright, my first teacher in ethics and philosophy, the University of Bristol's Peter Haggett, the doyen of medical geography, and the University of Manitoba's Joe Kaufert. All are now emeriti; all have educated and informed me across the years.

Finally, my thanks are due to Denis Wood, the cartographer-geographer whose work on maps and mapping is cited in various chapters. He has been my critic and friend (often, I admit, in that order) for more than forty years. And then there are the numerous acquaintances and associates, both in the fields in which I work and in my life, who have listened patiently as I tried to formulate the questions this book sought to address and the resolutions that, in the end, it attempts to present. My thanks to all.

1 Moral Stress, Distress, and Injury

Ask coworkers or friends (or yourself) if they're responsible in their work and life. Odds are the response will be, "Sure." Ask if they're ethical, moral people, and most will answer, modestly, "Well, I try." Then ask if they sometimes feel a bit queasy about an assignment, a directive, a policy they are required to implement that they think, if not wrong, then wrongish. Most people will shrug, admitting, "Uh, sure. It happens." In that case, you ask, have they hurt people they're supposed to help? Those who are honest usually cringe and respond with a troubled "maybe," if not a declarative "yes." How do they feel about that? "Terrible."

This book is about the queasy, inchoate feeling that arises when you've done everything right but know you've done something wrong. The result sits festering in the gut, waiting for a resolution that will not come. There is the sense of an ethic violated, a moral viewpoint denied by work we are directed to perform or policies we are supposed to promote. Social injunctions or professional strictures overshadow the personal in ways we do not like but cannot easily resist. The world is out of joint, its experience distinct from the way we thought the world to be. As a result, our days are troubled, and so, sometimes, are our nights. It's not about balancing choices or just working through a problem to an acceptable solution. It's about when every choice is bad and the *only* choice is between bad and worse. Philosophers call this "moral distress," a condition that occurs when "one knows the right thing to do, but institutional [or other] constraints make it nearly impossible to pursue the right course of action."[1]

It's not a new idea. For Georg Wilhelm Friedrich Hegel (1770–1831), this sense of conflicted moral dissonance was the stuff of tragedy. An irresolvable conflict develops between "two substantive positions, each of which is justified, yet each of which is wrong to the extent that it fails either to recognize the validity of the other position or to grant it its moment of truth."[2] The result is intolerable for the individual whose ethical perspective is at loggerheads with institutional or social imperatives. No happy

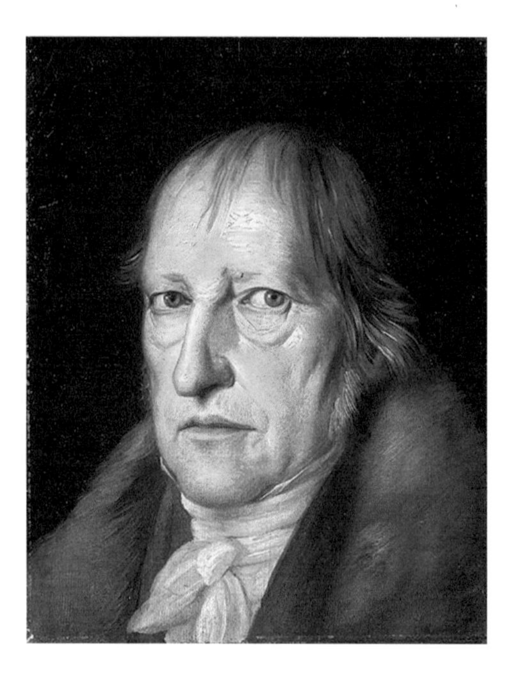

Figure 1.1
Jakob Schlesinger painted this portrait of Hegel in 1831, the year of his death. Wikimedia Commons.

resolution is possible. There is only soul-destroying guilt for accepting directions a person believes improper or punishing consequences if orders are resisted. "It is the honor of these great characters to be culpable," Hegel wrote. Swell.

He borrowed from Aristotle in this bleak setup, using the story of Antigone, and later Socrates' trial and subsequent death, as models of tragic moral conflict. For their parts, Kierkegaard and Nietzsche later weighed in with similarly gloomy, classically weighted variants on the theme. All saw this moral distress as inevitable when individuals are asked to behave in ways they believe wrong but society (or, more precisely, the powerful in a society) deems appropriate. Mostly, the classic tragedian lament focused on the grand hero or heroine, not the common person. The conflicts they presented were exceptional rather than mundane.

The problem, if ancient, is also very modern, a constant background ache for many. For some, the issues are more severe, distressful, and injurious. In 1986 the rocket engineer Bob Ebeling pleaded with his supervisors to delay the launch of the *Challenger* space shuttle because he believed the rubber O-rings would fail. "He collected data that illustrated the risks and spent hours arguing to postpone sending it and its seven astronauts into space."[3] Nobody listened, and the shuttle exploded soon after it was launched. Despite his warnings, Ebeling felt responsible. Somehow he should have done ... more. On the day of the launch, his wife dissuaded him from taking a gun to work to force coworkers to halt the launch. Ebeling quit soon after what in retrospect was a preventable disaster. He then turned to nature conservation work as a kind of penance, "to try and make things right."[4] A sense of guilt, of unrequited responsibility, stayed with him for the rest of his life.

A similar distress contributed to the suicide of Canadian Armed Forces Corporal Shaun Collins. After he returned from his second tour in Afghanistan, he was haunted by nightmares and flashbacks from the war. "Shaun seen and did things over there that were against everything we taught our kids to respect," his father told a coroner's inquest.[5] The morality he was raised with did not condone the realities Corporal Collins experienced; his sense of patriotism and duty came into irresolvable conflict with his sense of appropriately honorable behavior.

This kind of professionally grounded; "moral injury" is now "one of the core topics in clinical ethics."[6] its focus typically military or paramilitary personnel, police and other urban "first responders." David Wood nicely described the problem in a 2014 article, "The Grunts: Damned If They Kill, Damned If They Don't."[7] Soldiers like Corporal Collins, doing what they are told to do, afterward find the memory of their actions impossible to endure. The realities they experience in war intrude on their abilities to live as ethical persons in the civilian world to which they return. Nightmares and night sweats are the least of the symptoms that persons with this kind of post-traumatic stress endure.

Ethicists and moral philosophers tend to focus not on veterans or first responders but on doctors and especially nurses.[8] Alan Cribb,[9] among others, argues that medical personnel's "own sense of self as a moral agent" is continually challenged when personal imperatives to care conflict with institutional strictures.[10] From this perspective, moral distress is all about "scripts" (rules of behavior) we are instructed to follow as professionals. Moral distress results when, as Jonathan Hait and Jesse Graham put it, "We cannot excuse ourselves from the ethical judgments the scripts embody or the consequences of script following."[11] This literature's focus is always "the self as moral agent," the person's ability to accept the disjunction between personal morals and professional directives. It is rarely if ever the morality of the scripts themselves.

The problem is not limited to any single profession, however. We all like to think of ourselves as "moral agents." Nor can it simply be sourced to a malignant "managerialism" creating hostile environments for otherwise honorable working professionals.[12]

The Canadian Broadcasting Corporation (CBC) reporter Curt Petrovich was training for a half marathon on the day he got the call to travel to the Philippines to cover the devastation of Typhoon Haiyan in 2013.[13] Amid the overpowering stench of decomposing bodies and crowds of persons who had lost everything, "We weren't bearing anything other than the odd bottle of water that we could give to them. ... That's a difficult position to be in." No food, no water, no shelter: what type of person does nothing but record another's misery without offering to help? After returning to Canada, Petrovich was diagnosed with post-traumatic stress. "I learned that this feeling of helplessness that I had," he says, "was a conflict running pretty deeply in my conscious and unconscious brain."

The circumstances of our mundane ethical quandaries may be less extreme, but the result is the same in kind, if not necessarily in degree. How can it be otherwise? We are all mired in irremediable conflict. On the one hand, we are told that self-determination and individual choice are principal virtues, that autonomy is the keystone of modern social democracy. We are enjoined to think for ourselves, to develop and then follow our own moral compasses. In doing so, we are told that each of us is responsible for his or her actions. More to the point, we are responsible for their consequences. It is the soldier who pulls the trigger, the doctor who orders the treatment, the engineer who is responsible for the launch.

And yet we are also expected to put aside our personal predilections and ignore deeply held values when they conflict with an employer's demands, an insurer's mandate, a superior's injunction, a profession's dictates, or a nation's imperatives. We are ordered to do what is required even if we believe it is not what is needed or what is right. Our professional associations proclaim high-minded codes of ethics; our nations trumpet a set of high-minded ideals. Too often, however, what is proclaimed in the abstract we are directed to ignore in practice.

If we follow our own moral compass, the charge we face is reckless selfishness injurious to the common weal. Who are we to challenge a client's directions, a patient's wishes, a supervisor's insistence, or a government's mandate? In our intransigence, we are told, we promote harms greater than the good we seek to ensure. As a result, we are disciplined and perhaps fired. Some simply burn out and, like Bob Ebeling, quit work once loved to seek some other way to be. Others, like Corporal Collins, find the conflict more than they can bear. It is Hegel's tragedy refitted for popular consumption, a problem broadly chronic rather than exceptional and specific. The question becomes: Is conscience to be reserved for the quixotic, vainglorious rebel? On what grounds might it be empowered and, perhaps most importantly, unleashed: where might it lead and what can it teach us all?

Moral Philosophers

Nancy Berlinger, a medical ethicist at the Hastings Center, calls ethical distress an "avoidance problem" that occurs when there is "ethical uncertainty about how normal work should proceed in a complex system, one in which workers must continually adapt to changing conditions under pressures that include the need to keep themselves or others safe from harm."[14] For their part, Bruce Jennings and Fredrick Wertz describe it as a problem of "agency," of the individual's ability to respond to conditions of "ethical tension."[15] Among these and other writers, the central issue is a person's ability to conform to a set of procedures or rules that seem to him or her inappropriate, inhuman, or somehow unethical. Implicit in their work, and that of most others, is the assumption that these problems can be resolved handily and individuals can make, if not a good choice, then a best choice "under the circumstances."

But we cannot avoid injurious moral distress when there are no good choices, no way to reconcile the conflicting demands of integrity and outside direction. For engineers like Bob Ebeling, soldiers like Corporal Collins, or reporters like Curt Petrovich, there was no "fast thinking," as Daniel Kahneman calls it, that could make the problem go away.[16] It is the expectation of agency and its attendant responsibilities that lies at the heart of the irresolvable conflict. If agency is denied, then we are powerless. And if we are powerless, what does our individual integrity mean? The conflict is intransigent and unavoidable. This is not, as some suggest, about justifying one's actions to others.[17] Rather, the distress is located, festering, in the person him- or herself as he or she struggles to evaluate and understand his or her place as a moral being in a world revealed as, if not immoral, then amoral.

Moral distress and injury linger long after the causal event, long past any potential physical danger to the self. It is the opposite of what Alan Cribb calls a pervasive "ethical laziness," in which one simply gets the job done and then moves on, or the "ethical arrogance" that results from ignoring the rules on the assumption that you know best.[18] If we could simply ignore the claims and needs of others, then there would be no problem. If we could ignore the rules imposed on us and act without consequence solely as we see fit, then there would be no dissonance, or at least little inner conflict. But in all these cases it is the rules themselves that are in conflict—the person's and another's—and the result is consequential and can be life altering. In these cases, satisfactory, simple solutions are simply not possible.

At heart we are social beings hardwired to care for and think of others. "Human intelligence rests on a foundation of social cognition reflected in a unique capacity for empathy; for appreciating the perspective of others."[19] Our sense of self is bound to others in ways that make their relations with us integral; their denial is a kind of dehumanization that affects us and them together. At the same time, we are cultural beings enmeshed in a range of roles—familial, educational, national, professional, and religious—each defined by rules and their underlying, not-always-complementary rationales. To ignore them is to ignore our relation to those roles and the place they hold in the construction of our world. Ethical quandaries are thus rooted not simply in individual convictions but in the way we are to be in the world with others. Sometimes our varying roles—citizen, family member, neighbor, professional—conflict. The question then becomes: what do we do when the world we believe in and the one we live in seem out of joint?

Moral Injury: Social

The idea of "moral injury" entered modern literatures—medical and social—not as a problem of the person but instead as a descriptor of social harms by classes of individuals. In 1909, the earliest reference I have found,[20] Dr. Willard Bullard urged fellow physicians to forsake the care of "undesirables" assumed to be congenitally disposed to low moral character.[21] Attention to their continued well-being, he argued, perpetuated a burdensome, morally profligate population whose continuance would undermine both the social order and the economic fabric of the nation. The solution he recommended was a eugenic cleansing of society's "idiots" and "morons" (persons with Down syndrome, hydrocephaly, spina bifida, etc.). Parents might object, and physicians might insist on their Hippocratic obligation to care for all, but acquiescing to either parental love or a sense of professional duty, Bullard argued, resulted in a moral if not mortal injury to the greater social good. In 1927 Supreme Court Chief Justice Oliver Wendell Holmes invoked a similar, economically based morality in his famous opinion *Buck v. Bell*, authorizing the involuntary state sterilization of "idiot" women who presumably would in turn birth "idiot" children.[22]

A similar kind of social injury is argued today by those who insist allegiance to ideals like equality and solidarity constitute an injurious moral failure hampering the neoliberal mechanisms of supply-side economics.[23] They advance instead an ethical standard grounded in market-smart efficiencies powered by the unfettered activity of individual entrepreneurs.[24] Personal moralities grounded in antiquated values of mutuality are, from this perspective, no more than sentimental baggage damaging a nation's bottom line and its future potential. A general moral injury thus becomes the inevitable result of an allegiance to the Enlightenment ideals that are the rationale for programs of communal care and support. Two very different ethical paradigms based on different moral perspectives—one economic and the other social democratic—seem at perpetual loggerheads.[25]

In the first half of the nineteenth century there was a brief period in which it seemed possible to make the health and general welfare of average citizens a defining criterion of prideful nationhood.[26] The idea floundered by midcentury, however, as economic indices became the principal measure of national well-being and future health.[27] In recent years, some have tried to reinstitute a kind of social progress index, or one of general well-being, as at the least complementary to economic measures like the gross domestic product. Those noneconomic indices remain eccentric, however, and are given relatively little official weight.[28] It is therefore fair to say that, beginning at the latest in the mid-eighteenth century, practical ethics and practical morality *became* economic, their central metric the financial well-being of the nation defined by a utilitarian vision of the abstract greater good. We might proclaim allegiance to Enlightenment ideals, but in practice we apply an economic standard to our relations, one to another. It is along this fault line that many modern moral fractures exist.

To take one example, in bioethics born in the second half of the last century, the physician's imperative to care was devalued as financial growth and well-being came to dominate policy in many countries.[29] Who were doctors to disagree with the demands of the state?[30] Insurers paid the bill (in the United States) and thus should be permitted to set the health agenda. Public moralities of care floundered as a result. So, too, did the physician's earlier right to organize the best possible care for a patient. At another scale, individual autonomy and choice were promoted as ethical goods. But that was done (as chap. 8 argues) largely without regard to the person's ability to pay for care or necessary treatments. Treatment alternatives were the economic preserve of insurers or, in some countries, the state. Today similar clashes between ethical paradigms—personal, professional, political, and social—are rife across many divisions of society.[31]

Morals and Ethics

"Moral distress manifests itself as the principal component of psychological responses to social forces."[32] It is there, rather than the moral declaration of the individual isolate, that the problem is grounded. It is not about us or "them" but about how we stand as people in a society that demands specific attitudes, and thus resulting behaviors, of its citizens. For Hegel, the problem was what to the hero or heroine seemed a "profound identification with a just and substantial position" at irresolvable odds with another, equally substantial and broadly accepted.[33] Tragic failure is the only and inevitable outcome for the person whose moral perspective challenges what, at any given moment, is a generally accepted ethical worldview.

How can this broad class of chronic conflicts best be understood? To address that question requires, first, a distinction between ethics and morals, nouns and sometimes adjectives that are typically conflated in contemporary literatures.[34] Most assume each to be a synonym for the other. Here, however, morals are defined as a declarative set of values, definitions of right and wrong that brook no discussion. Every culture has a small set on which its laws, professional injunctions, religious declarations, and social codes of behavior are based. "At the heart of every moral theory there lie what we might call explanatory moral judgments," Judith Thomson wrote, "which explicitly say that such and such is good or bad, right or wrong … because it has feature *F*."[35]

Ethics are the means by which we attempt to apply those values, the *F*s, in our lives. "The ethical is presented as that realm in which principles [moral definitions] have authority over us," not independent of our attitudes but as their basis.[36] The result takes the form of a "practical syllogism" whose construction links a moral idea, the syllogism's major premise, with the specifics of the minor premise to say that a particular action, or kind of action, is required ethically. "If this is good or 'right' [by definition], then I/we must do … that."

The idea of a set of moral definitions, value statements that result in applicable ethical imperatives, is at least as ancient as Aristotle's writings. He made justice the *F* value and defined it operatively as requiring that equals be treated as equals. But are we all really equal (slaves and slave owners, men and women, Christians and Moors)? And how is equality to be defined? The apparently simple Aristotelian idea seems as if it could require an endless process of definition and redefinition until the syllogism is so proscribed it has no operative value.

Here R. G. Collingwood[37] and J. L. Austin[38] come to the rescue. In the 1940s, Collingwood argued a kind of linkage in which a proposition (the major premise of the syllogism) involves one or more *suppositions*. These assumed truths power the ethical proposition "*If* this is good (justice as equality), then I will do it." But because the supposition is itself open to question ("What is justice?" "What is equal treatment?"), each leads to a set of prior *pre*suppositions attempting to more clearly define the previously stated *F*.

The result is not endlessly recursive, however, like an M. C. Escher print. There is, Collingwood argued, a small constellation of *presuppositions* that do not answer to any question and are not open to debate. They are bedrock values whose definitions are accepted reflexively and without question as clear. In our discussion, these bedrock *F*s ground ethical propositions that are based on or follow from them.

The point, as Austin makes clear, is that speech is laden with associations and meanings that call forth action (or reaction). Roland Barthes presented another, related way of saying much the same thing. His semiology described a systems of "signs," used to present events or things that serve as "signifiers" carrying the values of an ultimately "signified" idea or ideal (patriotism, e.g.).[39] For Barthes, *any*thing—the Eiffel Tower, a map, a photograph, or a wrestling match[40]—can be "unpacked" (some would say "deconstructed") to reveal meanings, values, and traditions underlying this or that prosaic event or thing.[41] Where philosophers begin with the big idea and its construction, Barthes's semiology and Collingwood's linguistics rolled their analyses up from the mundane.

All of this sounds impossibly academic and, well ... philosophical. The point is first that everything is grounded in an *idea* about the world, at once realized and often simultaneously hidden. Second, those ideas are shared, communicated in one medium or another. Third, ideas about what is good or bad, right or wrong, stand not alone but within a chain of ideas ultimately grounded in a set of bedrock presuppositions I call here "moral definitions." In assessing the nature of distress, we can therefore track back from the initial proposition to the root idea that anchors our thinking in this or that situation. From there we can see mechanisms through which practical syllogisms are enacted, implicitly or explicitly.

Someone may hold to a personal, eccentric moral code, and thus a set of unique ethical propositions. But to be generally credited as grounding appropriate behavior an individual's "Well, I just believe" serves in neither ethics, law, nor the community at large. It is those moral presuppositions we share, and the suppositions they give rise to, that carry communal ethical weight. Identifying a set of broadly subscribed-to moral presuppositions—the *F*s—and their resulting suppositions is relatively easy. They are clearly stated in foundational documents (the US Declaration of Independence and various national constitutions), laws, and international conventions (e.g., the UN's Universal Declaration of Human Rights). They are referred to explicitly or implicitly in the ethical codes of most religions and most professions (e.g., the American Association of Advertisers).[42] All speak, to a greater or lesser degree, to ideals of community, care, honesty, truthfulness, and well-being for the person and society as a whole. They are about us, together, not simply each of us alone.

But here's the rub: the process of syllogistic construction and resulting action is dynamic, not static. The underlying suppositions and presuppositions that give us meaning are clarified, changed, or undermined through their application. Everyone believes in "justice," but one person's just cause is another's unjust action. It is in the actions we take that our ideas of justice are practically confirmed. By enacting an ethical proposition (we should do this because...), we affirm and simultaneously bring forth the moral definitions that seem, at the thin level of declarative principle, so clear. Refusing to act on that proposition, conversely, brings its moral grounding into question, if not potentially into disrepute.

Map Talk

This book is not about mapping but about how we talk (and think) about doing what is right or recognizing what is wrong. The map is just "a kind of talk," another language in which we construct active arguments (syllogisms) based on presuppositions and suppositions.[43] From this perspective, map-talk, you might call it, is a way to see all this philosophy in action. And from that perspective, maps are a rich field of ethical and moral investigation.

An advantage of the medium in this exercise is that maps are everywhere, a constant in the literatures of economics, demography, journalism, sciences (of all kinds), statistics, transportation, and so on. They are a daily presence in academic journals, popular magazines, and daily news reports (broadcast and print). All are first and foremost social documents arguing a particular view of the world. "A map is never just a map," as Timothy Barney puts it, "but a confluence of social forces that constrain a culture's sense of its relationship to, and in, the world."[44] In their construction, maps call forth what Daniel Callahan termed, in another context, a "vital background constellation of values,"[45] enacted through a set of general ethical injunctions grounded in one or another moral perspective.

At its most basic level, a map is a collection of what Barthes called organized signs signifying a worldly event (disease, draft, poverty, war) and, in its presentation, our values. Every map brings into existence an idea about something through a set of symbols (points, lines, rectangles, etc.) organized in a generally accepted, easily understood (and thus visually legible) manner. The logical form of the map, like that of ethics (If *F* is good, then we do that), is propositional: *If* this is important, *then* here is what it looks like; here is where it is found.[46] In other words, maps locate the subjects we believe to be important in a landscape we find familiar. What is signified, map to map, is this or that ideal and, implicitly or explicitly, a call to act on it. After all, if the mapped thing had no meaning, no ethical imperative, why make the map at all?

Objectivity and Argument

That a map is not an objective statement but an idea made to *seem* factual will be disconcerting to some. Until recently, the subjective nature of the map was simply ignored, where not positively derided, by most professionals. A discoverable, value-free reality was assumed to be the cartographic goal.[47] The idea was,[48] and for some continues to be, that "good" maps are "mostly" objective and thus truthful, although perhaps inevitably advancing an at-times "persuasive," authorial point of view.[49]

The distinction between the "objective" and the "persuasive" is an old one. In his *Inquiry concerning Human Understanding* (1748), David Hume distinguished between objective facts collected for critical consideration and those "influenced by taste and sentiment." He lauded the factual while condemning the persuasive to the degree it masqueraded *as* objective, choosing data to make an argument seem reasonable.[50] This echoed Plato's account of Socrates' debate with the rhetorician Gorgias, who boasted he could argue every side of any issue, convincing people of its rightness, no matter how limited or false the position might be.[51] Socrates saw that claim as mendacious, and thus dishonorable, because, for him, truths were things contributing to the social good (his presupposition). The alternative is the rhetorician's false beliefs grounded in the self-interest of an employer; his truths thus served a base, and extremely limited, end.

Maps are active, practical propositions *about* the world as we see it based on a sometimes complex set of suppositions. In every map, "thick" experiential statements and "thin" principled ideas are entwined.[52] The problem is that we *want* maps to be true. We want them to be objective because we want the world to be certain, its truths absolute and unbounded. Alas, knowledge isn't like that. Truths turn out to be malleable, and knowledge, the accumulation of data structured in a certain way, is no more than a set of sometimes shaky truths buttressed by ideas and ideals.

This is neither a book about cartographic ethics nor a learned treatise on the limits of knowable truths. It is instead an attempt to investigate problems arising at the intersection between sets of conflicting expectations and standards governing personal practice, professional ideals, and social policy. But because maps are a principal medium in this investigation, it makes sense to take a few pages to consider the map and the means by which its ethical propositions and moral suppositions are revealed.

Maps and Mapping

At the simplest level, mapping (like ethics) is about things together. It takes a set of individual cases, rows of data, and makes them into members of an event class located in relation to others in a more or less recognizable geographic field (political boundaries, streets, etc.) that we think of as approximating the real. The world thus brought forth is set at a scale, from very local to global, in which the map's argument is situated. In the mapping, the mapmaker proposes relations between event classes located *in* place, disease incidence and income by county, for example. *If* this is there *and* that is there, *then* this and that are related in a space we know. Beneath that conjunction lies an often hidden value proposition: If *x* (say health) is important, then we must look at it in a certain way. If *y* (say poverty) is bad, then we must look at it in a certain way. If poverty leads to ill health, and if the map shows areas of ill health are areas of poverty, then we argue that the ill health related to poverty is ... bad. Good and bad are moral conclusions implicit in the mapping of the potentially causal relationship between health, disease, and poverty.

Nothing surprising here. Data are *always* chosen on the basis of assumptions and definitions that determine their selection and the mode of their analysis. Whatever the medium, "people who formulate those facts have to use assumptions: patterns of expectation, within which they select arrange, shape, and classify their data."[53] The map's potential evidentiary power lies in this: it wraps a lasso around its facts, organizing them in groups of common characteristics, similarly symbolized, and then posts them in a space filled with other groups of things (landforms, jurisdictional boundaries, streets, etc.) in a manner insisting on their shared communal reality. It sets its constituents in a relational space whose elements synergistically interact to create a complex reality of things, together. In this way, maps concretize the abstract. The result invites a map's users to see an ideal and its argument *as* a geography, a thing made concretely real with real-world consequences set at a specific resolution and attendant scale.

A Simple Example

All of this is easier to see than to talk about. Figure 1.2 presents a vector version of a map by Dr. John Snow, the nineteenth-century British physician who famously argued that cholera was solely waterborne rather than primarily airborne, as many of his contemporaries believed.[54] The basic proposition was "*If* cholera is waterborne, *then* a water source must be at the center of any cholera outbreak." The first event class, whose members are symbolized here with small triangles, posted the location of the homes of almost six hundred persons who died from cholera in the first weeks of an outbreak in Snow's London neighborhood. The mapped circles symbolize local wells that served as the principal water sources for residents of the affected area. Both exist together in what Snow called a "topology" of disease, a geography of streets and landmarks (a pub here, a poorhouse there) that constituted the context of the outbreak. Snow believed that the obvious centrality of a single pump nestled among a dense circle of deaths proved his proposition.

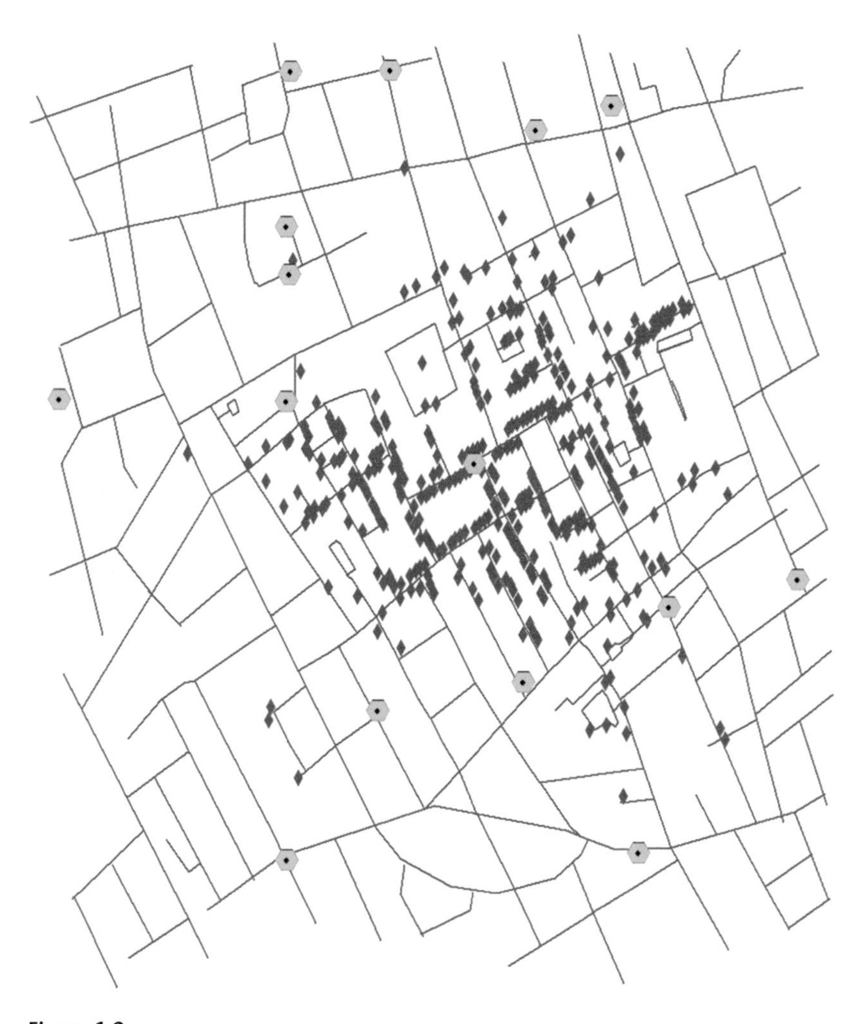

Figure 1.2
In mapping a ferocious cholera outbreak in his London neighborhood in 1854, John Snow layered a series of event classes (deaths from cholera, streets and some shops, water sources) to argue that cholera was a waterborne rather than airborne disease.

The map is an ecology in which the individual datum is sited in a class of similar events interacting with—defined by and defining—a complex environment (biogeographic, human built, political). In that dynamism is a propositional relationship between event classes: *If* we see x (cholera deaths), then it must be in proximity to y (water sources). *If* we see y (water sources), then we may expect to see x (cholera). If this is present, then that will occur. The meaning in the map grows with the complexity of the event classes it presents, the completeness of the geography to which they are indivisibly joined, and the propositions that argue their presumably causal relationships, one to the other.

In his map (fig. 1.3), Snow used data on reported deaths from cholera collected by and made publicly available by the Registrar General's Office. Barthes would say that the diamonds (deaths), circles (water sources), and lines (streets) were signs that

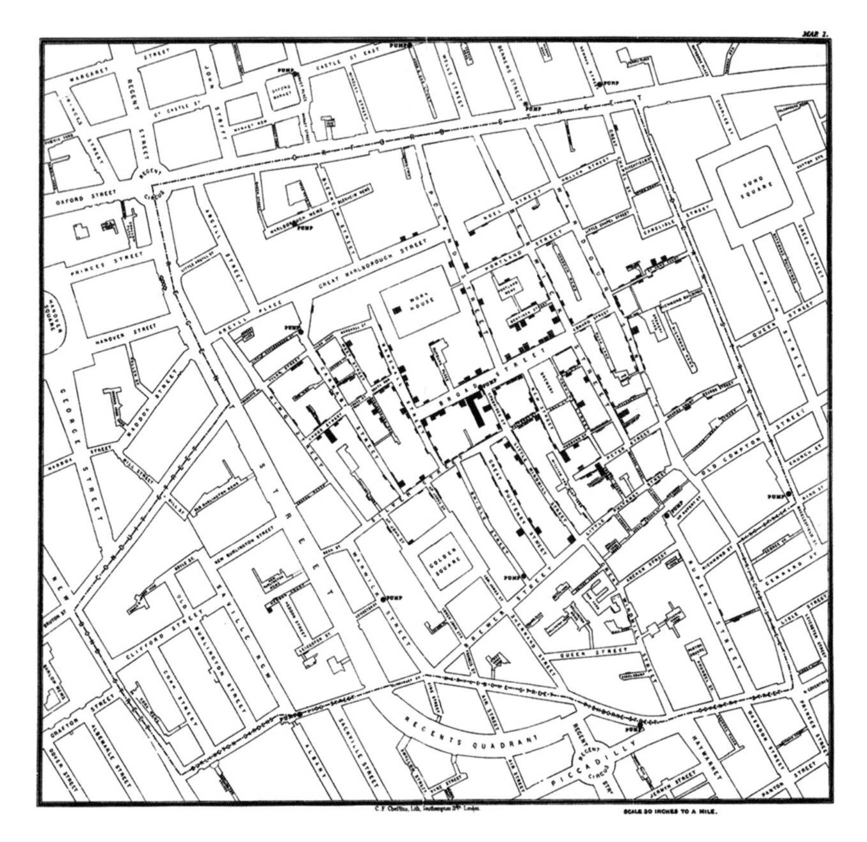

Figure 1.3
Detail of John Snow's map of neighborhood cholera in the 1854 outbreak. If cholera is waterborne, the map argued, then a water source must be at its center.

together signified the cholera outbreak in Snow's Broad Street neighborhood. The real signified, however, was Snow's *idea*. In the mapping, Snow left out the sewers whose foul-smelling airs ("miasmas") many believed were the cause of the outbreak. And, too, in this map he neglected the old plague burial site that others believed was the likely origin of those airs (in another map, he included it, positioning it incorrectly). The map presented Snow's *idea* of cholera as a waterborne disease and not the complex ecology (including sewers and old cemeteries) others believed cholera presented.[55] Others who had different ideas about cholera mapped the neighborhood and its cholera differently.[56]

Ethics and Morals

Implicit in Snow's maps and explicit in his writings was an ethical syllogism: *If* we wish to save persons from cholera, and *if* its source is unclean water, *then* we are obliged to ensure clean water for our citizens. Famously, Snow argued this to the local parish committee when he recommended disabling the central Broad Street pump, the suspected source of the outbreak. To define cholera as waterborne thus implied a practical demand that clean water be provided to protect the lives of London citizens. Because the constituents of health in this case were thought to be broadly public rather than individually determined, Snow's map argued the ethical insistence that officials—civil and religious—do everything in their power to tame the disease by attending to its environmental cause. Implicit in this argument was a moral presupposition defining human lives as something valuable to be protected. This moral-ethical definition-injunction of public health as a civil (and, in Snow's day, parish) responsibility had been asserted ever since the Romans built aqueducts to ensure clean water for their citizens.[57] So Snow's map argued the ethical necessity of public officials to provide clean water for citizens.

Not everyone agreed with Snow, of course. In 1831 a group of unnamed authors published in the *Lancet* a review of cholera's progress from its origins in India through the Middle East to Russia and then western Europe.[58] They argued against quarantines and other restrictive measures as not only likely to be ineffective but, more importantly, injurious to national trade. Better a bit of cholera, the authors concluded, than a set of policies that might harm the economics of the nation. From their perspective, the death of some from cholera was less important than the maintenance of industry, trade, and the profits that resulted from them.

We know a lot about John Snow, his ethical posture, and its origins from his writings.[59] At a professional level, Snow was enjoined by a set of moral declarations and practical injunctions that instruct physicians not only to treat disease but, in the

'In consequence of what I said'
the handle of the pump was removed...

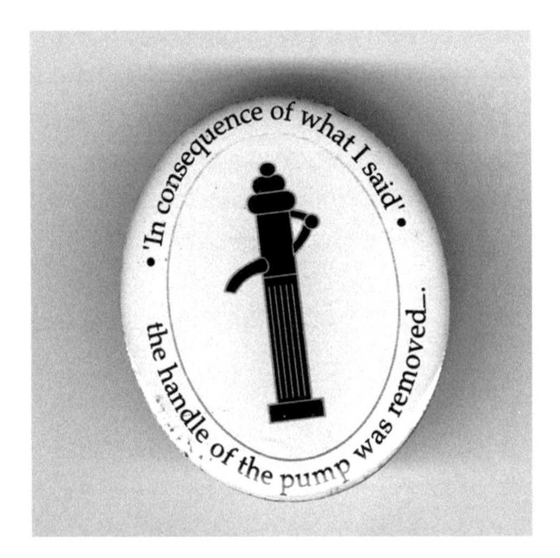

Figure 1.4
A simple lapel pin from the John Snow Society showing the Broad Street pump that Snow proposed to disable to stop a local cholera outbreak in 1854.

Hippocratic tradition, to prevent it where possible.[60] This created a clear imperative to public action by physicians.[61] In that tradition, preventable deaths are ethical "wrongs" violating the moral raison d'être of medicine, the preservation of life. Moreover, since governments had in theory developed for the care and advancement of citizens, there was a similar injunction toward health protection for nonmedical public officials.

Snow's focus on cholera in the 1850s was also deeply personal, however. As an apprentice apothecary, he had served mining communities near Newcastle that in 1831 were decimated by cholera in its first British outbreak.[62] His best efforts did little to save the miners. The result was a traumatic experience he described repeatedly in his writings on cholera from 1849 until his death in 1858. The deaths he could not prevent weighed on him in the same way that Bob Ebeling was tormented by the shuttle deaths and Corporal Collins by his wartime patriotic service.

Finally, Snow wished as a scientist to definitively describe the nature of cholera and the manner of its diffusion. The goal was not pure knowledge but applicable knowledge that could be used to save lives. And here he learned the essential fact: Science is not just about being right. It is about convincing others of the truth of an argument based on data that all accept and a methodology others find convincing. Snow didn't do that, at least not to the satisfaction of his contemporaries. His failures—what was not mapped—were as important to them as the strengths of his argument were to him. Snow's major premise (cholera is waterborne) was disputed, and so his proposition and its ethical conclusion (we must clean up water sources) lost much of its immediacy and power.

What was not contested was the ethics of his search, the moral goal of preventing cholera deaths. *Everybody* wanted to control its spread. Physicians worried about death and sickness; bureaucrats about the health of productive, tax-paying citizens. Merchants worried about their customers and their own health. So behind the map and its debate were both a broadly shared moral stance and a set of highly practical concerns. A similar argument can be found in figure 1.5, where the "signs" are children and adults with water pails, the pump from which they draw the water, and the image of death as its operator. The signifier is the idea that contaminated water causes deaths

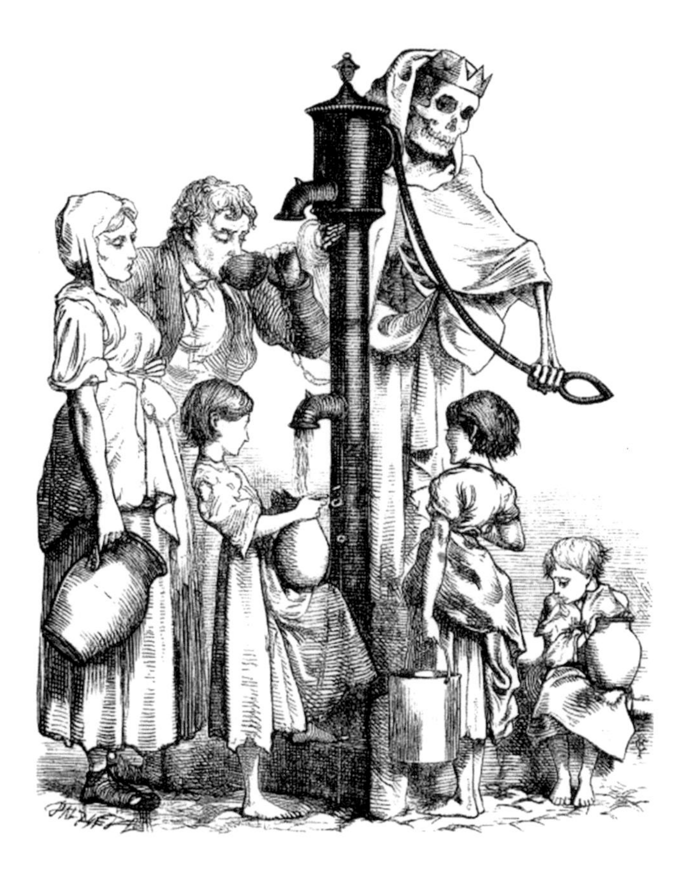

Figure 1.5
In this mid-nineteenth-century illustration, Death is recruiting local children by pumping contaminated water from a communal pump, the kind that provided household water for most residents of London.

(in this case, cholera). What is signified—the message—is the necessity of clean water to preserve the children by removing Death's hand from the pump.

I am neither an ardent semiologist nor an analytic philosopher. Throughout the rest of the book's chapters, I will only occasionally use the language of those professions: enough is enough. It is sufficient here to describe the means by which maps (and charts, graphs, tables, etc.) carry ethical propositions based on moral definitions of what is or should be seen as a good. The example of John Snow makes clear how one can be in liege to a set of moral definitions and ethical propositions that are consequential. He was, after all, at once a practicing physician, a superior researcher striving for recognition, and not coincidentally a citizen of the neighborhood and city whose cholera outbreak he mapped. In all that follows, it is important to remember that complexity lies not simply in the culture at large, or the structure of a particular discipline or profession, but also within the lived life. Like Snow, we all bring to our daily world an experiential history that is as deeply personal as it is professionally enabled and socially embedded. Moral stress lies not only in a simple conflict but more often in a conflicting set of ideals and principles we attempt to hold simultaneously.

I An Ethnography of Ethics

[Ethnography's mission] is to gain access to other minds and other ways of life so as to represent what it is like to be a different situated human being … in pursuit of differences that make a difference for the way lives are lived, developed, and experienced, and for the way competence, excellence, virtue, and personal well-being are defined.

—Richard A. Shweder, *True Ethnography*

2 Ethics, Geography, and Mapping: The Failure of the Simple

At the Beginning

Weighty thoughts about ethical distress and moral injury were not on my mind when I attended the October 2005 meeting of the North American Cartographic Information Society (NACIS). Ethics and mapping were separate areas of my work, and until then, I had never considered their conjunction. That spring, Esri Press published my first book on the history of medical mapping, *Cartographies of Disease*,[1] and, honestly (and isn't that a virtue we seek to advance?), I was going to NACIS to promote its purchase among conference attendees. And since I then was coteaching Geography 381 ("Spatial Data Analysis Using GIS") at the University of British Columbia, I was curious what graduates of programs like ours were doing and saying.

And then there was the conference location itself. Salt Lake City, Utah, is the home of the great Mormon Tabernacle Choir and its extraordinary organ. I desperately wanted to hear it. Rebuilt and expanded several times since it was inaugurated in 1867, the organ's 11,623 pipes arranged in 267 rows produce an extraordinary congress of potential sounds managed by a complex combination of stops toggled in various combinations. These give precise character to the notes played on any of the organ's five keyboards and pedals. NACIS was an opportunity to hear and see if not perhaps play this behemoth in its home auditorium, one so large it takes, guests are told, 1.5 seconds for sound to travel from the auditorium wall stage left to the opposite wall, stage right.

Great organs fill the air in a visceral way. The largest pipes produce undertones that vibrate through the walls and floor into the wooden pews. You can *feel* the sound. Depending on the choice of stops, notes played on the organ console become the whispered call of a bird flying in the midst of a thundering storm or the energy of the storm itself. In Salt Lake City the organ is played every day at noon and again at 5 p.m. During the conference, I attended almost every recital.

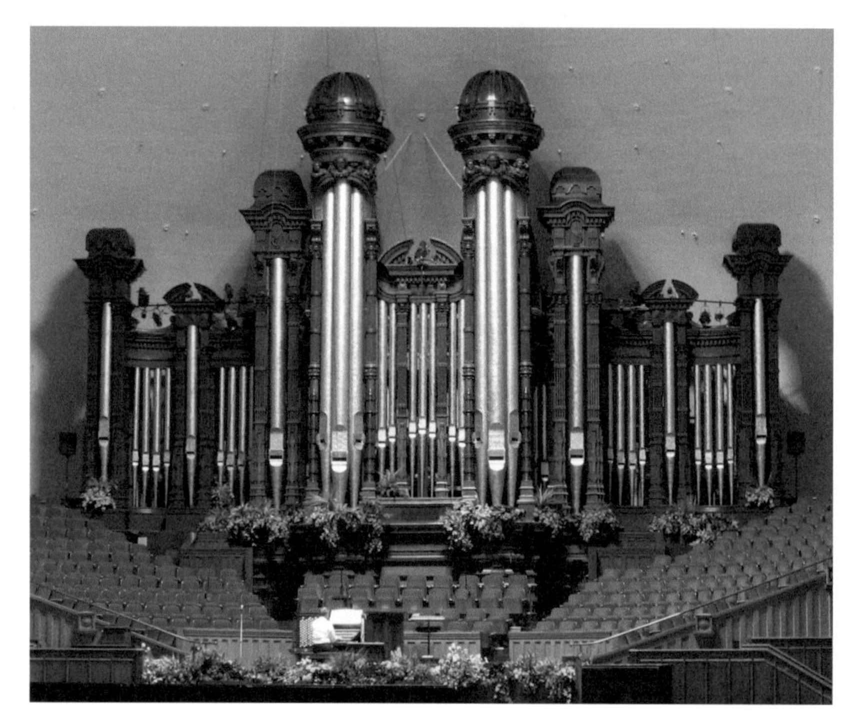

Figure 2.1
The Salt Lake Tabernacle organ provides a metaphor here for the complex relations that pervade issues of ethics, science, and their mapped presentations. Wikipedia/Common Use.

For me, the organ is a metaphor for the complexities of the world. Even an apparently simple musical idea can be transformed into something elaborate and grand when transposed across three simultaneous lines of notation performed at once with both hands and both feet. For me, nothing so exemplifies the broadly connected complexities of the world, or the way we choose among them, than the organ.

That complexity, multiple choices within a seemingly simple system, is what I have always found to be the reality in medical ethics. Apparently simple diagnostic "facts" become complex points of deliberation when treatment options are transposed through the scales of fear and hope expressed by the desperately ill and their families. Medical ethics are easy if you never have to meet with the patients, their families, or the sometimes exasperated medical staff whose members too often have little patience with either doubt or hope.[2] In practice there are always complex negotiations between personal, professional, and social values. The result is rarely a simple, "objective" certainty of what is "right" but rather a set of tentative conclusions open to interpretation and discord when interpretations diverge and essential values differ.

Mapping similarly presents a congress of choices ordered around apparently simple themes. So many decisions go into their making that the map's proud declarative, "It is," is better expressed as "This is how I think it might be." Just as I wrestle with how to play a Bach sonata (or a Lennon-McCartney song), so I struggle with the sometimes-conflicting potentials that can be distilled in the imaging of what seems, at first, simply described. What are we really saying, and to whom are we speaking? What speaks which idea best?

NACIS and Ethics

Although I attended the conference as a geographer, I found that ethics were in the air. Participants worried in different sessions about what they perceived as the problematic ethics of subcontracting work offshore to countries where mapping expertise and printing processes were cheaper than in Canada or the United States. Yes, it made business sense, members said, but wasn't it unethical, or at least unpatriotic, or somehow un*something* to deprive fellow citizens of badly needed work? And, in other matters, some asked, what was the appropriate response to a job whose stated goal seemed biased in its assumptions and limited in the data the mapmaker was given to promote a particular cartographic conclusion?

The conflict, to me, was obvious. Were these largely independent contractors grounded solely in an economic ethic whose bedrock presupposition made gain their sole objective, or was their ethical perspective grounded in a morality of community and social good that extended beyond personal benefit? How could they feel proud of work whose message they denied, about business deals that helped them but hurt those who were their confreres?

Map-Off

The high point of the NACIS meeting that year was a more or less friendly competition called "Map-Off" in which five or six volunteers presented maps on a subject assigned by officials five days before the meetings began. The results were then publicly judged in an open, studio-style critique by an expert panel. After that, conference attendees commented and then voted with a show of hands for their favorite. In 2005 the subject was Hurricane Katrina.

By every measure, the worst submission was by a mapmaker employed by a major US newspaper whose entry, she later admitted, was produced not for the competition but on assignment weeks before. It was an ugly and to my eye flawed map of a section of flooded New Orleans (little contrast in its deep browns, as I remember, and a curious scale) with a curling Mississippi River snaking through the city. It had something to do with the area where the levees were breached but the point of the map was far from clear. It was not only inferior in its production but also ... a cheat. It had been submitted *as if* constructed for the competition and therefore in compliance with NACIS Map-Off rules. In fact, it had been completed at the direction of her news editors weeks earlier and then slipped into the NACIS mix.

Maps presented by other participants were more honest (their creators did not violate competition rules) but less than enlightening. As a group, they proclaimed a woeful lack of even a modest knowledge of the complex interplay of biogeographic and socioeconomic factors that made Katrina so inevitably devastating. In 2001, for example, Anuradha Mathur and Dilip da Cunha reviewed literatures on the Mississippi Delta as a dynamic entity in which hydrologic forces and human activities interact unceasingly.[3] That turned issues of hydrology (and thus its mapping) into an intensely interactive subject as complex as any organ fugue.[4] The problem for me with the Map-Off entries was that they presented the storm as a presumably unforeseeable, natural, and thus simple, one-off meteorological event. In a more theological age, it would have been called, with a shrug, an act of God. The devastation that resulted therefore was nobody's fault.

Natural and Unnatural Events

During the general discussion, I suggested that since earlier in the day folks had raised questions of business ethics—subcontracting work offshore—ethics might be a way to think about the contest maps. I pointed out that the newspaper cartographer's map was a self-conscious violation of the competition rules. What, I asked rhetorically, are the ethics of flouting policies of fair engagement? I then questioned the ethics of mapping Katrina's path and its resulting urban destruction without attention to either the history of recurrent gulf hurricanes or repeated reports of the inadequacy of local levees in a city where major storms are an almost annual event. After all, detailed histories of those hurricanes have been accumulating for more than one hundred years, and the wholesale destruction resulting from breached levees has been detailed at least since the 1920s.[5]

At the least, a poster-style map set of historical storm tracks (fig. 2.2) would have said much about the inevitability of Hurricane Katrina and thus its probable effects. The US National Oceanic and Atmospheric Administration (NOAA) has published detailed data on the path of every hurricane reported since the 1860s.[6] More recent

Hurricane Katrina: One more time

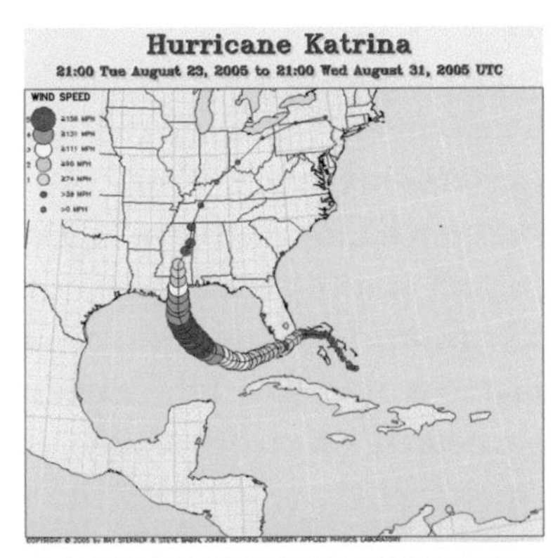

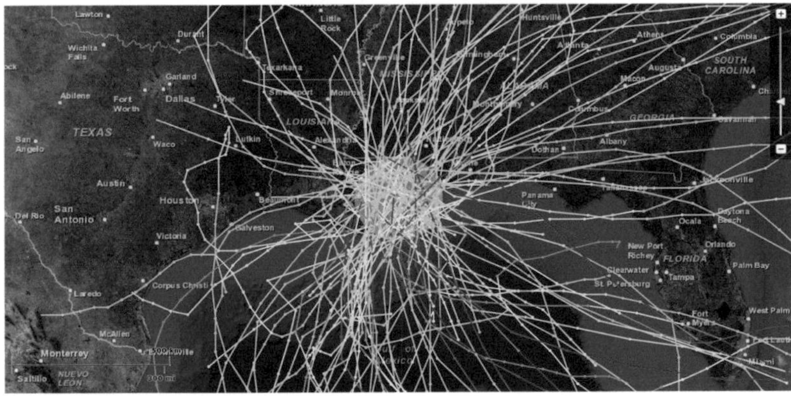

NOAA Map of hurricane storm tracks and New Orleans: 1655-2012

http://csc.noaa.gov/hurricanes#

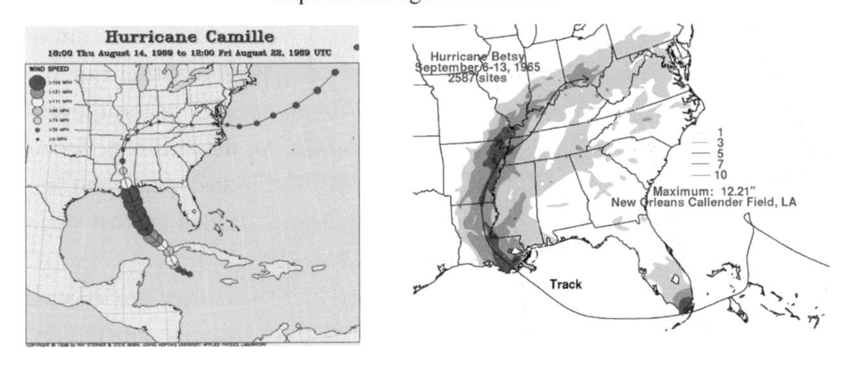

Figure 2.2

The NOAA map shows the centrality of New Orleans in hurricane tracks recorded over the last 160 years. Author/NOAA data.

storms mapped include, in a partial list, hurricanes Betsy (1965),[7] Camille (1969), Bret (1999),[8] and Wilma (2005).[9] Mapping Katrina as if it were a unique event denied that history and its potential lessons.

Similarly absent in the Map-Off entries was the wealth of then-available data detailing the city's many physical vulnerabilities.[10] A map of roads and streets of New Orleans, and their links to the rest of the state and country, would have been an important contribution to understanding what turned the hurricane into a human disaster.[11] New Orleans's evacuation protocols, such as they were, assumed that citizens would flee in private cars and, further, that Louisiana highways could handle the outflow volume. No one had tested those assumptions or predicted the traffic chaos that might result. And, more ethically central, the assumption of independent evacuation meant people without cars were likely to be stranded if the levees failed and the city flooded.[12] By far the greatest losses in Katrina occurred among the fragile who because of age, illness, or poverty were stuck in place.[13] As June Isaacson Kailes and Alexandra Enders would argue in 2007, attention to those with "diverse needs" serves not only the "disabled" but also a range of persons living in or near disaster sites (earthquakes, fires, hurricanes, landslides, tornadoes, and so on).[14] None of this, however, was lodged in the maps of the Map-Off participants.

The most devastated wards with the greatest loss of life, the Lower Ninth and North Bywater,[15] were the poorest in the city and the ones in which lived the highest percentage of African American residents (78 percent).[16] In the weeks after Katrina, Mathew Ericson, deputy graphic editor for the *New York Times*, and his team together traced the extent of the flood on a map of New Orleans wards and then added socioeconomic data to demonstrate the relative effect of the hurricane on poor and rich, black and white, New Orleans residents (fig. 2.3).

In 2005 issues of poverty, race, and levee safety in the Ninth Ward and Bywater were an old and familiar story. In the 1920s, the old Ninth Ward was bisected in the name of commerce so that the Industrial Canal could be deepened to permit increased deep-water shipping. In theory, adjacent wards were protected by levees, but their adequacy was repeatedly questioned. After they were breached and the ward flooded by Hurricane Betsy in 1965, President Lyndon Johnson, who toured the resulting devastation, promised it would never be allowed to happen again. Before Katrina, federal engineers had recommended remedial action for at-risk levees—they knew the potential for disaster—but the necessary repairs were never funded and thus never carried out. Without them, and given the virtual certainty of a category 5 hurricane, sooner or later (the levees were designed to withstand, at best, category 3 storms) the human disaster that was Katrina was not merely predictable but inevitable.

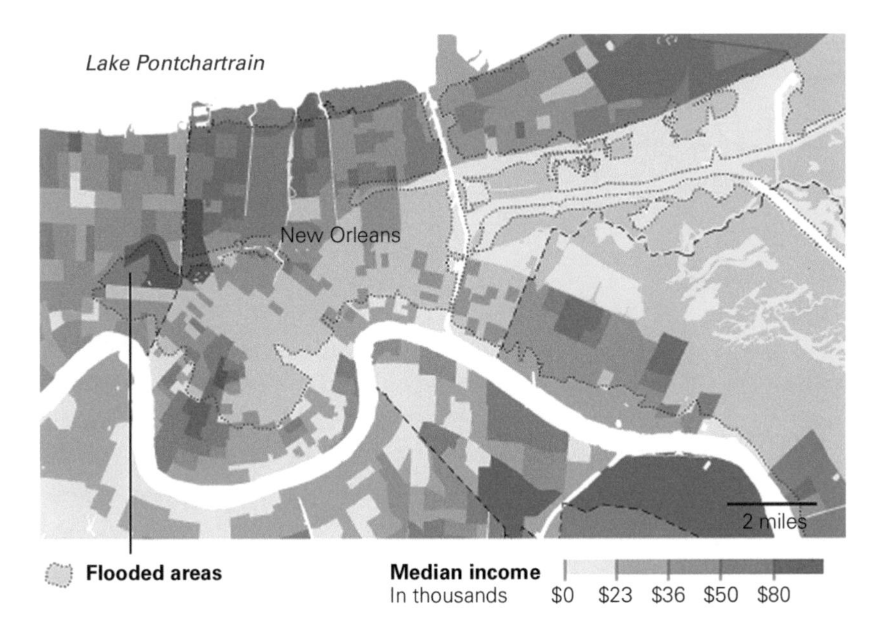

Figure 2.3
In the weeks after Katrina, Matthew Ericson of the *New York Times* attempted to map the relationship of income levels and residence in the city's most decimated wards. Ericson, "When Maps Shouldn't Be Maps."

Similarly inevitable was that the brunt of the storm would fall upon the poorest wards, the Ninth and Basewater. A *New York Times* map of affected areas was embedded in a page that gave the average income, general demographics, and population of each ward (figure 2.4). This "epi-text" in which the map was placed gave to each area a sense of population and the relative effect of the storm on poorer versus richer citizens living farther from the most vulnerable levees.

All of this, I suggested, had a lot to do with ethics and responsibility in mapping. The hurricane was natural, but the extraordinary loss of life and property was not. Rather, it was the result of a long history of local, state, and federal inaction. To present maps of the storm and its effects as if they were an unavoidable and unexpected "natural" disaster denied the histories that transformed predictable occurrence into destructive human catastrophe. It let everyone off the hook. Where were the ethics in *that*? If this was the best that North America's cartographic experts could do, what did it say, I asked, about us as citizens and professionals?

That created quite a stir and a lot of discussion that continued long after Map-Off ended. First up was the newspaper's mapmaker, who took heated exception to my

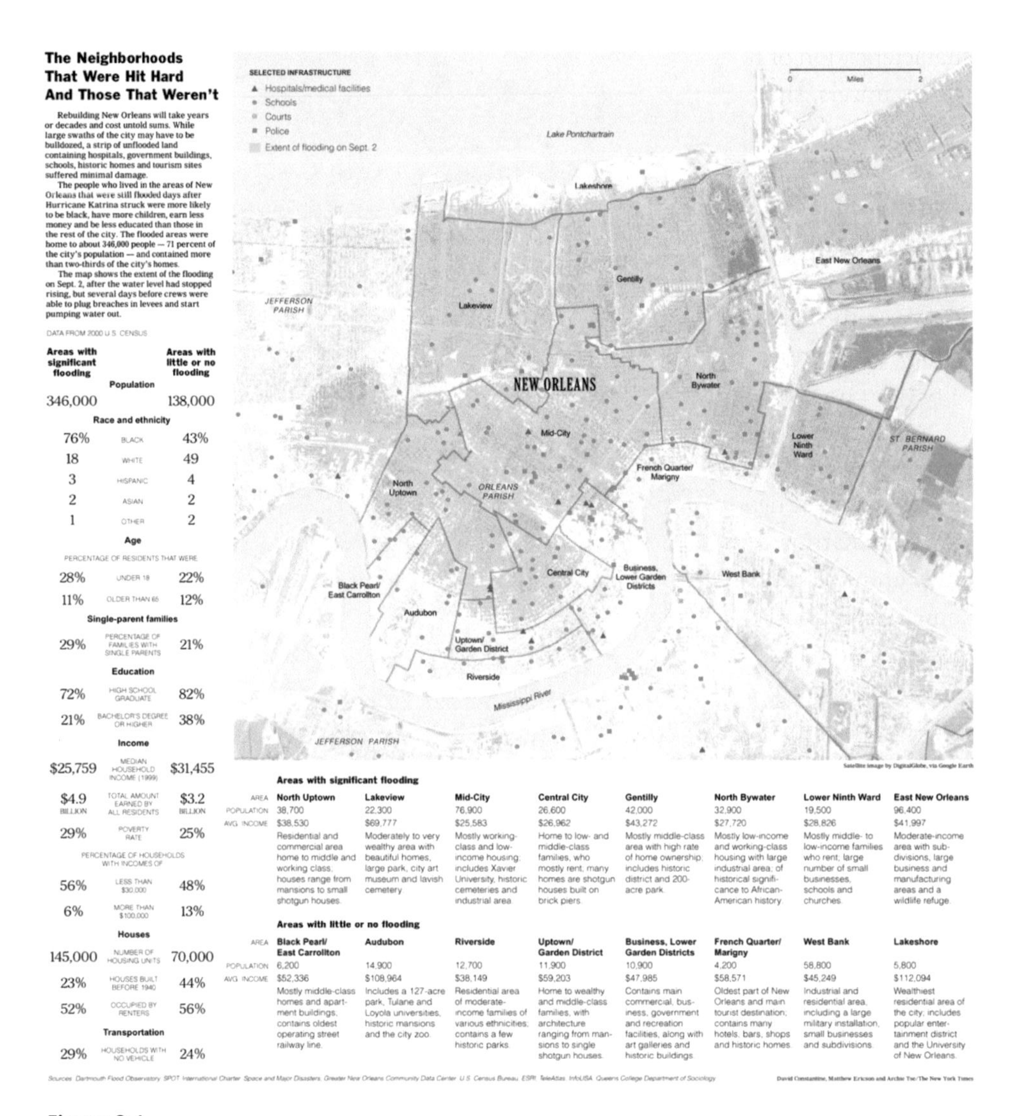

The Neighborhoods That Were Hit Hard And Those That Weren't

Rebuilding New Orleans will take years or decades and cost untold sums. While large swaths of the city may have to be bulldozed, a strip of unflooded land containing hospitals, government buildings, schools, historic homes and tourism sites suffered minimal damage.

The people who lived in the areas of New Orleans that were still flooded days after Hurricane Katrina struck were more likely to be black, have more children, earn less money and be less educated than those in the rest of the city. The flooded areas were home to about 346,000 people — 71 percent of the city's population — and contained more than two-thirds of the city's homes.

The map shows the extent of the flooding on Sept. 2, after the water level had stopped rising, but several days before crews were able to plug breaches in levees and start pumping water out.

DATA FROM 2000 U.S. CENSUS

Areas with significant flooding		Areas with little or no flooding
	Population	
346,000		138,000
	Race and ethnicity	
76%	BLACK	43%
18	WHITE	49
3	HISPANIC	4
2	ASIAN	2
1	OTHER	2
	Age	
	PERCENTAGE OF RESIDENTS THAT WERE	
28%	UNDER 18	22%
11%	OLDER THAN 65	12%
	Single-parent families	
29%	PERCENTAGE OF FAMILIES WITH SINGLE PARENTS	21%
	Education	
72%	HIGH SCHOOL GRADUATE	82%
21%	BACHELOR'S DEGREE OR HIGHER	38%
	Income	
$25,759	MEDIAN HOUSEHOLD INCOME (1999)	$31,455
$4.9 BILLION	TOTAL AMOUNT EARNED BY ALL RESIDENTS	$3.2 BILLION
29%	POVERTY RATE	25%
	PERCENTAGE OF HOUSEHOLDS WITH INCOMES OF	
56%	LESS THAN $30,000	48%
6%	MORE THAN $100,000	13%
	Houses	
145,000	NUMBER OF HOUSING UNITS	70,000
23%	HOUSES BUILT BEFORE 1940	44%
52%	OCCUPIED BY RENTERS	56%
	Transportation	
29%	HOUSEHOLDS WITH NO VEHICLE	24%

Areas with significant flooding

AREA	North Uptown	Lakeview	Mid-City	Central City	Gentilly	North Bywater	Lower Ninth Ward	East New Orleans
POPULATION	38,700	22,300	76,900	26,600	42,000	32,900	19,500	96,400
AVG. INCOME	$38,530	$69,777	$25,583	$26,962	$43,272	$27,720	$28,826	$41,997
	Residential and commercial area home to middle and working class; houses range from mansions to small shotgun houses.	Moderately to very wealthy area with beautiful homes, large park, city art museum and lavish cemetery.	Mostly working-class and low-income housing; includes Xavier University, historic cemeteries and industrial area.	Home to low- and middle-class families, who mostly rent; many homes are shotgun houses built on brick piers.	Mostly middle-class area with high rate of home ownership; includes historic district and 200-acre park.	Mostly low-income and working-class housing with large industrial area; of historical significance to African-American history.	Mostly middle- to low-income families who rent; large number of small businesses, schools and churches.	Moderate-income area with subdivisions, large business and manufacturing areas and a wildlife refuge.

Areas with little or no flooding

AREA	Black Pearl/ East Carrollton	Audubon	Riverside	Uptown/ Garden District	Business, Lower Garden Districts	French Quarter/ Marigny	West Bank	Lakeshore
POPULATION	6,200	14,900	12,700	11,900	10,900	4,200	58,800	5,800
AVG. INCOME	$52,336	$108,964	$38,149	$59,203	$47,985	$58,571	$45,249	$112,094
	Mostly middle-class homes and apartment buildings; contains oldest operating street railway line.	Includes a 127-acre park, Tulane and Loyola universities, historic mansions and the city zoo.	Residential area of moderate-income families of various ethnicities; contains a few historic parks.	Home to wealthy and middle-class families, with architecture ranging from mansions to single shotgun houses.	Contains main commercial, business, government and recreation facilities, along with art galleries and historic buildings.	Oldest part of New Orleans and main tourist destination; contains many hotels, bars, shops and historic homes.	Industrial and residential area, including a large military installation, small businesses and subdivisions.	Wealthiest residential area of the city; includes popular entertainment district and the University of New Orleans.

Sources: Dartmouth Flood Observatory; SPOT; International Charter: Space and Major Disasters; Greater New Orleans Community Data Center; U.S. Census Bureau; ESRI; TeleAtlas; InfoUSA; Queens College Department of Sociology

David Constantine, Matthew Ericson and Archie Tse/The New York Times

Figure 2.4

The *New York Times* combined mapping, statistics, and text to argue the relationship between socioeconomics and storm damage. Ericson, "When Maps Shouldn't Be Maps."

characterization of her efforts. She had accepted the assignment as a favor to the Map-Off organizers, she told me, but hell, she was a very busy person and had a map she had already produced for her employers, so … where was the harm? The rules were crafted to ensure all contestants a level playing field, I replied. Submitting her map as if it were made for the competition, and thus in accord with Map-Off rules, I replied, was simply dishonest. The harm was to her fellow mapmakers, also busy professionals, who had obeyed the rules, spent the time, and given their best effort to the competition. Moreover, the harm was to other NACIS members who expected participants not only to play by the rules but also to do their best work. If honesty is an ethical virtue she subscribed to, I said, shouldn't she be ashamed of her false pretenses?

Another mapmaker complained that he had carefully mapped the storm's track through the Gulf, and what was wrong with that? Nothing, I said, except that we had all seen scores of nearly identical maps on TV and in newspapers during and immediately after Katrina. Mapping the storm's track yet again was at best repetitive and certainly uninteresting. What did he want us to *learn* from his map that we did not already know? What, precisely, did he want to *say*? Why make a map at all, I asked, if it only tells us what we think we already know, if it merely repeats what has already been said? A map that argued the disaster was socioeconomic and cultural, not simply natural, would be both more informative and more interesting to produce.

What most people wanted to talk about, however, was the *idea* of ethics as a practical thing. What did I mean by ethics, they asked? How might ethics be understood in relation to people whose livelihood is based on contractual assignments from clients—academic and commercial—requiring they formulate graphic statements based on data the mapmakers did not themselves either choose or collect? Wasn't it enough to be "professional," by which most meant competently completing an assignment on time and to a certain standard of aesthetic and cartographic excellence? And, really, aren't maps just the transposition of a dataset into a graphic? Was it *really* their business to question an assignment, critiquing the relevance of the data they were given? Was it somehow their responsibility?

That Queasy Feeling

The philosopher Mary Midgley declares that "people avoid thinking about things which would stop them from doing what they wish."[17] But NACIS members *were* thinking about such things, not shying away. Their "moral intuition" wasn't a sudden impulse or instinct but a recurring problem for which they could find no answer.[18] Most of the NACIS members I talked to said they knew what it was to be uncomfortable with an assignment, either its general subject or the adequacy of the data they were asked to map. They had experienced that queasy feeling when a job is competently completed but, in its aftermath, they can feel little pride in the result. Most could describe an incident in which they did everything right but knew that, somehow, what they had produced was somehow wrong (or at least wrongish).

Something was missing. There was, they said, nothing in their training that prepared them for this sense of ethical unease incurred while mapping other persons' stories and subjects. Some said they had taken a course in philosophy in college, but reading Aristotle, Plato, and Kant had been of little relevance, and less guidance, in confronting the mundane choices they encountered in their roles as professional mapmakers for hire.

I told the NACIS members that, as a bioethicist, I had worked with nurses, doctors, and hospital officials who expressed a similar sense of ethical unease and moral uncertainty. I had heard such concerns from graphic artists illustrating work they thought at least somewhat inappropriate, and from academic librarians whose research they believed was used selectively to create incomplete and thus if not biased then at least limited reports. I suspected but wasn't sure the distress, or at least discomfort, NACIS members were describing was similar. I promised to try to figure out how they corresponded and to write an article from the mapmakers' perspective that might speak to their concerns.

Moral Philosophy

I first turned to moral philosophy, whose practitioners seek to systematize potentially applicable notions of good and bad, right and wrong, in their crafting of "normative" frameworks potentially (but not necessarily) applicable to practical questions of conduct and behavior.[19] There are four major approaches, and a quick reference to any of them might have served had I chosen to fashion a superficial answer. As I worked on this problem, talking to cartographers and then demographers, journalists, and statisticians (as well as ethicists), I would see one or another of these general frameworks enacted time and again by people who had never read works in the field.

Consequentialists focus less on the act (what we do) than on its resulting effect, good or bad. Consequentialism is typically invoked to emphasize the "big picture" of outcomes rather than the smaller field of individual actions. A soldier's performance on the battlefield is judged by its result (take that hill, hold that town, and thus win this war), even if the killing required to achieve that objective seems morally problematic to the soldier him- or herself. If the war is deemed just, then so, too, are the actions of the soldiers who in its prosecution follow the "rules of engagement" their superiors have laid out.

Deontology, on the other hand, presents a kind of more or less rule-based ethics. For a deontologist, mapmakers have an obligation to complete their contractual obligations. Like most citizens, mapmakers are expected to tell the truth as best they can. They have an obligation not to steal another's work or to manipulate data in a manner that is self-consciously untruthful. Those are the rules. The NACIS news cartographer, for example, broke faith with her fellow members by not following the rules designed to give Map-Off contestants an equal playing field. Whether rules are just or unjust, capricious or carefully wrought, may be another issue.

That NACIS members cared at all about such things spoke to the third main branch of moral philosophy. Virtue ethics' neo-Aristotelian theme focuses on what motivates persons to feel good about their lives. A sense of well-being comes from living in accord with a set of shared social virtues. So from the start it is about the person in relation to society and its values. "But what virtue is, and what constitutes a good man, have always been matters of conflicting opinion."[20]

Alasdair MacIntyre attempted to create an Aristotelian, virtue-based ethic but found it rough going. "Every action is the bearer and expression of more or less theory-laden beliefs and concepts, every piece of theorizing and every expression of belief is a political and moral action."[21] And since those are open to dispute and disagreement—suppositions seeking clarification—what is correct is rarely immediately clear. The result, MacIntyre said, is that "it begins to appear implausible to treat moral judgments as factual statements." But if everything is subjective, then how do we choose?

Finally, there are the so-called moral realists, who insist there is no fundamental, ironclad moral truth. For followers of William James's pragmatism, the values we promote and the ethics we embrace are the result of an ongoing mix of experience and reflection.[22] We kind of make it up as a society as we go along, in other words. We do this based on a broad base of historical values—religious and secular—that set the context of contemporary values. The result is the virtue we proclaim through the rules we apply to behavior whose presumably ethical results are things we can feel good about promoting. The result may guide individuals whose judgments consciously exist within the context of a great social value set.

By putting these branches of moral philosophy together, I found I might describe moral stress or distress as an inevitable condition of people trying to do right (virtue ethics) while playing by the rules (deontology), but who know or suspect their actions have consequences that are somehow injurious, misleading, or just plain wrong. They can't feel good about that. As virtue ethicists, the nature of their character is tarnished.

Queasiness exists, therefore, at the intersection of a number of vectors: a person's sense of self-worth and social standing, constricting behavior-governing rules (deontology), and a scale of consequences (individual, cultural, social) they believe likely if not inevitable. The result is a morass in which pragmatic solutions do not easily answer complex underlying questions.

Geography and Ethics

For the average mapmaker, ethics is primarily deontological. The rules are simple: don't lie (falsify the data being mapped) and don't steal (plagiarize another's work). The objective of mapping is to produce a value-free, factual representation of the world (or at least an employer's vision of it). To do less is to break faith with map readers (a moral violation) because, as Judith Tyner put it, "map users tend to place inordinate faith in maps and accept them as true and complete representations."[23] Failing those expectations, mapmakers fail their readers, violating their trust, offering what seems true and complete but is not.

But as Tyner acknowledged, *all* maps fall short of that goal because they are abstractions whose promises of completeness and objectivity are bounded by the limits of the data sets selected and the means of their presentation. As Brian Harley put it, "To present a useful and truthful picture, maps must tell white lies."[24] A truth built on lies seems, however, problematic. Complete truthfulness is an unobtainable, default standard,[25] because all "scientific geovisualization" is biased, or at least influenced by the mapmaker's aesthetic and his or her point of view.[26]

So the real message has been that maps promise what they can't deliver. Looking for objectivity and truth is something of a mug's game. Mark Monmonier says the problem is that a two-dimensional map is just too small a canvas to capture the real.[27] Even atlases—map collections focused on a single subject—can't do the job, however. "Powerful narratives often underlie the seeming objectivity" of atlases, wrote Bieke Cattoor and Chris Perkins in 2014.[28]

This was all pretty much a riff on David Hume (1711–1776), introduced briefly in the previous chapter, perhaps the greatest philosopher ever to write in English. "Reject every system," Hume advised those seeking the critical and objective, "however subtle or ingenious, which is not founded on fact and observation," and "hearken to no arguments but those which are derived from experience."[29] The problem is that observations *always* are based on and bent around a set of ideas that define the search for relevant data, determine the method of analysis and then the medium in which its conclusions are presented. So at best, maps (and by extension, as we will see, charts, graphs, tables, and other graphics) are only as "objective as possible" within the framework of a given authorial point of view.

That was a basic message of Denis Wood's *The Power of Maps* (1992), which concluded that, in the end, maps *re*present nothing. Instead, as Jacques Bertin later put it, maps present ideas about things in the world through a system of signs employed to craft a view of the world *as if* it were complete, objective, and therefore true.[30] Truth, objectivity, and the ethics that promote them are merely tracings of a system of presentation ordered around an idea about things and their importance.

Complexities

None of this is unique to cartography. It is instead a general limit to our knowing. Journalism, for example, similarly promises an "objectivity" whose "truth" is always limited and at best only partial. *The Reporter's Handbook* describes the news reporter's job as being "to accurately report what is said, heard, or seen by an individual at a place and time."[31] That the attributed description or statement may be fantastic puffery is irrelevant. Simple deontology rules: reporters accurately reproduce a subject's statements in an objective manner. The consequences of correctly attributing this or that fantastic assertion are of little relevance.[32] The newsperson's ethical allegiance is to neither the veracity of the attributed statement (that it is true rather than simply truthfully reported) nor its completeness but primarily to its repetition. The new story thus promotes a small truth (she said, he said) but remains agnostic about the greater truth value of the statement itself. The same is true of statisticians (as I later demonstrate) who analyze data collected by others and then distill those numbers into a conclusion.

This was made clear in 2016 and 2017 with the accusations of "false news" trumpeted by a new president who, across his candidacy and after his inauguration, issued a series of duly reported statements whose factual basis was largely nonexistent. The news reportage was factual, however, in the sense that it was an accurate restatement of his utterances. The news was real, but the content, when considered impartially, was not.

Riding beneath the ethics pervading cartography, journalism, and most "knowledge industry" professions is a belief in the world as a simple place where unassailable facts exist like Lego blocks, which, correctly assembled, accurately mirror the objective real. One needs simply to fit them together to produce a disinterested, rational presentation of events. But complexity rules at every stage and in every field: "On the one hand there is an order that simplifies, and on the other there is an elusive and chaotic complexity expelled, produced, or suppressed by it."[33] In our maps, charts, graphs, graphics, statistics, news stories and reports, we present the simple without attention to the elusive and chaotic. Sometimes we then feel uneasy about the result.

The Project

Two things were clear. First, if the NACIS meeting was typical, a lot of working cartographers were sometimes uneasy about the ethics of their work. By this I understood them to be unclear about the role of their mapmaking as a social good (and remember, for Plato, truth *is* a social good) in which they could take pride. Second, neither cartographers nor geographers possessed a clearly articulated moral paradigm that might be transposed into a daily ethic of practice. From the geographer Immanuel Kant,[34] whose philosophical writings form the bedrock of modern ethics,[35] to the Marxist musings of a young David Harvey in his 1973 *Social Justice and the City*,[36] geographers (and cartographers) have been grand at high-toned moral pronouncements but (with a few notable exceptions) generally deficient in their practical application to the urgent if pedestrian issues facing average citizens seeking informed answers about good and bad practices, about how to assign values like right and wrong in their daily lives.

Welcome to the complexity that rules us all. One person's virtuous whistle-blower is another's chatty, untrustworthy tattletale. One person's fact is another's fake news. One profession's exemplar is another's villain. One person's data trove is another's toxic data dump. What was needed was a map through the mire of ethical platitudes and presumptions whose general fault lines were, in the end, basically unchanged since the days of David Hume.

The goal became to use cartography as a laboratory in which to investigate the lines between ethical pride and distress, moral comfort and discomfort, good and bad, right and wrong. Hume repeatedly warned against any approach that begins with grand truths that "fix beyond controversy the foundations of morals, reasoning and criticism."[37] That is still good advice, because ethics, at least as they are understood here, exist *in* controversy over how things are to be evaluated, interpreted, presented, and then judged. One must look at actions *and* consequences, rules *and* results, in evaluating a map (or story or statistic) and our responsibility for and to it.

Michael Dobson summed up the general problem nicely in a 1991 roundtable on ethical problems in cartography: "If we want to serve the public well and not be at odds with our inner drives, [then] our objective and subjective responsibilities must be closely aligned."[38] Three assumptions are buried in his seemingly simple proposition. First, public service is a universal and recognizable good, something everyone believes in to a greater or lesser extent. If we are to be ethical, we must serve the public and not simply ourselves and our employers. Second, public service can potentially conflict with personal beliefs, needs, and limits. Third, "external demands and requirements" impose practical constraints that create problems of ethical unease.

The morals of the map, and of everything else, thus reside in what Andrew Pickering called "the mangle of practice," in which the world we perceive, and our place in it, is an often conflicted series of interactions in which public statements, personal convictions, and pragmatic realities abut like sliding tectonic plates.[39] The question became how to make this clear, how to set it in a context that would serve the needs of NACIS members who had challenged me to help those for whom moral distress, or at least moral stress, was a part of their daily life.

The Problem

It took me a year to craft a serviceable example that would reflect these complexities in a simple way. The result, "False Truths: Ethics and Mapping as a Profession," was published in the NACIS magazine *Cartographic Perspectives* and serves as the basis for the next two chapters.[40] Craftily, I think, it presented (without naming them) an opportunity for consequential, deontological, pragmatic, and virtue-based approaches to ethical problem presentation. Depending on the reader's point of view, any or all of those approaches could be deployed to give different answers to what I called "the Tobacco Problem."

For several years, I presented the problem in classroom and conference lectures and exercises. In those venues, participants asked questions I could not answer, although, like any good lecturer, I could finesse them with a quip. Is the map a unique ethical environment? How does the map differ from the database of incidents on which it is based? Why can't a general ethic assumed to prevail in society simply be applied to problems of mapping? Might the ethics of mapping provide a way to critique the general ethics of modern (which is to say postmodern) business and culture? And most importantly, how does one seek the answers to these questions?

The result was a kind of evolving anthropology of ethics, an ethnography that "confronts us with alternative worlds of value and meaning" and whose goal is a consideration of the "differences that make a difference for the way lives are lived, developed, and experienced, and for the way competence, excellence, virtue, and personal well-being are defined."[41] Ethnographers focus on the way people talk about and reflect on their lives. Going deeper, seeking the roots of those reflections, reveals the substrata on which we build descriptions of our place in the world.

3 The Tobacco Problem

Think about this: You and your partner are the owners and operators of a struggling cartographic and statistical firm, Map-Off Ltd. You're scraping by, barely paying the monthly mortgage installment or the bill for the kids' hockey lessons. The hypothetical American Tobacco Consortium (ATC) offers you a highly lucrative contract. You are asked to generate a map of healthy long-term smokers over sixty-five years of age in the United States. You can use US census data as a basis for your work. In fact, they provide a link to the data. You are encouraged to find and use graphics (a bar chart, for example, or a photograph) or anything else that will make your map the best possible statement of the existence of long-lived tobacco users in the United States.

The map you produce will be used in an advertising campaign targeting tobacco-using senior citizens. You are told, informally, that if ATC likes your work, more and equally generous contracts will follow.

Do you take the contract, knowing that tobacco is a carcinogen responsible for the deaths of some but not all users, as well as the deaths of nonusers affected by second-hand smoke? Do you proudly send the map to your father if your mother died of a tobacco-related cancer?

Thinking about ethics and their underlying morals is hard stuff. As Socrates famously said in *The Republic*, "The argument concerns no casual topic but one's whole manner of living."[1] And while it's personal—what *you* believe, and how you choose to act—it is far more than that. "Ethics requires us to go beyond 'I' and 'you' toward a universalizeable judgment," writes the contemporary philosopher Peter Singer, "somehow perceived from the standpoint of the impartial spectator or ideal observer."[2] The problem is that the idea of impartial spectators pronouncing on a "universalizeable judgment" is one of philosophy's enduring great fictions. Over the centuries, its precise identification has proved to be, like complete scientific objectivity, an impossible dream. Wholly impartial spectators are phantoms we seek but can never find.

There are no ironclad tests that a thing is moral; no statistical certainty will ensure *A* is always ethically appropriate while *B* is always bad. Morality is always bounded by the mores of the society in which it is defined and the means by which its ideals are first understood and then applied in a particular context. Ethics may enforce, but cannot prove, the correctness of the underlying moral definitions—the bedrock presuppositions—on which they are based.[3] This does not necessarily lead to moral anarchism or untrammeled relativism. It does, however, limit discussions of ethical alternatives from the search for universal bedrock truths (all cultures and all times) to a more limited social (and thus legal) framework.

Every culture has a small set of moral definitions used to justify laws, professional injunctions, and social codes of behavior. When stepped down to the scale of individual activities, these create the framework of a shared practical ethic. Ethical actions therefore, at least as understood here, are only as universal as the moral suppositions and resulting declarations grounding propositional if-then syllogisms. *Y* only follows if we accept the antecedent *x*. Truthfulness is defined as a moral good, for example, because without it, civility would suffer in a society dependent on honest exchanges between citizens. If social civility is important, then truthfulness is an important good. *If* that is accepted, *then* self-conscious lying must be seen as a danger to the civility and openness of society. Ethically, therefore, we should aim to promote truthfulness and condemn deceit.

Taken this way, ethics is morality's conditional operand, the mechanism with which we evaluate actions based on a small set of broadly accepted moral presuppositions. Put another way, ethical propositions are action statements based on moral definitions reflecting the "manner of being" of good individuals in communities acting in the shared world.

Ethics is therefore from this perspective a communal thing, enacted individually within a shared morality. Its moral groundings can better be described as a set of cultural ideologies rather than as philosophic immutabilities. To call the resulting ethos ideological is not to demean it. Ideologies shape our perceptions and our judgments everywhere, in science no more or less than in philosophy.[4] There is *always* a set of definitions, declarations, and attendant suppositions directing our focus in one direction while inhibiting thinking in another. From that ideology comes a set of conditional and unconditional values.[5] Our shared truths grow from shared agreement; it is consensus that makes them powerful. The only test in the end, therefore, is whether a demonstrable consistency exists between moral declaration, ethical program, and resulting social action.

Consider the fictional tobacco company assignment that begins this chapter. Ask: *Is this assignment ethically problematic? Is it morally questionable?* In calling forth a graphic argument, the question becomes: why does it make us, or at least some of us, feel so queasy?

The Map

If the map of long-lived smokers (fig. 3.1) is no more than a graphic presentation of data compiled by others, then the mapmaker has no greater responsibility for its content than has the person who laid out this page for my argument. The typesetter didn't read the whole manuscript; nor did the book's designer. They probably didn't read it at all. They simply took edited .docx files and transposed them into a publishable form, electronic or paper based. The designer's job, and that of the printer, was to ensure that the result is legible and as attractive as possible, not that its argument is comprehensive and compelling.

At Map-Off Ltd., you are not asked to critique the data on long-lived smokers, to judge its accuracy or completeness. You are not called on to consider its potential public effect on viewers. The employer, ATC, does not invite your concerns about the relation between sustained tobacco usage and various cancers. The mapmaker's charge, like the page designer's, is simply legible and hopefully persuasive presentation. The sole task is to transform a select set of data into a graphic argument composed of spatial (the states of the United States), illustrative (coloration, border width, etc.), and typographic (numbers and words) elements.

From this limited view, the mapmaker *is* simply a mindless drudge.[6] The *only* issue is whether the map meets a professionally acknowledged, generally accepted aesthetic standard. If it does, then the employer must fulfill his or her promise of payment in exchange for a piece of work whose commercial value was agreed on in advance. To do less would be a breach of contract and thus an act of bad faith, a violation of the general ethics of responsible commercial exchange (the moral supposition that agreements must be honored).

The map that results is not a representation of reality, "the world-as-it-is," or even a reality necessarily known to the mapmaker. Rather, the map presents as if certain and true a particular reality in a geography selected to advance the employer's point of view. It is how he or she would *like* the world to be perceived. At this level, mapmaking is an ethically vacuous, thoughtless, thoroughly pedestrian, if persuasively potent, craft. Social responsibility and greater truths are off the map.

Still Smoking: After all these years!

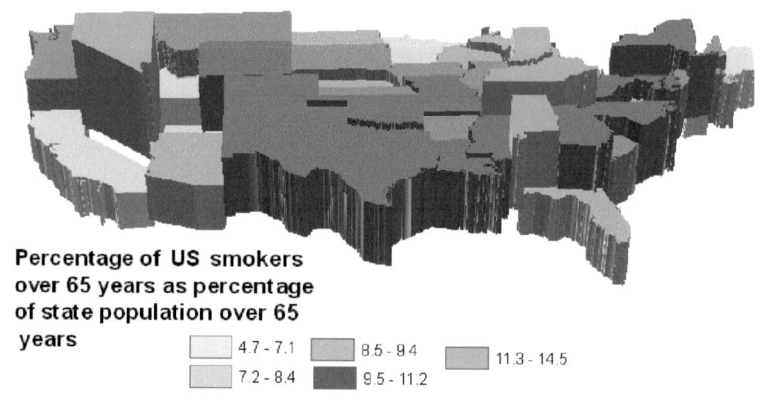

Most people begin smoking during or shortly after adolescence. While many smokers of all ages choose to quit, including seniors (see chart) some continue to use tobacco products. This includes seniors who have smoked for most of their lives.

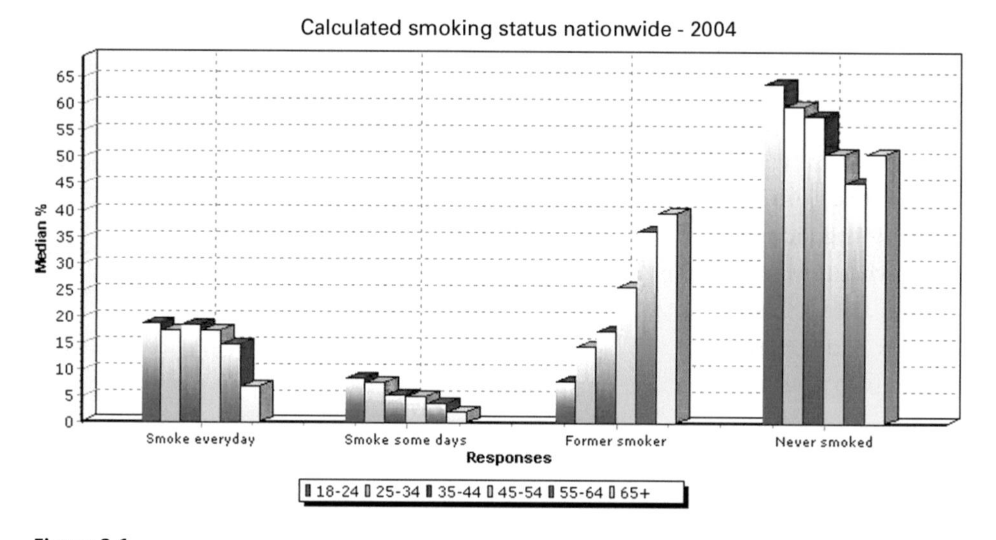

Figure 3.1

"Still Smoking: After All These Years!" A potential response to the hypothetical ATC contract for a map of data on smokers over sixty-five years of age in the United States. Map by author.

The Problem

Cartographers do not like to think of themselves as morally vacuous, ethically empty-headed people. Nor, of course, do analysts, demographers, geographers, graphic artists, statisticians, journalists, and other members of the graphic designing, number-crunching professions. Most workers in what today is sometimes called the "knowledge industry" prefer to see themselves as intellectually rigorous professionals whose skills contribute to a society that values their expertise and judgment. Like most of us, mapmakers want to be proud of the work they do, and that means proud of its public service. The idea is as old as the guild system[7] and was a mainspring powering the rise of professionalism as an ideal in modern society.[8]

The problem is that it will be hard for most of us to be proud of "Still Smoking: After All These Years!" At issue is the message the map presents. "In every map made by a professional cartographer [and by every amateur, too]," wrote J. B. Harley, "some sort of judgment has to be made as to how to represent the world."[9] In this case, the map asserts a positive correlation between longevity and tobacco use. At the least, the map implies smoking is certainly no barrier to longevity. In "Still Smoking," the implicit judgment is that smoking will encourage longevity, and thus health and life.

A bedrock moral presupposition defines human life as the ultimate good, as something precious. The ethical result enjoins life's protection. The proposition behind the map is this: "*If* life is to be preserved (morally), and *if* smokers live long lives, *then* smoking is good for longevity. It is good for life." That, Barthes's semiologists would say, is what is signified by the signs embedded in the map.[10] Its components (blocks of colorful states) promote a falsely positive correlation between tobacco use and the good of an extended lifespan.

The map does not lie. In its lower right-hand corner, it credits the US Centers for Disease Control for the data it deploys; and isn't the CDC the closest thing we have to Singer's impartial observers? That the map does not lie does not mean it tells the truth, however. While the data are official, the conclusion is not. For decades the CDC and almost every other health-related federal agency have been at pains to demonstrate the degree to which tobacco use is a causal factor in a range of cancer and cardiopulmonary fatalities.

We *know* with all sorts of certainty that long-term tobacco use directly or indirectly contributes to the death of thousands of people every year. Current figures suggest there are 480,000 annual deaths related to extended tobacco use in the United States, and about 47,000 in Canada.[11] So the mapped association of smoking with longevity is a "false truth,"[12] mendacity wrapped in a cloak of objective facticity. The map of long-lived smokers is therefore ethically problematic because it presents as factual and complete an equivalence that is unsupportable. Longevity may occur *in spite of* long-term tobacco use, but never *because* of it. The map implicitly advocates as a life-enhancing good a behavior that is injurious and perhaps life threatening. The result is not only a lie but one that violates a moral standard of life promotion and protection.

The mapmaker-as-drudge doesn't care about any of that. He or she, in philosophical terms, is a simplistic deontologist who has followed the rules of commerce: this is the job, those are the figures, take the money and be grateful for the work. Consequently his or her engagement stops there and does not extend to the potential effect of the map campaign on readers. But for some and perhaps for many, the contract would create a conflict in which deontological rationalization conflicts consequentially with the self-image of a would-be virtuous person. Map-Off Ltd. principals know that some smokers, especially the young, may see the map as a rationale encouraging the use of tobacco products. Older addicts (and the addictive qualities of tobacco are firmly documented) may see the map as permission to continue to smoke. It is hard to be a virtue ethicist when the consequences are so harmful, whatever the rules.

Professionally the job should be completed ("I need the money!"), but socially the contract should be rejected. After all, aren't we all charged as citizens with, if not self-consciously promoting health, then at least refusing to present as complete what we know to be a potentially injurious half-truth? Taking the contract, won't we be at least a bit responsible for the seventeen-year-old who shows the map to his parents and says, "See, folks, I can smoke and live long, too." It's a mundane but practical example of Dobson's conflict, described in chapter 2, between private needs and public responsibilities. And then there is the thorny issue of freedom of expression (who am I to censor others?) and, pragmatically, the need for Map-Off Ltd. to make enough money to pay its employees so that they can pay their bills.

We can immediately draw two conclusions from this simple but not simplistic example. The first is that the ethics of mapmaking does not reside solely in the veracity of the facts a map purports to present. Second, a map's ethical quotient does not depend on the excellence of its design. Indeed, to the degree the map's design is persuasive, it only makes the problem more serious, the false truth ("To live long, light up!") more convincing. Instead, the ethics of the map—and our discomfort with it—resides in the proposition it enacts, the conclusions it is crafted to present, and the means by which our morals (MacIntyre's virtues) are challenged (or confirmed) by the result. The map and its graph together present an idea about the world, using data that power (some would say "concretize") a proposition in a landscape that seems "objective" and therefore "truthful."

Representation versus Presentation

The idea that well-constructed maps are technically precise, unambiguous representations of the objective world was a broadly accepted notion until quite late in the twentieth century. This idea was implicit in the work of the doyen of post–World War II cartography, Arthur Robinson, whose *Elements of Cartography* was for decades and through successive editions the teaching bible of the discipline.[13] Maps were to be judged on the manner in which they accurately and aesthetically ordered spatially grounded, objectively impartial data.

Robinson did not urge his students to consider the uses to be made of the maps they constructed. Nor did he advise them to question unduly the data they were asked to map. Given his history, this approach is not surprising. Robinson headed the US military department of cartography, whose members mapped Allied bombing runs in World War II. "They would come to the office," Robinson later said of his years of military mapping, "the main office, my office, and be assigned to a cartographer. He would go over all their needs, establish what data they had and what data we had to provide."[14] Robinson's mapmakers would use those materials to plan bombing runs for air force personnel.

The ethics of Robinson's cartography began and ended with the resulting map's military utility. If the bombing run he was asked to plan would destroy a church, school, or orphanage, it was not his concern. Consequently he did not agonize over the tens of thousands killed in the sorties he helped plan, or the hundreds of pilots carrying his maps who died on missions he and his team scripted. The towns destroyed were not to him the homes of civilians but dots on the target maps he and his staff constructed. For him, and then for the generations of students he taught, a cartographic ethic was in the main an ethic of moral disengagement.

That began to change by the 1990s, when a group of "critical geographers" challenged the idea of the map as a value-free objective presentation of anything.[15] In 1991 J. B. Harley called for mapmakers to consider the "rightness of the social consequences of map-making," recognizing that "every choice that goes into the making of the map has an ethical effect."[16] In 2008, Denis Wood and John Fels redefined the map as a propositional argument with an "if-then" form.[17] And so attention to the predicate clause, the "if" ("if this is true," "if this is important," or "if this is ethical") becomes the fulcrum on which a map's argument might be judged. Queasiness results when mapped results violate a conditional belief in, say, health as a moral good or "truth" as more than a narrowly defined, self-serving rhetorical tool. As we will see, it is the very idea of truth as a simple, objective fact that in the end is challenged as well.

The Map as Story

The problem is not cartographic but general, arising for many people employed in today's knowledge industries. Journalists, to take only one example, face the exact same problem. "We are chroniclers of, rather than participants in, the society around us."[18] Beyond broadly accepted social injunctions against self-conscious lying or theft (plagiarism), the rules of ethical reportage are similarly colored in "shades of grey"[19] and "cannot be cast in stone," as one Canadian journalist proudly put it.[20]

Consider the hypothetical case of a reporter for the Raleigh, North Carolina, *News and Observer* assigned to cover a press conference called by (fictitious) ATC president and well-known local philanthropist Thomas J. Crawford. Upon entering the room, reporters are given a high-resolution color copy of the Map-Off Ltd. tobacco map, "Still Smoking!," and a printed version of Mr. Crawford's prepared talk. The newspaper's cigar-smoking city editor budgets the story for the front of the Metro Section to run with the Map Off Ltd. map graphic under a 36-point headline: "Long-Lived Smokers." Perhaps the page on which it is to be printed carries an ATC product advertisement.

Here is a part of the resulting story:

> "Tobacco use is not a death sentence," Thomas J. Crawford said Thursday. The president of the American Tobacco Consortium was in town to promote a new advertising campaign focused on seniors. "While anything can be deadly in excess," he said, most things—including tobacco—can be pleasurable and even beneficial in moderation." After all, he continued, the human body has natural nicotine receptors, and they obviously are there for a purpose. They are ... natural! Crawford urged North Carolinians to "think for yourselves ... see the CDC data we've mapped here."
>
> Members of the American Cancer Agency (another made-up name) said that they, too, want Americans to think for themselves. "And when they do," said Nikita Kwan, the ACA North Carolina director, "they'll know tobacco is a health risk to be avoided."

During his talk, Mr. Crawford used a laser pointer to emphasize the six-point type at the bottom of the map identifying the data source, http://apps.nccd.cdc.gov/brfss (a link no longer active), the cartographic equivalent of the journalist's "he said" or "she said" attribution. In doing so, the ATC president assigned responsibility for the mapped data to the US Centers for Disease Control, which, as Crawford told reporters, is about as objective and unbiased a federal organization as can be found. The CDC's findings are to be trusted.

The balancing quote from the imaginary American Cancer Agency spokesperson is supposed to make the story objective and neutral, but it does not. Indeed, it reinforces the credibility of Mr. Crawford, who first encouraged his listeners to "think for themselves" and, hey, just look at the map. The ACA official is thus transformed into a support voice urging independent thought that, on the mapped evidence and the story's text and they together seem to embrace long-term tobacco use as an aid to longevity.

The story is "true" in a limited way—Mr. Crawford said this, and statistics on long-lived smokers can look like that—but the result is nobody's greater truth. Mr. Crawford's "think for yourself" invokes as a moral good autonomy and individual choice. That, in turn, echoes the call to rational philosophy and Singer's dispassionate observation. Mr. Crawford's "look at the data, look at the map," neatly subverts any greater body of other public health data detailing the hazards of sustained tobacco use.

Map Stories

Every day thousands of such stories are broadcast or published. Correctly attributed quotes lead to conclusions that are questionable at best if not, upon consideration, nonsensical. During my news career, I wrote hundreds of them. A story's limited facticity—based on the attributed quote—is what brings into being a story's seeming value-free objectivity. From the day of their first byline until their last day on the job, reporters are instructed simply to report: question, perhaps, but do not debate. As one well-known reporter once told me, a reporter should seem to be without opinions, without a personal point of view. There are exceptions, of course, including editorial writers. But they are just that: exceptions.

It therefore should come as no surprise that maps are staple tools accompanying and buttressing news stories. The US-based Investigative Reporters and Editors (IRE), an organization to which I have long belonged, periodically hosts seminars on mapping as a way to both build and buttress news stories. Esri Press, whose parent company produces the popular computer mapping software ArcGIS, has published case studies of news maps.[21] In 1999 Mark Monmonier published *Maps with the News*, a history of progressively accurate and ever more truthful, if sometimes limited, cartographic journalism.[22] Monmonier's book contained no discussion of ethics, or morality, or anything resembling the problems discussed here, however. Maps represented the world through the graphic presentation of data. It was as simple (or as complex) as that.

Maps often serve not simply as an illustration to a news story but as the story itself. In 2005, for example, US wire services carried a map sourced to the software mapping company ESRI (Environmental Systems Research Institute)—the parent company of Esri Press—titled "War with Insurgents Ramped Up." It ran as a stand-alone graphic in some North American newspapers and in others as part of a broader news package.

On November 9, for example, the *Reno Gazette-Journal* included the map with a *Los Angeles Times* wire story on the Baghdad drive-by murder of the defense attorney Adel

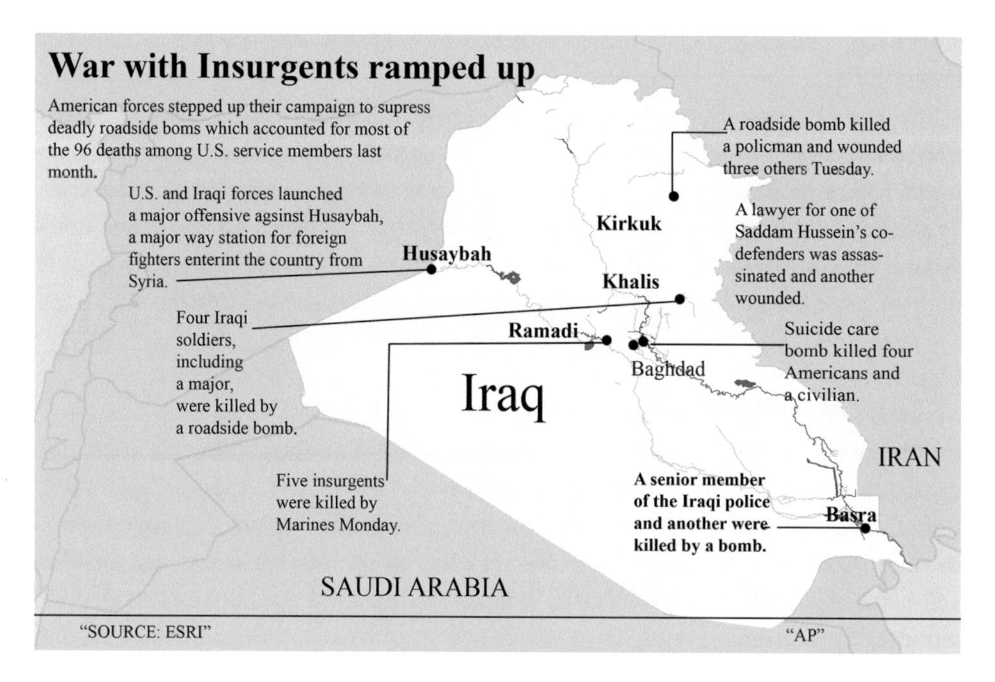

Figure 3.2
A near facsimile of a map produced in 2005 by ESRI (or at least using ESRI materials), with content added by and distributed by US wire services. By author.

al-Zubeidi. Zubeidi had represented Iraqi vice president Taha Yassin Ramadan, then a codefendant at the trial of Saddam Hussein.[23] While the *Los Angeles Times* copy made clear that no one knew who had killed the former vice president or why, the map linked—by means of both its text and its "epi-text," its positioning in the newspaper with the story—the defense attorney's murder to the then-ongoing and righteous battle by US soldiers and their allies against "insurgents."

The original map was one of thousands generated by and for journalists during the US invasion. Many were based on, or simple reproductions of, one or another of the 35 million maps generated by and for the US military in support of its campaign in Iraq.[24] Many of those maps were given to the tens of thousands of US troops (and their embedded journalists) for way finding. Thousands more were used, à la Robinson, in the planning and assessment of military sorties. Military and State Department officials used still more maps in both internal discussions and press briefings (where, I suspect, this map or at least its data originated).

On the map, its source is given as ESRI, which at that time provided map products and expertise both to the US military and to news agencies. The map was carried by the

Associated Press news service and perhaps by others, as well. The map included in this book is a "near facsimile" an "almost but not quite right map" because AP refused permission for its "commercial" use here. Although ESRI was the map's "source," company officials said that because text may have been added to their map product (by the AP or the military; nobody knows), it could not license the map's use here. Whoever made and then modified the ESRI map, its data almost certainly originated in a military press briefing where either the map itself or its summary data were given to reporters. The map included here has the same data and a slight but sufficiently different presentation to avoid legal stricture.[25]

The maps—both mine and theirs—identify locations, posted as black dots, where US troops and their allies had been killed. Those dots are linked by gray lines to explanatory text boxes. One, for example, locates US-led attacks at Husaybah, "a major way station for foreign fighters entering the country from Syria." As in the case of the fictional *Raleigh News and Observer* story with its "Still Smoking!" map, we are seduced by the map's concreteness, its apparent facticity. And certainly the map tells a small truth: US troops and their allies were killed in places identified on the map. They in turn mounted offensives against supposed insurgents in other places like Husaybah.

What would Peter Singer's independent observer think about this? When we read the map, we see insurgents killing virtuous US troops and their allies, who in turn are defending Husaybah, a "way station" for foreign fighters. The map thus ignores the inconvenient fact that US troops were themselves foreign fighters in a country where at least some insurgents were Iraqi-born nationals who saw themselves as patriots defending their homeland against foreign invaders, the US troops. "In fact, the insurgency was made up of a complex mix of forces" who turned Iraq into a terrorist center after, and in no small part as a result of, the US invasion.[26] The result is a small truth (bombs here and battles there) enfolded within a series of polemical postures.

There was nothing exceptional in this. Even the august *New York Times* "based their analysis of the war in Iraq on Pentagon talking points, mostly lies."[27] *CNN* news officials acknowledged "with some pride" seeking Pentagon approval for the hiring of a general as their principal military commentator.[28] It's hard to question a story quoting a general. They are assumed to be authoritative and knowledgeable, if not necessarily impartial. What makes the mapped argument so useful here is that its ideology is at this remove so obvious and its argument so questionable.

The Iraq map continued a long tradition of Cold War–era mapping and news writing that, while publicly proclaiming objectivity, were fashioned to present the idea of a virtuous nation defending values in a dangerously uncivil world.[29] That era's mapping, in turn, followed upon an older tradition in which maps and news stories were self-consciously fashioned to advance this or that militarily enforced, political objective.[30]

The resulting maps and reports were (and are), you might say, "objective propaganda," employing carefully culled sets of data selected to promote a limited, partisan view of the world and its conflicts. In this case, the right to self-defense was the moral declarative justifying the US military's "ramping up" its forces. The proposition was simple: if Americans are attacked by outsiders (foreigners), and if their lives are precious, they then are permitted and indeed obliged to defend themselves. Virtue therefore resides with the US troops fighting for values (democracy, for example) that the virtue ethicist would applaud. Ramping up the military response to foreign insurgents thus was presented as a morally justified, consequentially sound, ethical act.

Did the mapmaker feel queasy about the map he or she was asked to turn out? We don't know. Probably not. In the constant press of deadlines I suspect that he or she didn't think about it at all. Had the cartographer or perhaps a news subeditor said, "Hey, boss, this is bogus!" would he or she have been lauded or told to shut up? Again, we don't know, although my guess, based on years of newsroom experience, is the latter. What is clear is that the map raises ethical questions that go beyond simplistic "he said, she said" truths.

Maps as Science

But, some might say, that's just journalism. Science, on the other hand, is *about* objectivity, its charge Hume's impartial accumulation of value-free facts and Plato's imagined world of nonpersonal, more general truths.[31] There at least is a bastion of impartial presentation rather than a complex and evolving negotiation between argument, bias, fact, and fancy.[32] And yet scientific maps and stories can be as misleading as any produced for commerce or the news. Like all other areas of social knowledge, science is a constructed and tentative argument about a proposed reality it seeks to justify. We saw this in chapter 1 in the story of Dr. John Snow and the London cholera outbreak, and it remains true today.

Consider, for example, the two maps of waiting times for graft liver transplantation shown in figure 3.3. Both were included in a 1999 report prepared by national Institute of Medicine (NIM) scientists charged with evaluating the ethical propriety and the organizational efficiency of the US national graft organ allocation program.[33] The data they used were collected by the United Network for Organ Sharing (UNOS), a nonprofit, arms-length agency created in the 1980s to supervise the US graft organ collection and distribution program under the supervision of the US Department of Health, Education, and Welfare (HEW).

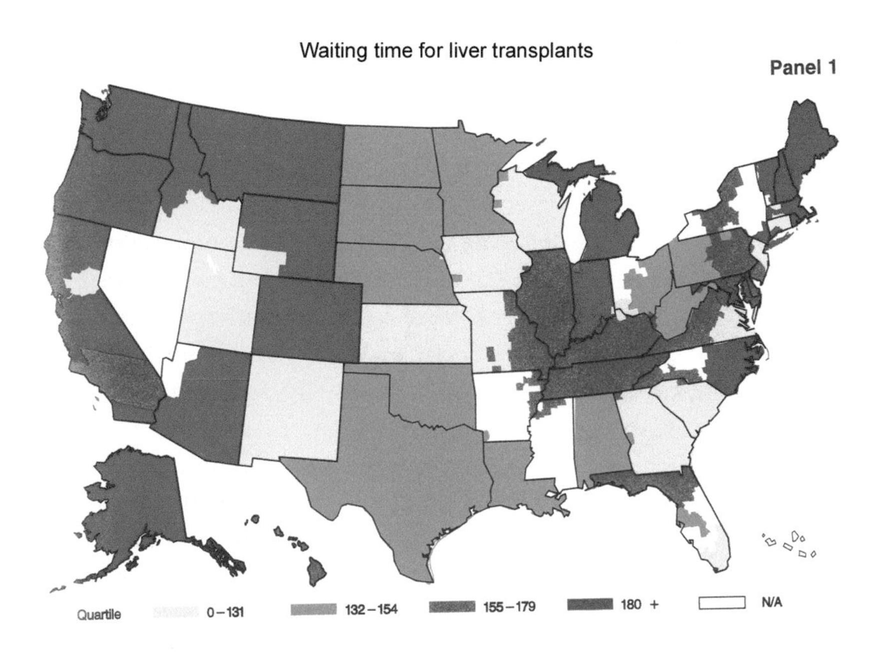

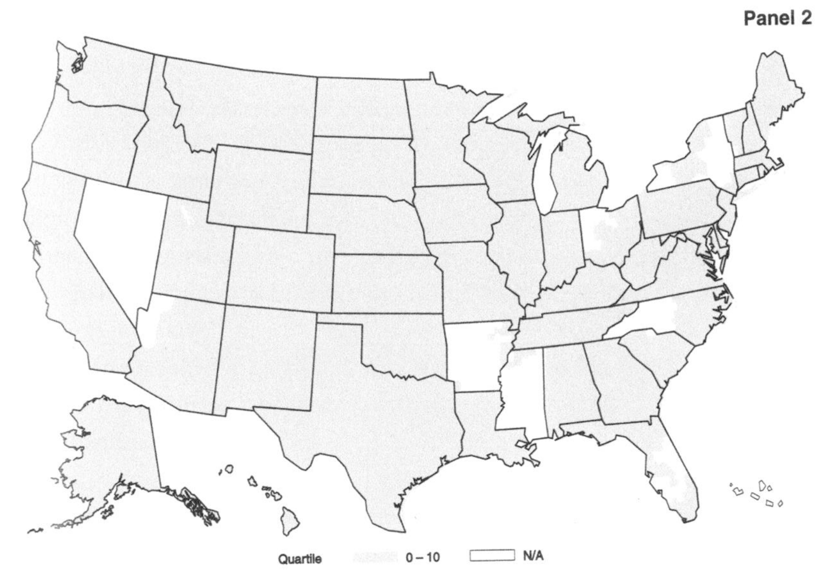

Figure 3.3

The medical status of all patients with liver disease who will require transplants (top) compared with those in urgent need of a liver transplant (bottom). Source: Institute of Medicine, *Organ Procurement and Transplantation,* 58a.

The maps presented state-level data on the wait times of 68,000 persons diagnosed with progressive liver disease. The first map posted a fair amount of geographic variation in the waits experienced by persons on the UNOS registry of potential recipients with chronic but not yet end-stage liver disease. The second map's uniform yellow coloration concluded that when their disease became truly life threatening, people in every state got what they needed and, we assume, were saved.

The study was ordered because, in the 1990s, Health Education, and Welfare secretary Donna Shalala argued the necessity of reforms to correct what she described as serious geographical inequities in the UNOS system of graft organ distribution.[34] If demonstrable, those inequities would have violated the enacting legislation's promise of equal treatment for all potential organ recipients.[35] That promise was based on moral ideals of "equality" and "reciprocity," around which the service was to be ethically organized. The virtuous goal of the system was thus to ensure the equal treatment of all potential recipients.

There was a practical rationale as well as an ethical injunction. Organ transplantation depends on the free donation of organs by families of deceased persons. Presumably people would donate because they believed they or their loved ones had an equal opportunity to receive an organ if one was needed. If they believed that to be untrue, then the rationale for donation in a community of sharing would be restricted.

Hidden in both maps was a series of inequalities and, some would conclude, inequities. I discuss these more fully in chapter 8, but a brief review here makes sense. In 1999 the national organ transplant system included no transplantation centers in thirteen states. Patients in nonserved states who needed a liver (or a kidney, heart, or any other organ) were required to register at and then travel at their own expense to transplant centers in other states, where they might be required to wait for months in hopes of a graft organ becoming available.

That system imposed a number of burdens—familial, financial, and personal—potentially inhibiting the participation of patients who lacked substantial financial resources.[36] Moreover, at least in some cases, those geographic inequalities and their costs presented a potential obstacle to both organ receipt and for those receiving a transplant to the postoperative care and support of patients separated from community and family support systems.

More critically, the UNOS data that report researchers studied included *only* patients who had been accepted as candidates for transplantation. It thus ignored the manner in which socioeconomics—a polite way of speaking about economic, racial, and social disparities—limited potential graft organ receipt.[37] "Although the procurement system is national, patients' access to it is not. Patients must generally either have health insurance that will pay for transplantation or be able to pay for it themselves."[38] Few if any of the more than 40 million citizens who in 1999 lacked health insurance could afford the cost of a transplant and its often equally expensive aftercare. "Few doubted that the barriers of socioeconomic difference were deeply embedded [but hidden] in the maps."[39]

So the UNOS list of potential liver recipients hid, at least potentially, the existence of not only geographic but also socioeconomic disparities affecting a citizen's ability to receive a lifesaving or life-extending graft organ. Legislated ideals of reciprocity and equality were violated. The poor and their families were encouraged to donate organs, but as potential recipients, many were simply ... off the map.[40]

Race and Ethnicity

Researchers for the Institute of Medicine were firm in their insistence that "no significant effects of race or gender were observed, indicating that the system is equitable for women and minorities once listed [as potential recipients]."[41] The key phrase, however, was "once listed." The researcher thus avoided having to think about all those who never made it onto the waiting list. By focusing only on those "once listed," report researchers were able to ignore the effect of race on income, home location, and the ability to afford health insurance on transplant eligibility.[42] The real question should have been, in law and ethics, not simply the performance of the UNOS system for those "once listed" but, more importantly, the reality of those in need but not listed because of location, poverty, race, prejudice, and so on.

In an attempt to show exactly what this meant, in 2001 I produced two maps of Southern California.[43] In figure 3.4, the upper map posted the Southern California counties by population. In the lower map, counties were resized to reflect only the estimated population of health-insured persons. These figures were calculated by subtracting the percentage of uninsured citizens from the total mapped population. In 1998, 35.1 percent of Hispanic Americans were uninsured, and 24.8 percent of African Americans were uninsured, compared to 15.2 percent of white Americans.[44] As a result, the map of Southern Californians eligible for organ transplantation (but not, of course, donation) was changed dramatically. The equity of the system was questioned as a result.

Like the map of Iraqi insurgents, the Institute of Medicine authors' map was truthful in its presentation, but at best incomplete in the conclusions it sought to argue.[45] The error resided in the assumptions that, first, all in need were admitted to the UNOS waiting list irrespective of ethnicity or income, and, second, the relation between

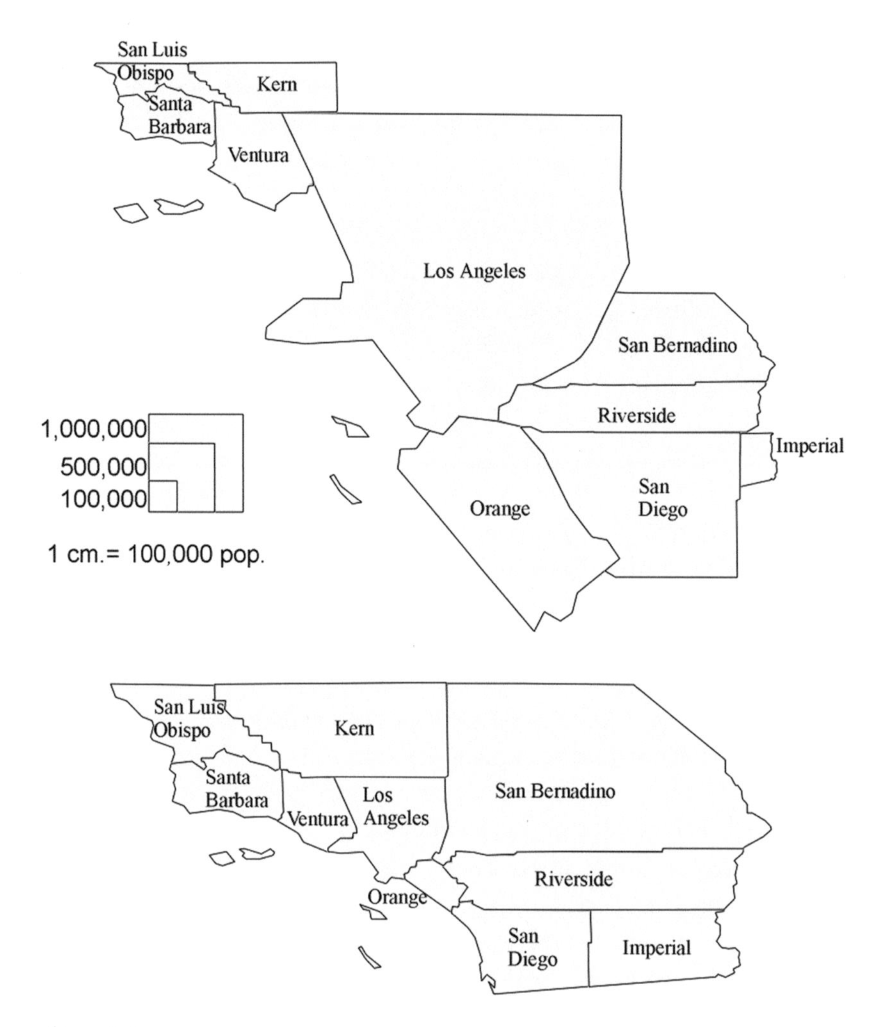

Figure 3.4
Two views of Southern Californian political boundaries in 2001. The first reflects the general population, the second only the health-insured population. A lack of health insurance would result in many persons being unable to afford a graft organ transplant. Maps by author.

home and hospital center locations would make no difference in patient eligibility or treatment.

Like the fictional Raleigh reporter, the transplant study researchers did not independently generate the data they mapped. Instead they used UNOS-collected data for analysis. A UNOS official might say the organization's mandate is to provide an efficient system of graft organ retrieval and distribution and not to resolve structural inequalities in American healthcare or society. But the National Organ Transplant Act of 1984 defined transplantable organs as a national resource to be made available to all in need on an equitable basis. Equal access for all in need was enshrined in law as a moral necessity. And if equality is a moral necessity, and if there were disparities in graft organ distribution, then the system was in violation of its ethical mandate. That was what HEW Secretary Shalala argued and what UNOS officials vigorously (and successfully) disputed.

Reputation

So what? Shouldn't the ethical weight of false or at best partial truths fall on the shoulders of those who order the map? Was it the fault of the Institute of Medicine's cartographers and statisticians? "We took the UNOS data, and if it's incomplete," the mapmakers might have said, "that's on them." And yet wouldn't *you* feel a bit queasy if these were *your* maps, if this was your study? What if it were *your* father who, laid off from his factory job, lost his health insurance and thus his chance for a necessary life-prolonging transplant? If we construct the maps (or charts, or graphs, or pictures, or stories), then we are either mindless drudges—or complicit.

Because ethics goes "beyond 'I' and 'you,'" as Singer put it, this is about more than individual self-esteem or self-interest. To ask about the ethics of an act—analytic, cartographic, statistical, or any other—is to ask about our role in society, our allegiance to its ethical framework and moral values. It is about our actions or inactions as citizens in communities. As Erving Goffman put it in 1959, ethics becomes sociology in a different frame (or perhaps sociology is ethics in a different frame) when a person wants others to take seriously the persona he or she sets forth as responsible and "good."[46] When we dig through these and other examples, however, the work resembles more an anthropology of ethics rather than a sociology of morals. And as an anthropology, it is grounded in the concrete and experiential, as the next chapter attempts to demonstrate.

4 The Morals in the Map: Stress and Distress

Over the years, I have used the Tobacco Problem as both a flexible lesson plan and a tool to investigate how cartographers, geographers, and statisticians (students and professionals) think about the work they do, or hope to do in the future. In a one-hour class or a two-hour seminar, the problem is presented and persons are asked whether they would make the map for ATT or turn down the commission. They are then asked if they would accept a similar assignment for far less money from a cancer-fighting agency seeking to develop a smoking cessation program targeting persons sixty-five years and older. If we have time, the question becomes what the difference would be between those two maps.

Other scenarios were created for special groups. In one, participants were asked to assume they were members of a religious group opposed to abortion. Would it be sinful, and thus inappropriate, to accept a contract to create a map of abortion centers whose purpose was to identify underserved areas where new facilities could be added? Would the map's ethical posture be different if, still as members of that group, they were hired to create a map identifying sites where antiabortion protesters could stage effective demonstrations? What might be the differences, if any, between the maps they produced?

In these and other, similar scenarios, the goal was to introduce the idea of practical, applied ethics in a manner that would seem pertinent to the working lives of those in the classroom. The goal was to encourage participants to think about how mapped content reflects not simply an objective image of the world but the mapmaker's assumptions about it. How might Harley's observation, cited earlier, that all maps (and all studies) present eccentric worldviews, each with potential ethical consequences, be made concretely meaningful? What would be the consequences that participants might see for themselves as people who liked to think of themselves as ethical and upright?

Sometimes, but not always, the discussion ended on a consideration of the limits of "truth" as a realizable ideal and "fact" as an objective standard that required little consideration.

My agenda was as much anthropological (or ethnographic) as it was instructional. I wanted to understand the distinctions participants would make. Would they feel, as did the NACIS members, a tension between Dobson's inner and outer drives, between social responsibilities and the immediate priorities of a person responsible for the success of a business that pays the rent and feeds the family? If so, would they see this as a personal conflict, something inherent in the nature of their profession, or a more general social problem?

In most classes, I would begin by loosely defining ethics as "the evaluation of human conduct, a practical set of ideas of right and wrong." The rules that ethics imposes in evaluating any act, I would say, are typically derived from broadly general moral definitions. For example, if equality is defined as a human good, then it is grounded in the moral declaration that "all men [and all women] are created equal." Ethically, we apply these declarations ("presuppositions" sounds so formal) in if-then propositions (practical syllogisms). If we believe all persons equal, then, all else being equal, it is ethically wrong to advance programs that promote inequality *among* persons. Maps and statistics that hide evidence of inappropriate inequalities can be criticized as ethically inappropriate, as "false truths."

In undergraduate classes in both applied ethics and philosophy, definitions of ethics and morality would first be parsed and then carefully critiqued, their respective etymologic pedigrees discussed over several weeks of dense readings and lectures. But for students in other disciplines, "morality" is a big, big word, one that scares them. It's personal and to be avoided *because* it refers to beliefs that brook no discussion. For most, the idea of ethics seemed a more manageable, and certainly more malleable, judgment category. That a discussion of propositional ethics (if and then) might necessarily involve moral suppositions was not something most participants had considered.

Undergraduates in geography typically found it unsettling that dilemmas might be inherent in applying the basic cartographic techniques they were being taught, that they might have to make difficult ethical choices. They had been taught to think of mapmaking as a technical craft or trade in which hard, objective data representing worldly realities are transposed to the two-dimensional, graphic plane. Professionalism, they assumed, was nothing more than making the most legible map possible using available data. Presenting those data in a visually pleasing graphic form was a technical, and at its higher levels aesthetic, exercise. Most assumed that the nature of the data and the manner of their manipulation were an incontestable given. That statistics are partial and "facts" are bounded by bias and authorial perspective was for most students a matter of some unease.

At first, most undergraduates did not know how to answer a question about their relation to, or responsibility for, their work. That they might be required to make a principled decision that would affect their income, and perhaps their careers, was deeply disconcerting for many. Even more unsettling was the realization that their work might adversely affect the lives of others in their community. The central question—"Would you take the contract?"—personalized ethics (and morality) into a concrete choice in which practical goals and professional aspirations seemed potentially to conflict with a sense of one's place in society as a "good" person. And because these classes were interactive exchanges, not normal lectures, all participants had to announce (and sometimes defend) their choices. In most classes, the discussion followed a similar progression.

First, one or another student would say that his or her major was "commerce," and "in commerce" there would be no question: you do the job you are hired for. Ethical responsibility for the content resides with the employer. That one might, on ethical or moral grounds, *refuse* a contract on grounds of conscience was simply not on these students' radar. Those in prelaw would opine that if the offer from the tobacco interests was presented as a legitimate contract, there should be no problem. After all, Map-Off Ltd. is a business in the business of making maps for others. One student at the University of British Columbia simply shrugged when asked, replying rhetorically, "How could I *not* take the contract?"

Deontology ruled in classes whose students saw mapping as just another tool of commerce. To ask about the ethics of a map's application made as much sense to those students as asking carpentry students about the ethical use of a hammer. The difference between a good map and a bad one, a map to be proud of and a map that was not an object of pride, rested not in its content but in the aesthetics of its presentation. Did the color ramp in a choropleth map adequately and clearly distinguish the categories of data? Was the title's typeface appropriately chosen and correctly sized? At best, some students might ask if the state level of data was the best for "Still Smoking!" (fig. 3.1). Perhaps county-level data should have been employed. Which would yield a better image? How could the noncontinental US states (Alaska and Hawaii) best be included given the projection that was being used? Perhaps a different projection would be better. Maybe Alaska and Hawaii could just be ignored.

Sooner or later, someone would disagree. Sure, "The map is a tool," as one student put it. "The question is how we feel about what's being built. ... Is it good or bad?" At this point, another student usually jumped in to argue that saying maps are just tools "is like saying a gun is *just* a tool and, hey, guns don't kill people, people do." Thus the map would be equated with a gun, and its use in a smoking campaign targeting seniors was seen for the first time as potentially deadly. The analogy typically led someone to extend the analogy, asking if, since guns *do* kill people, then why can't maps kill, too? Even if maps are just tools, they are tools with a purpose. And in this case, the purpose is to promote tobacco use.

And if maps can kill (I would mention here Arthur K. Robinson's military history, described in chapter 3), or at least contribute to killings, are mapmakers at least partially responsible for those deaths? If we blame bartenders who serve drinks to drunken patrons who then commit vehicular homicide, shouldn't we blame mapmakers for maps whose effect is at least as deadly, albeit at a greater remove? Finally, someone would make the point that "everybody knows" prolonged tobacco use causes cancer. We blame tobacco manufacturers for the effects of the carcinogenic products they make and promote, so wouldn't a map that promotes tobacco use be culpable, too?

At this point, someone else would nod and say, "My uncle [or aunt or grandfather], a smoker, died of lung cancer last year [or last month]." Thus the discussion then becomes personal. Taking the contract means supporting something that kills relatives, just as promoting guns, especially certain guns (the Uzi, the Kalashnikov, automatic weapons with overlarge magazines), promotes the killing of people. The equivalence, false or not, is established. "How can you live with that?" one student asked another who said the assignment would be "just business."

Then the bell would ring to signal the end of class. In these classes, the best that could be offered was the beginning of a discussion. In a one-hour class, we rarely got to the question of the nature of the data, the choices the data reflected, or their presumed objectivity. When the classes ran longer, the discussion would get progressively more detailed and even more interesting.

University of Regina

Perhaps the most revealing of these sessions occurred at the University of Regina, where I was hired for a one-week seminar on mapping medicine. Previous annual summer sessions had focused on crime reportage and its mapped statistics, but declining enrollments required program supervisors find a more attractive and thus more remunerative subject. Health and medicine seemed a good choice, and subscriptions for the new seminar were strong. The almost forty paying attendees were professional cartographers, demographers, and statisticians. Some had university appointments. Others worked at one or another level of government, and, in one case, for an independent health agency.

I was hired to deliver a plenary on the history of medical mapping and to teach a two-hour introductory class in computerized mapping using ESRI's ArcGIS software. Across the program's five days, attendees were introduced to at least eight different computer-based programs variously employed to promote data collection and organization, statistical analysis, and, finally, data mapping. On the penultimate day, a scheduled instructor was called away, and I was asked to fill in with another class. "They've had enough software for a year," I said. "Let me do the ethics problem instead of another mapping session with more software most never have used before."

In presenting the Tobacco Problem, I did the normal setup, distinguishing ethics from morality, before dividing attendees into working groups of three or four with at least one mapmaker and one statistician in each group. "Each of you is a member of a company, your group," I said. "Each group is offered this highly lucrative contract from ATC to produce a map titled 'Still Smoking: After All These Years!'" I then added that at the same time (in previous classes, this was a second problem), the Canadian Cancer Prevention Agency offered a far less lucrative contract ($10,000 versus, say, $100,000) for a map targeting long-lived smokers to be used in a smoking cessation campaign. "Take ten minutes or so and decide, as a group, if you take a contract and, if so, which one."

Soon I was approached by one participant, who asked if group decisions had to be unanimous; and without much thought, I replied, "Ideally, and if at all possible." Then I was asked if the majority in a company could fire a dissenting member. I said yes, but only if he or she could find another group to join. Then another asked if she could quit the company in which she found herself, one whose majority position she rejected as "ethically, morally … what*ever*" insupportable. Again, I said yes, but only if she could find another group in which to work. After ten minutes, most of the groups had fired one of their own, a cartographer or statistician who, with others who had been similarly discharged or quit, then created new groups of like-minded persons. Each group elected a speaker to present its decision, and the reasoning behind it, to the class.

Several of the groups said they would take the commission, no problem and no questions asked. It wasn't illegal, and they needed the money. As the representative of one group, a statistician proudly said, "My job, well, *our* job, is data and statistics. I work the numbers, and all this ethics stuff is irrelevant." *Forget* consequentialism; virtue lay in a well-performed contract. The woman behind him leaned forward and asked loudly, "So, if they asked you where to locate a concentration camp, you'd just 'crunch the numbers' and give them a prime location, you fascist?" The statistician turned to her and with equal force replied, "Who is going to decide which numbers are good and which are too hot to handle? Who is going to tell me what jobs to take? Is it going to be some muddy-headed liberal earth mama like you?" This was, he said, about *freedom*: you take the data you want and make the maps you want. If someone doesn't like it, well, let him make his own damn map.

The statistician saw his work as deontological, based on the rules of commerce and contract, and thus could simply work the numbers he was given without any qualms. His critic was clearly consequential in her thinking at the societal level, concerned about the greater effect of the map and the data's analysis. For her, his attitude was amoral if not actually despicable, ignoring the effect of the work he does. Had she been a classicist, he would have been Gorgias, and she would have been Socrates. For him, her judgments were an imposition on his rights and thus on his moral preserve (where freedom is the defined value). For her, his freedom imposed upon values she believed to be general, societal, and morally explicit. Both obviously had very different ideas about the nature of the virtue ethics they individually sought to promote.

After enjoining civility (too little and too late), I noted that both persons had raised fair points and fair questions. German concentration camps, I said, were precisely located, mapped to maximize the use of rail systems that brought in prisoners as forced workers and then carried out whatever war materials the inmates produced. The camps' placement was a technical problem in locational analysis that drew on a range of spatial data in the formulation of an optimal solution. So Auschwitz, Dachau, and other camps were indeed examples of "just data" applied to a purpose that most students in the class, I assumed, would think repugnant. So it was fair to ask if data are *always* neutral, and if so, if the purposes to which data are put are therefore similarly free of ethical constraint. Did the statistician really mean *any* data … irrespective of purpose or source?

Had I been better prepared, I would have asked both students if they would have happily participated in the statistical analyses and subsequent mapping that, beginning in the United States in the 1930s, were used to identify poor areas where banks would not invest (fig. 4.1).[1] This practice was called "redlining" because the cartographers drew red lines around poorer neighborhoods where data suggested that investment would be least likely to generate "safe" returns. In those areas, the price of services might be increased to discourage borrowers or denied altogether.

The resulting US "residential security maps" were made at the behest of the 1935 Federal Home Loan Bank Board in a directive to the New Deal's Home Owners' Loan Corporation (HOLC).[2] They were thus federally inspired and carefully constructed, applying the best available numbers to the solely economic definition of neighborhoods (best to worst) in cities like Baltimore, Buffalo, and the Bronx, New York.

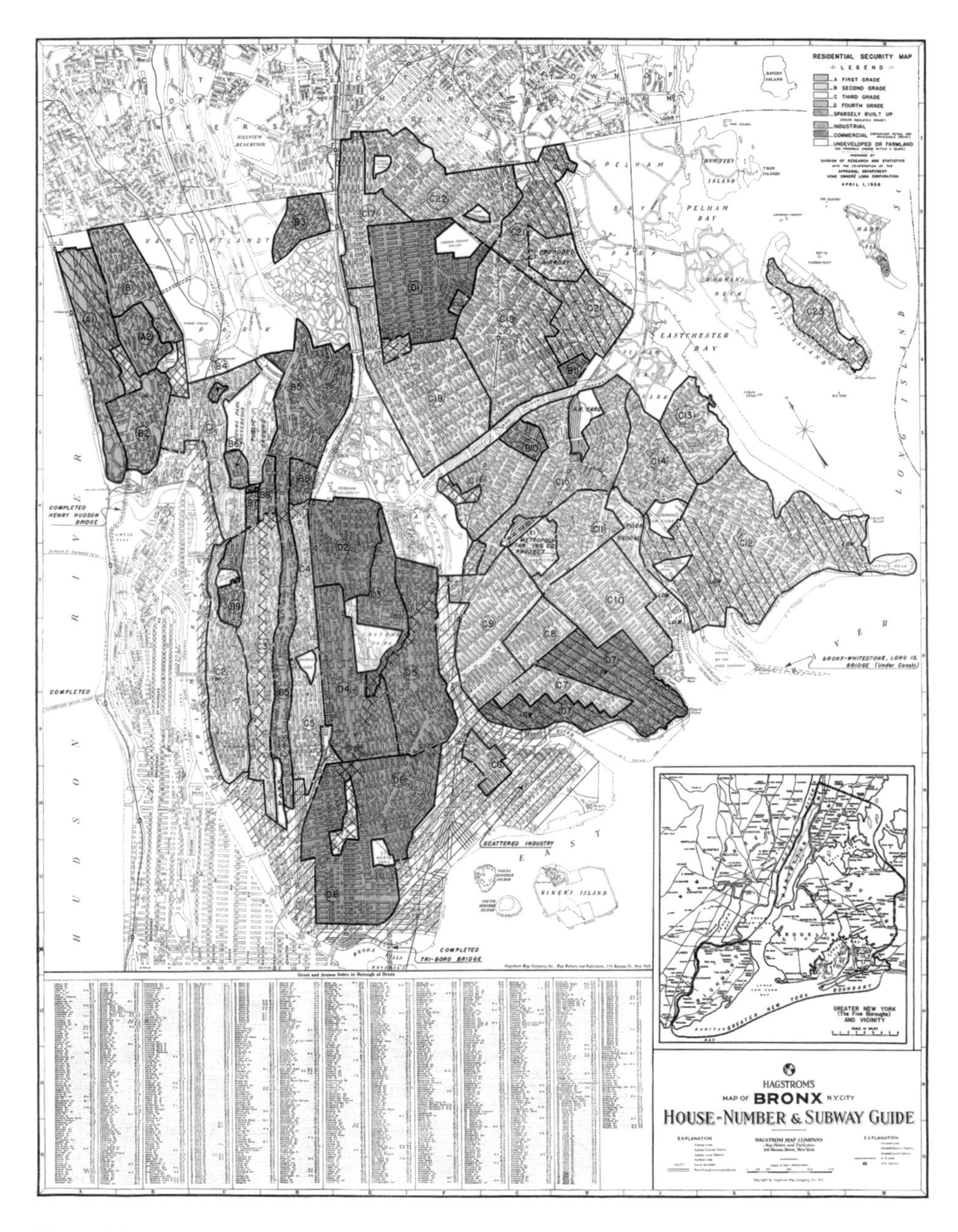

Figure 4.1

In this 1938 residential security map of the Bronx, neighborhoods were constructed and then ranked on the basis of an economic index. "Good" neighborhoods could get bank loans denied to others.

Here is a wonderful example of the general problem. In times of economic distress, wouldn't it be insane to refuse a government contract? The numbers in the map just reflected the way things were. No big deal.

But as a commentator pointed out in 2016, the maps were as much about racial segregation as they were about economic neighborhood divisions.[3] They *created* a no-go, segregated area whose mostly African American residents were denied the money they would need to build a business or sell a house and move. The result contributed to the construction of underserved, poorer African American neighborhoods that since the 1930s have been continually disenfranchised economically. The effects of this redlining can be read in the landscape of many American cities today.

Here we have at least three ethical imperatives in conflict. The first assumes racial equality is the issue and that redlining violated its promise. The second is purely economic or at least business based. Banks are obliged to do whatever is needed to maximize their returns for shareholders. If African Americans or any other group are a poor financial risk, well, numbers don't lie: too bad for them. Finally, there is the question of the role of the government and the manner in which it enacts its moral suppositions.

Finally, this whole question challenged the very ideas of neighborhood and of local communities: how should they be defined, and by what standard should they be disavowed or supported? If neighborhoods are seen as aggregations of people who deserve equal treatment within the city, state, and nation, well, then redlining was a bad thing. Redlining was neutral at worst, sensible at best, if neighborhoods are merely economic districts whose potential is defined by the possibility of safe loans providing adequate returns to the lenders. Either way, an ethical stance based on practical definitions with moral underpinnings is advanced.

At this point, the interplay of broad economic patterns, general morality, personal ethics, and social policy comes together. For the statistician, numbers are abstracts whose analysis and manipulation rarely carry ethical weight. It is not his or her job to challenge the assignment, not even for a Nobel Prize. Officialdom sets the policies; the practical programs that result are theirs to judge. Simple ethics requires only that numbers not be falsified and analyzed using acceptable statistical techniques. Simple economics insists that money comes first and banks need to focus on the bottom line. Society may decide some outcomes are undesirable, or unacceptable (concentration camps, racial ghettos), but that's for officialdom to decide. It is not for the cartographer, demographer, geographer, or statistician to question.

For others, however, the redlined neighborhood maps are ethically bad maps, albeit well drawn. In other classes, I would introduce, here, the idea of a "public goods problem." Public goods are things held in common, shared resources like streetlights in cities and good air or water for urban residents. Redlining was a public goods problem if, but *only* if, one thought of neighborhoods as public, shared goods—communities to be nurtured in common—rather than mere economic zones to be mined for financial gain. Since the idea was federal, one could say the US government was advancing a set of moral definitions that was economically biased rather than socially responsive. The result barred the poor from the assistance they might need and otherwise legitimately seek.

Here an interesting question was raised. Was the mapped division of cities into economic zones good business? It was the insistence that the poor are worthy of microcredit financial support (even without collateral) that earned Muhammad Yunus and Grameen Bank the Nobel Peace Prize in 2006.[4] Lending money in grade 4 neighborhoods can be, we now know, good banking, good business, and a benefit to society. Certainly the disenfranchisement of redlined African American communities has had long-term, costly effects. Might the "security zones" have simply been renamed "opportunity zones" for small-loan programs?[5] And more deeply—but still practically—are neighborhoods no more or less than the average or mean income level of their residents? Is that how we wish to measure the places where we live, the urban areas we seek to preserve and promote?

Introducing redlining in other sessions was merely another way to introduce the idea that the Tobacco Problem was designed to present: how we analyze the data we choose to collect reflects not simply objective facts but social perspectives that result in concrete actions with human consequences. If people believe economic exclusion to be ethically wrong (violating common moral definitions), demographers and cartographers *should*, as ethical citizens, argue against the production of maps that promote such a practice. If we believe in freedom and equal opportunity, then anything that inhibits their fulfillment is, as one participant impatient with my academic language put it, "just plain, you know, like, duh, bad."

Later iterations of this kind of lecture would include maps of world poverty and global income inequality (figs. 5.7 and 5.8). In undergraduate classes, I once added reading materials about the collapse of the illegally constructed Rana Plaza in Bangladesh, where more than 1,100 persons died in 2013.[6] Those killed and injured were low-paid garment workers producing clothes for, among others, Canadian department stores. In maps of global inequality and world poverty, one sees that Bangladesh is one of the poorest countries in the world. Foreign clothing manufacturers (including Canadians) see the country as a business opportunity, a fine source of cheap, nonunionized labor.

As Canadian purchasers of Bangladeshi-made, Canadian-labeled clothing, should we be proud of supporting Bangladesh's garment industry, and thus providing work to its impoverished citizens? Or should we be ashamed to wear clothes (inexpensive and good looking though they might be) produced by Bangladeshi people living lives of abysmal poverty while working ill-paid jobs in dangerous factories? Aren't we in some part responsible?

This was a way to ask if there was a scale of diminishing responsibility as we moved from neighborhood to city to state to nation to world. Do our moral definitions extend to humanity at large, or is equality limited to those with whom we share a legal compact (a constitution, for example) and a shared daily social environment? I tried this scenario only once, and the general result was mixed. Sure, most said. We feel bad about the Bangladeshi folk. But hey, the world is a big place, and we can't worry about everyone in it.

A Practical Solution?

Returning to the Tobacco Problem and its Regina presentation, one group thought it had the answer. "Our group has a solution," said a participant, "at least to the Tobacco Problem: We take the ATC money and produce the map of long-lived tobacco users. Then we take *that* map and rework it for the cancer prevention folk at a discount. We make money. We don't have to make uncomfortable ethical choices, and everybody is happy." Perhaps, she continued, there *is* harm in the tobacco map, but the benefits of using the ATC monies to subsidize the Cancer Prevention Agency work would outweigh that harm.

There was a lot to be said for this thoroughly pragmatic solution. Not the least of its benefits was that it removed the mapmaker and statistician alike from the need to make a principled choice that might be financially ruinous. They could in good conscience collect the money that ATC offered and which their struggling company certainly needed. Working for the antismoking campaign, they then could transform the first map to create a socially responsive second map. Public morality might condemn tobacco use, but public morality also called for impartiality of service and treatment. Voilà! Problem solved.

I had not anticipated this answer and was tempted to prevent its inclusion by introducing an exclusivity clause in the ATC contract. Then I realized the proposed solution was perfect because it introduced a fundamental misunderstanding. It assumed that it would be easy to turn the ATC map "Still Smoking: After All These Years!" into a new map with a new title, perhaps "Still Smoking? After All These Years?" Changing the title would not change the fundamental message, however, because the map would still propose a correlation between smoking and longevity. *Any* map using this dataset would *always* present a positive correlation between longevity and tobacco use.

Data are collected for a purpose. A map designed to urge long-lived addicts to quit would need a different data set, perhaps one tabulating tobacco-related deaths as a percentage of an addicted cohort population in relation to the population of active smokers who have yet to die. That map might be titled "Bad Odds: Two-thirds Die, One-third Survives."

Wittgenstein: "A Picture Is a Fact"

It was the idea of supposedly objective facts serving *as* realities that Ludwig Wittgenstein was criticizing with his famous aphorism "A picture is a fact."[7] He did not mean to suggest that the inverse is true, however: that "a fact is a picture" and thus a firm reflection of the objective world. For Wittgenstein, a fact was *made* real, brought into being through the lens of our perceptions, our picturing, our speech.

The idea came to him during courtroom reconstructions by witnesses using toy cars to model an automobile collision. It was in the physical imaging of the accident that it became comprehensible and thus real. Often, drivers of different cars reconstructed the accident both were involved in very differently. The recitation of those distinct, after-the-fact versions of a shared event remembered differently was each witness's "objective" truthful statement. Each was a memory made distinctly real through the act of modeling.

The facts we picture, Wittgenstein argued, are themselves meaningless in the sense that there is no absolute static, Platonic plane in which "truth" resides, assured and independent and therefore beyond our construction. We imagine and then image (in words or pictures, in charts or graphs or maps) the thing-in-itself in a context establishing its being and thus its seeming truthfulness in the world. It was this thinking that would inform later authors, cited in chapter 1, including Austin, Collingwood, and Roland Barthes.

Denis Wood and John Fels hammered home the same idea in *The Natures of Maps*. Everything changes, they argued, once the map is seen as a field of concepts rather than a barnyard of facts; everything changes once statistics are seen as concept fields rather than firm and complete number sets describing an objective reality. In their telling, concepts are first and foremost ideas about the world whose result "is the social manifestation of what the map [any map] presents as its 'intrinsic' and 'incontrovertible' factuality."[8] Similarly, charts, graphs, and tables *appear* to be factual and thus ethically neutral. But that factuality is based on prior choices (what dataset for what purpose? How is it organized?).

Wittgenstein did not write about maps, statistics, or even "pictures" as things-in-frames. Like Austin and Collingwood later, he was interested in language and logic as tools of understanding. But the idea serves here if the map is a Wittgenstein picture, a construction or reconstruction of an idea about things we put together to create a world we wish to present. We saw this in the news map (fig. 3.2) and its proposition that US military personnel are always native, everywhere local, and universally righteous. The redlined residential security maps (fig. 4.1) created an economic city in which residential areas are nothing but economic zones with a racial bias. The effect on affected populations and the long-term effects on the greater city are simply ... *off* the map.

So the redlined maps are true and accurate presentations of data supporting the notion of the neighborhood as nothing more than a potential opportunity for banks and mortgage lenders. But by other measures of community and community cooperation, the maps falsely divided neighborhoods on the basis of a definition of neighborhood worth and economic opportunity.

The Nature of Things, Together

All of this cuts to the very heart of our concern. Because we can't think of a photograph, a map (a dataset, or anything else), as if it existed outside its context, its point of view, Wittgenstein insisted we couldn't judge accuracy or truthfulness as if it were a thing that just *is*.[9] If Wittgenstein's point was that knowledge is secondary to thinking and to its mode of presentation (speech), then every analysis—cartographic, graphic, journalistic, statistical—is secondary to the inaction of grounded propositions determining the elements that are collected and considered together. Taken from this perspective, mapping is, again, a kind of speech.[10] Various cartographic techniques (color ramps, projections, symbology, text size, etc.) are the rhetorical tools that make real—effectively or not—the mapped proposition and its ethical predicates; algorithms make real the statistics we generate about how we think of things in place. Implicit in the proposition's syllogistic form is an ethical view of us in the world.

"If everyone, or even a substantial number, assent to a map's vision of the world ... then that *is* the world."[11] Realities, as Wittgenstein might say (or Austin or Barthes or Collingwood), are dependent on us and not independent of our efforts. Our prejudices direct our work. Think again about the residential security map of the Bronx (fig. 4.2), in which divisions ran down, between, and across individual streets, separating

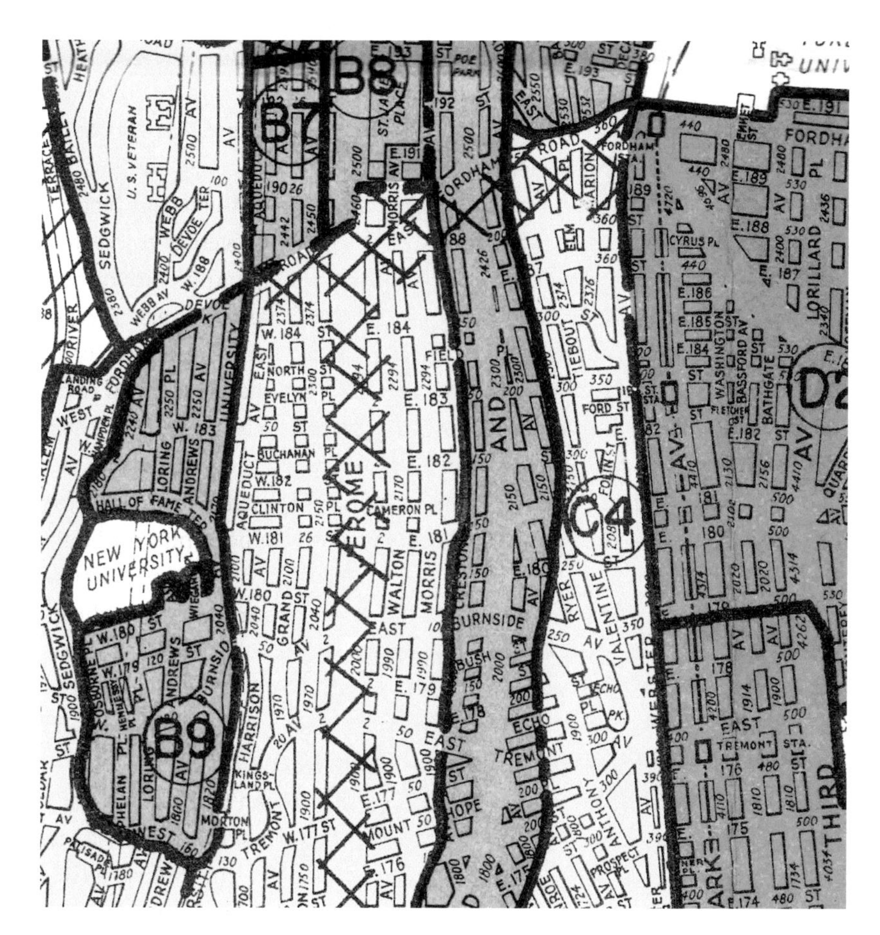

Figure 4.2
Detail of the 1938 Bronx security map in which green (grade 1) neighborhoods are distinguished from poorer blue (grade 2), yellow (grade 3), and red (grade 4) neighborhoods.

the best areas (green) from their blue (grade 2) inferiors and both from the even-less-desirable yellow (grade 3) as well as the undesirable red (grade 4) neighborhoods. The boundaries were not physical realities but cartographic imaginings carving up the city into better and worse economic ghettos. Mapping made them real.

The results were certainly fantastic to those who lived in the yellow zone at East Fordham Road near Tiebout Avenue in the Bronx, one short block to the west of a "blue" neighborhood and one block to the east of the "red." Aqueduct Avenue was not magically transformed into a new street at West 184th Street and University. Webster Avenue was not divided by barriers to the east and west. Driving down Webster, one would see just one more street. But in the map, it is yellow on one side and red on the other. The facticity of the map, the picture of the city it created *as if* it presented an objective reality, was the statistical result of propositions imposed on urban (a city of streets) and political (a city of political jurisdictions) geographies.

The neighborhoods created in the map's areas were not neighborhoods in the sense of communities defined solely by specific populations (racial or ethnic), unique geographies ("the Heights," "the Bluffs," "Riverside") or historical permanence ("Old Town"). They were not even official political designations. They were fictions created by functionaries who defined "neighborhoods" as simple economic zones. Those definitions in turn were based on a presupposition that made economics the central moral focus and ethics no more than efficient financial stewardship guaranteeing adequate returns on investment. Redlining cartographers and statisticians enacted the proposition that the city is a collection of investment opportunities to be promoted (with loans) or investment traps to be avoided. Consequential results focused on the lenders, not the people.

To say the city pictured in this way was imaginary does not mean it was not real. The result—call it "bankers' city"—took on an enormous reality for people who lived in red zones and thus could not get loans, and those in yellow zones for whom bank loans might be difficult even if, just across the street, blue-zone neighbors had an easy time of it. To live in a red zone meant that house prices would forever after be depressed because people would rather live where home loans were easier to get and social prestige certainly greater. In the relined zones, money for improvements would be unavailable.

The Cancer Example

A final map, or in this case an atlas, may drive home the point that maps and statistics are about ideas (and prejudices), and underlying those ideas are ethical propositions. In 1975 the US Department of Health, Education, and Welfare's Public Health Service published the *Atlas of Cancer Mortality for U.S. Counties: 1950–1969.*[12] For the first time, US health officials presented the geography of almost two decades of cancer deaths occurring within the forty-eight contiguous states. Basing their statistics on death certificates, researchers calculated the mortality rates of various cancers at 95 percent confidence levels across the nation's 3,056 counties. These data were then aggregated to the level of "economic area populations," what today we would call major metropolitan areas. The maps were based on tables, included in the atlas, for different cancers, each with separate mortality rates for males and females.

The goal was to identify areas with higher incidence of specific cancers in hopes of discovering causal factors influencing geographical variations in disease incidence:

"The maps should serve to identify counties, or clusters of counties, with elevated cancer rates which in turn may provide etiologic clues."[13] Other countries had engaged in similar studies of variable cancer rates, beginning with Alfred Haviland's pioneering nineteenth-century work in Great Britain.[14] By the first decades of the twentieth century, statistics of cancer incidence were being calculated and then mapped in England and across Europe.[15] Life insurance companies were particularly active participants in developing these materials.

The ethics and morality of this work were seemingly straightforward. Physicians and public officials are charged with combating disease because the health of the population is their responsibility in societies where life is declared a moral good. If environmental or social causes of cancer can be identified, they must be addressed. Because Americans believe the lives of citizens are precious, cancer is to be combated. From this perspective, the *Atlas of Cancer Mortality* was a virtuous achievement. More practically, insurers needed to know something about the lifespan of people seeking their policies. The atlas and its data on cancer deaths were, for insurers, good business.

Consider figure 4.3 and note that it mapped *only* the biliary and liver cancer mortality of white American females. African American, Asian, Latin American, and Native American females with these conditions were ... off the map. All the other maps and their supporting tables were similarly exclusive. In this manner, the atlas presented cancer in the United States as a mortal, whites-only threat to well-being. The conclusion was that a meaningful portrait of national cancer incidence could occur within a context of racial division. In the introduction to the atlas, the authors stated that there were practical reasons for the racial division but did not elaborate on what those might be. Instead they promised a future study (and presumably mapping) of cancers in nonwhite populations.

The stated goal of the atlas was to promote studies based on local and regional data that might identify cancer "hot spots" and, hopefully, then discover their causes. "Once the data was mapped, people saw clusters and said, 'Aha! I know what's there.'"[16] And it worked. Researchers found, for example, higher rates of pulmonary cancers among shipyard workers exposed to asbestos in World War II. In another example, the maps revealed unexpectedly higher rates of oral cancers in white women using snuff and chew tobacco in regions where, later investigation revealed, cigarette smoking was assumed to be unladylike. But those "hot spots" were whites-only cancer areas, and so the segregated picture was, at best, incomplete.

Had cartographers or statisticians complained that the racial division was ethically unacceptable—if all persons are equal, then segregation like this is simply morally wrong—they might have proposed cancer as a general, rather than racially explicit,

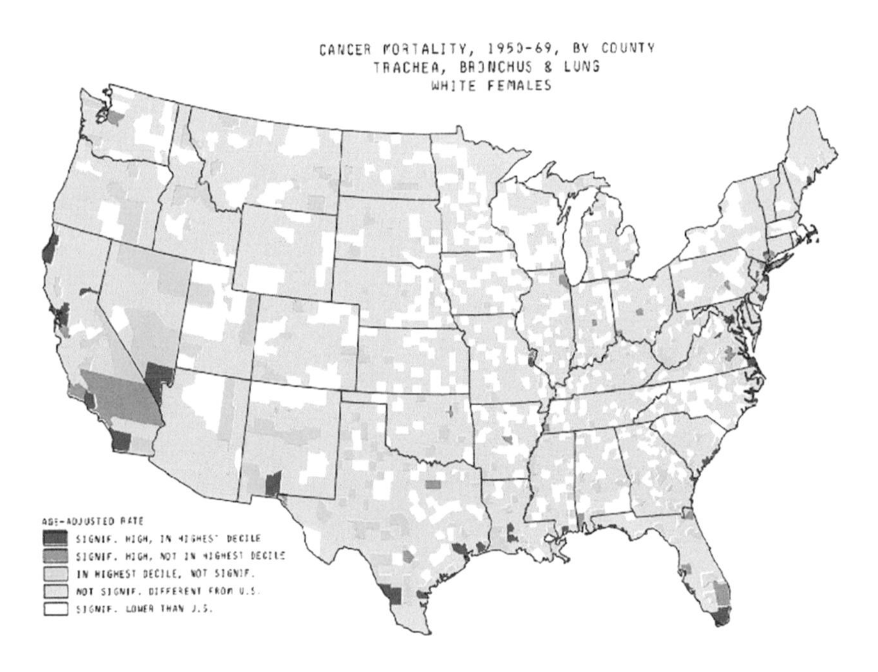

Figure 4.3
This map of biliary and liver cancer mortality in white females was one of a series of maps that attempted to distill county-level mortality data to create a national portrait of cancer incidence. US National Institutes of Health.

phenomenon. They could have argued that mapping the total cancer population would be a more effective way of identifying cancer hot spots. What about African Americans exposed to asbestos in navy shipyards during the war? What about women of color who used chew or snuff? Add them to the national picture, and the result at the least would have been more complete.

Eventually, a "separate but equal" cancer atlas was produced in 1999: *The Atlas of Cancer Mortality in the United States, 1950–94.*[17] In it cancer mortality rates were standardized for forty forms of cancers and then calculated by race (whites, blacks) and sex. The segregation can be justified on various grounds, both epidemiological and social. Some ethnicities may have a greater tendency to one or another cancer. Records for some may be better than for others. But still there is the stated goal of the atlas: to find areas of high incidence. Where those are environmental (and increasingly we know most are), racial divisions diminish rather than enlarge the relation between citizens, cancers, and their environmental (biogeographic and social) causes.

Truth and Lies

Anybody can lie with maps,[18] in news stories,[19] or with statistics.[20] It is easy to quote Mark Twain, who famously railed against "lies, damn lies, and statistics" (he credited Benjamin Disraeli with saying it first). Perhaps the most popular book about statistics in the second half of the twentieth century was Darrell Huff's 1954 *How to Lie with Statistics*.[21] More recently, Joel Best's *Damned Lies and Statistics* promised "to untangle numbers from the media, politicians, and activists."[22]

None of these works were fashioned as how-to manuals for the mendacious. Articles and books about lying with maps or statistics are really about how to tell the best truth possible (fig. 4.4, for example). It is no great trick to self-consciously choose a scale or perspective that promotes what we may wish to argue but know, upon reflection, to

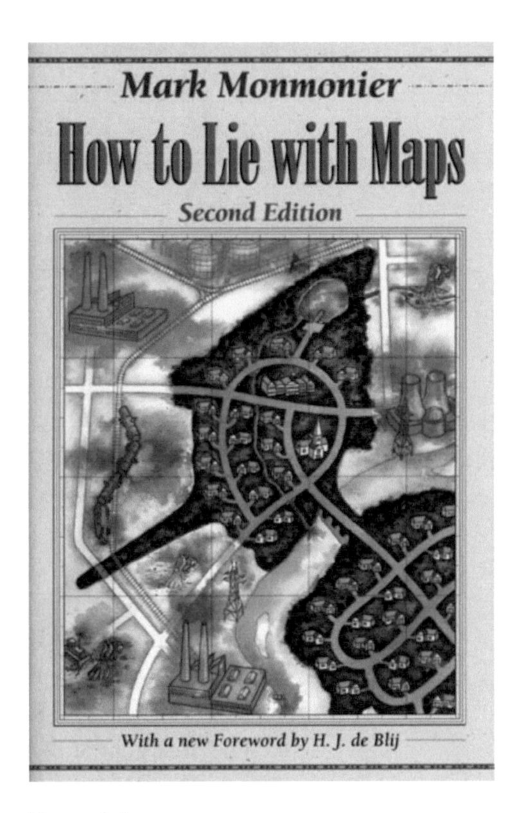

Figure 4.4
Most books on how to lie with maps or statistics (or rhetoric) are really about how to tell the best truth possible. After all, self-conscious mendacity is easy.

be uncertain or untrue. It is easy to find a dataset that will argue almost any point of view. Change the confidence level of a dataset, or select one that is exclusive rather than inclusive (whites only, for example), and voilà! The result is what one desired. The challenge is not how to lie effectively but how to identify and assess the rather bounded truths we choose to tell.

The Tobacco Problem was a fiction created to serve as a teaching example. But if the case was fictional, the lessons were as real as the "security maps" of the 1930s and the US cancer atlas based on exclusory incidence by segregated race.

Readers and Users

In presenting the Tobacco Problem to various groups, I was surprised at how quickly students and seminar participants engaged the issues and how their sometimes disparate ideas of practical ethics and their underlying morality were engaged. I had thought it would be harder to raise these issues than it was. As I thought about the issues and people's responses, I began to wonder why, and how, as readers and producers we so often ignore the conflicts inherent in a map or a table; why and how we can read uncritically the news stories whose flagrant statements are so easily questioned—if, of course, we choose to consider them critically. Are we simply lazy in our ethics and sloppy in attending to our moral definitions? Are we just uncritical readers and thus easy dupes? I did not want to believe that, and I do not believe it today.

In the next part of the book, the focus shifts from the mapmaker to the map reader and the means by which we all are so often blind to the moral failures embedded in the public artifacts we share on a daily basis as readers and reviewers. Daily we accept reflexively the limited truths in maps and stories whose arguments are, on a moment's consideration, clearly spurious and often ethically problematic. How does that happen, and what is the effect?

II Cultural Realities: Ethics, Values, and Morals

Culture is a reality lit up by a morally enforceable conceptual scheme composed of values (desirable goals) and causal beliefs (including ideas about means-ends connections) that is exemplified or instantiated in practice.

—Richard Shweder, *True Ethnography*

5 Mapping Poverty: Ethics and Morals

Consider figure 5.1, a map of poverty across the counties of the United States in 2008. It was made by Alexandra Enders, then at the University of Montana, for a study exploring causal relationships between poverty and citizen disability. It is well understood that physical and sensory limits often cause poverty in affected individuals.[1] But would areas where systemic poverty is greater show a larger number of persons with disabilities? If the correlation between poverty and disability was demonstrable, that would violate moral declarations of equality—we should all have a level playing field—and invoke the ethical corollary of mutual assistance for those who are less able through no fault of their own. After all, this was the idea behind the Americans with Disabilities Act of 1990 (ADA): a level playing field for all citizens irrespective of individual characteristics.[2] In bioethics the moral referent might be "beneficence,"[3] a moral duty to care and its broad social resonance as an ethical injunction.

At first, I did nothing more than glance at the map. I had seen others that were similar in subject treatment. Visually, the map insists on the reality of a singular geography within which poverty is posted as a defining feature of the American landscape. That poverty is located in 3,007 distinct US counties whose thin gray boundaries are themselves contained within black lines identifying each of the fifty US states. An inset map aggregates county-level data into a portrait of poverty as a state-level characteristic. Neighboring countries are neutral nonentities in both. Canada's northeastern coastline is evident in the map's upper right; northern Mexico is grayed into insignificance in the lower left. Both regions are blank areas serving only to locate and frame the continental United States and its poverty.

The poverty posted in the Enders map is drawn from the US Department of Commerce Census Bureau's "small area income and poverty estimates" (SAIPE).[4] SAIPE poverty is a conclusion derived from a statistical regression model using data from the Census Bureau's American Community Survey (ACE), Supplemental Nutrition Assistance Program (SNAP), and tax reported income.[5] So SAIPE poverty is a kind of

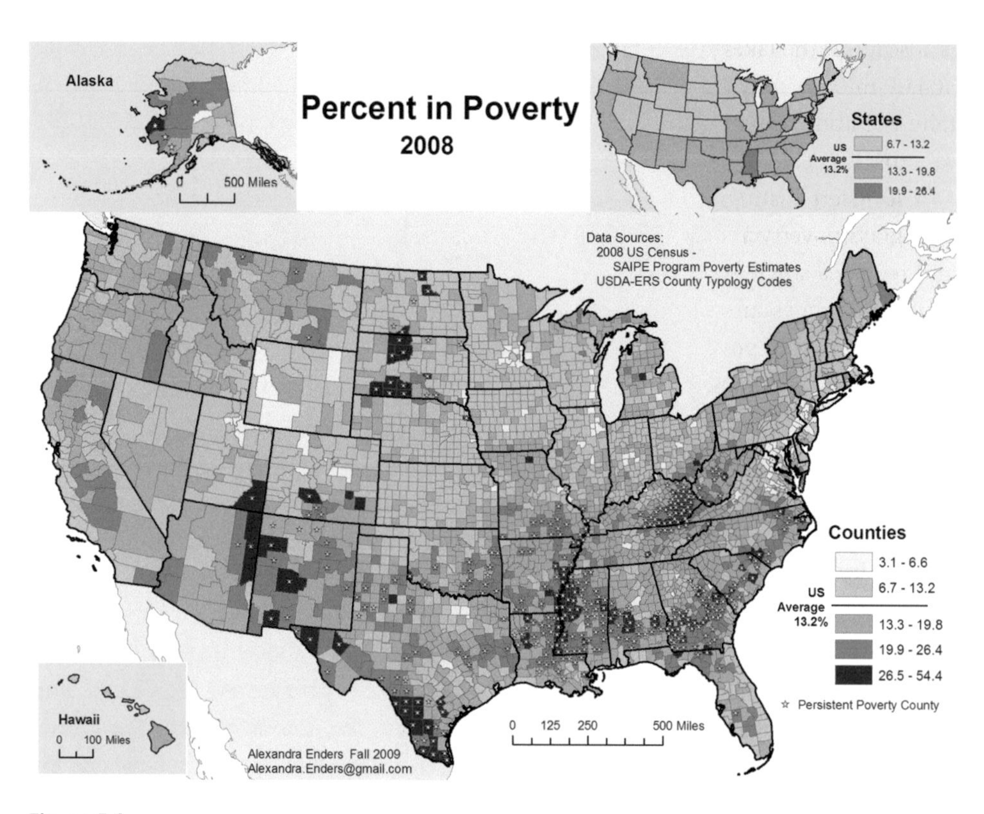

Figure 5.1

Alexandra Enders's map of poverty in US counties based on 2008 US census data. Reprinted with permission.

"poverty plus," a community measure that presents in the rows and columns of its data set an index of relative deprivation.

A color ramp (light blue to deep purple-red) creates a scale descending from the wealthiest and richest quintiles (blues) to the poorer and then poorest quintiles in ever-deeper shades of red. In the few wealthiest, light-blue counties, poverty rates range from 3.3 to 6.6 percent of the population; in the darkest counties, poverty pervades in a range from 26.3 to 55.4 percent, a quarter to more than half of all residents. Counties with persistently high poverty are starred. Dividing blue and red—and thus by implication good and bad, have and have-not—was the calculated *average* percentage of all US citizens living in poverty in 2008: 13.2 percent.[6]

The map thus presents the statement that more than one in eight Americans live in SAIPE-defined poverty. It seems as natural (and thus acceptable) a feature of the landscape as the lakes and mountains of the land. In 2008 the national population was 304.09 million, and 13.2 percent of that population was 40.14 million, not coincidentally the approximate number of Americans reported that year to be without health care insurance.

The insert distinguished relative state-level poverty using only three categories: blue-gray (poverty at or below the national average), pink (13.3–19.8 percent poverty), and red for a single state, Mississippi (19.9–26.4 percent). Aggregated at this scale, the county extremes are averaged into oblivion, resulting in a relatively homogenous, benign portrait of poverty in the United States, with Mississippi the only real outlier.

Because it is a map, the argument is not simply about the statistical incidence of poverty but rather about *relative* poverty among US counties and states. Because it is "factual" and objective, the map makes no judgment on poverty's prevalence or income inequality's national extremes. They just ... are.

Poverty Indexes

When one looks at the Enders map, the usual reaction is neither surprise nor outrage but a simple shrug of the shoulders. Why was the map not a call to national action to help 39.8 million impoverished fellow citizens? Why did it not immediately invoke a sense of moral outrage? One reason is simply that it is not an easy read. There are so many counties and so much variation between them that nothing in the map really moves the reader to cry "help" or "shame!"

Of course, it might be different for a map reader living in one of the starred, dark-red counties. But even if he or she did see the map, its poverty is not absolute but relative, a deficit "here" compared to abundance "over there." Perhaps the relative poverty presented is merely an inconvenience, driving an old pickup rather than a new Ford F-250 ($65,000–$75,000) or a Chevy Colorado ($21,000–$28,000). Maybe poverty means a night out at Boston Pizza rather than chicken cordon bleu at the local French bistro. It is hard to get excited about an abstraction mapped on a landscape so varied in its characteristics and so vast in its geographic range.

SAIPE Poverty Maps

There was nothing particularly innovative or remotely radical about the Enders map. The official SAIPE website provides an automated tool allowing users to generate their own maps.[7] Figure 5.2 shows a SAIPE website map that, for the sake of consistency, also presents 2008 data. The web-generated result gives up any pretense of international

PERCENT IN POVERTY, 2008
Total Population
Poverty by County
29.9 to 54.4
22.8 to 29.8
18.2 to 22.7
13.2 to 18.1
10.1 to 13.1
3.1 to 10.0
U.S. percent 13.2
State
MODEL-BASED ESTIMATES
The data provided are indirect estimates produced by statistical model-based methods using sample survey, decennial census, and administrative data sources. The estimates contain error stemming from model error, sampling error, and nonsampling error.
Source: U.S. Census Bureau, Small Area Income and Poverty Estimates (SAIPE) Program, Nov. 2009
U.S. Department of Commerce Economic and Statistics Administration U.S. CENSUS BUREAU
SAIPE08-1 1

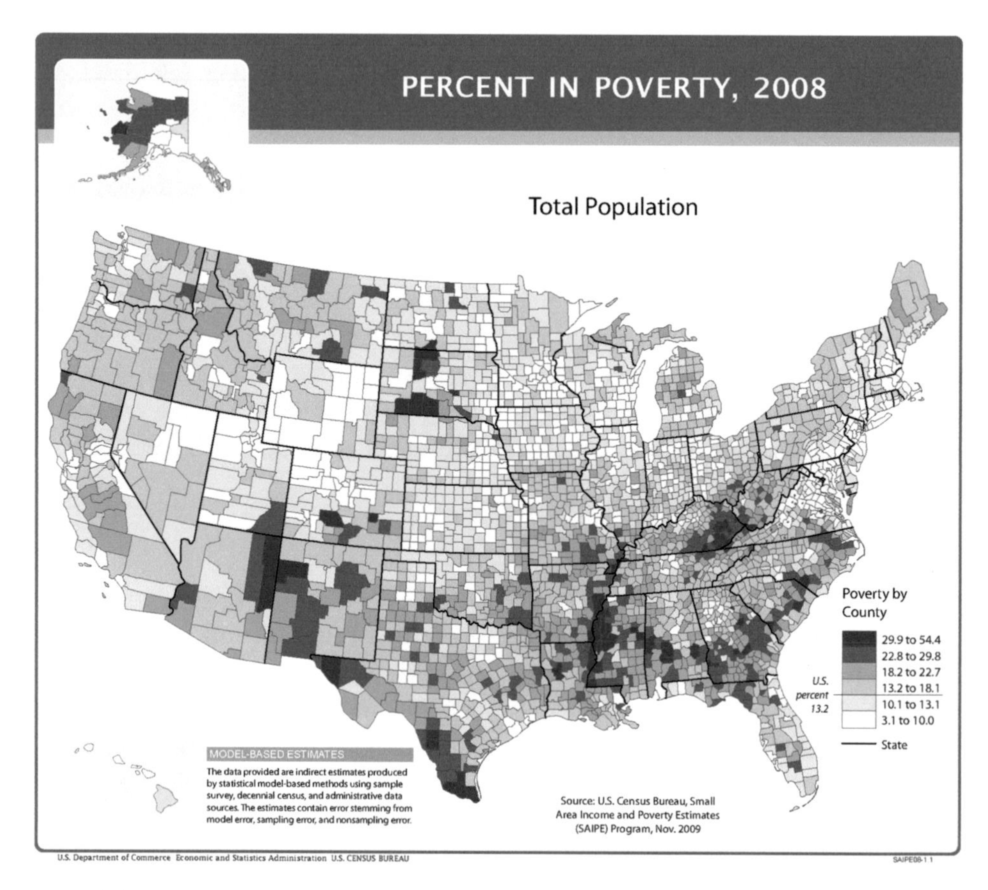

Figure 5.2

This map of the total percentage of Americans living in poverty was produced by the automatic mapping program of the US Census Bureau's SAIPE website.

neighborliness, eliminating even the gray ghost of Canadian or Mexican borders. It is America alone and independent, its neighbors hidden. Where the Enders map used a five-color ramp, the web-generated map automatically used six more muted colored divisions. Like the Enders map, the SAIPE website map accepts a 13.2 percent county poverty as a natural divisor between haves and have-nots across the US landscape in 2008.

Both maps share the conclusion that poverty exists at an uneven rate in the counties of the United States. Both serve as statements of federally calculated, statistically defined economic inequalities. Both present without comment counties where the percentage of persons without sufficient "threshold" income for life's daily necessities—the SAIPE definition of its poverty—is relatively high. One difference between the two maps is their respective color ramps. The more vibrant blues and reds in the Enders map make a stronger visual statement. The dull blues and purples of the SAIPE map, automatically imposed by the online program, mute the map's message and thus the importance of any but the most extreme variation between counties.

Less obvious is the difference in the construction of the respective maps' categories of poverty and wealth. In the Enders map, the light-blue coloring marked the least-impoverished counties with no more than a 6.6 percent rate of impoverishment, whereas the SAIPE map included in its wealthiest county category all those with less than 10 percent impoverishment. This gives the SAIPE map a larger number of first-tier counties. The poorest, dark-red counties in the Enders map were all those with 26.6 percent or more of the population living in SAIPE-certified poverty. The SAIPE mapping program painted its poorest counties beginning at 29.9 percent of the population, thus reducing by 3.3 percent the count of poorest counties. Thus the SAIPE map's categories diminish by statistical fiat the prevalence of the very poor. The result is that dark-purple counties are less evidenced. Nor in this color ramp are the divisions so visually accentuated as poverty increases, step by step.

There is nothing nefarious here. Students of cartography are taught the many ways in which the statistical pie can be efficiently divided. One can use an equal interval between all the cases, set a defined interval between classes, or create divisions with a formula creating natural breaks in the data. For a more comparative method, simply calculate a set of standard deviations from the arithmetic mean. And so on. All are legitimate choices, although some serve better than others depending on the map's focus and purpose. Finally, map data can be categorized in two, three, four, eight, or more statistical divisions. There is nothing sacred about the quintile, although, as a general rule, the larger color ramps (six to eight divisions) are harder to read.

What most radically distinguished the two maps was Enders's starring of dark-red counties in which high levels of poverty are endemic, occurring year after year. Adding that level of historical data made hers not only a map of relative income inequality among US counties but also a map of attendant poverty as a recurrent and structural reality in at least some counties. Whatever poverty means to communities, the Enders map argues, it must be seen as a recurring feature of the social landscape, at least in the red-starred counties.

The map can be reconstructed to emphasize the presence of relative poverty in the United States. Changing the number of statistical divisions or using more dramatic color ramps to present them might do the trick. That will not, however, change its basic message. Figure 5.3 uses the same 2008 SAIPE data as the previous two maps and the

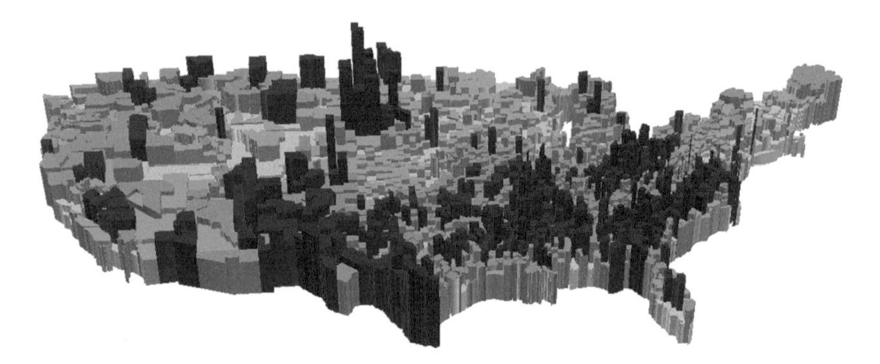

Figure 5.3
A 3-D extruded map of SAIPE poverty (2008) emphasizes the levels of poverty shown in earlier maps but does not change the message that poverty and wealth exist together across the US landscape. Map created by author.

same quintile divisions (and color ramp) as the Enders map. It extrudes the data, however, adding height to the counties based on the percentage of poverty found in each. It is certainly more dramatic. Still, it makes few imperative demands on our sense of moral justice or ethical propriety. Our eye is drawn to one or two tall, brown clusters—skyscrapers of poverty. But without more data, those clusters don't really mean very much to the average map reader.

As the percentage of American citizens living in poverty has increased over the years, the SAIPE statistician's divisor has shifted. The first "statistically significant" increase in the average national poverty rate after 2004 (12.5 percent) was implemented when the average percentage of Americans living in federally certified SAIPE poverty rose to 12.7 percent from 12.5 percent. From 2008 to 2013, the poverty bar was set first at 13.23 percent, and then more recently (2015) the dividing line between blue and red counties was set at 15 percent of a county's or state's population living in poverty (closer to one in seven Americans). From this perspective, the maps of SAIPE-defined poverty in 2008 are pictures of the good old days when *only* about one in eight Americans lived in federally certified poverty.

The Impoverished Landscape

Some may see all this as normal, natural, and anything but problematic. There are always winners and losers in a dynamic economy; income inequality is no more than the inevitable result of dynamic capitalism at work. The real issue is the general wealth of the nation (its gross domestic product, perhaps), not the plight of individual counties or the individual citizens residing in them. There is nothing wrong with extreme wealth existing adjacent to relative poverty so long as that wealth is legally obtained.[8] The result is simply free market economics at work.

Good for those living in Enders's light-blue places! Too bad for those in the darkly colored, starred counties. Nobody owes anyone anything because America is about individual freedom, the inalienable right to fail or succeed. Residents of the poorest counties can, as president Ronald Regan once advised, "vote with their feet" and move to richer, light-hued counties where they might (or might not) better their situation. If they decide to remain in place, well, that's what liberty is all about, and anyone who thinks otherwise is a damn socialist.

The Ethics of Poverty

The US Census Bureau calculates poverty by "comparing annual income to a set of dollar values called poverty thresholds that vary by family size, number of children, and the age of the householder."[9] Those "dollar values" are based in part on the consumer price index. Because the CPI is about buying power, the federal poverty threshold is about the monies a person or family has to spend on life's necessities (rent, food, etc.) and, if there is a surplus, nonessential but desirable things (designer clothes, good wine, etc.).

If before-tax income is less than the consumer threshold value set by official statisticians, then people can't afford the officially calculated basket of necessities. Posting the average poverty rate thus gives a general sense of the ability of the citizens of a county population to provide for themselves. As significantly, counties where incomes are low receive lower tax revenues and thus cannot afford the infrastructure (in education, health, job training, etc.) required if their poor are to improve their situation. At the other end of the tax line, the revenues of state and federal governments are similarly reduced. So poverty is about not only individual but also collective circumstances. It's about people, families, and government haves and have-nots.

The US Census Bureau collects this data because "poverty rates are important indicators of community well-being and are used by government agencies and organizations to allocate need-based resources."[10] Thus the data are collected to identify communities whose level of deprivation is such that government agencies and organizations are or should be obliged ethically to "allocate need-based resources."

Underlying this supposition is the moral presupposition that the federation is based on cooperation, on mutual assistance and support. As the preamble to the Constitution of the United States makes clear, the purpose of government is to "form a more perfect union" by promoting a "general welfare" that ensures the "blessings of liberty" for all. Mapped poverty describes an imperfect union in which that general welfare is denied to some. The map identifies a geography in which those promised blessings are selectively distributed and all individuals are not equally free to excel.

We have two opposing ethics here. First there is the "freedom to fail," in which poverty is a natural thing and everyone is on his or her own. Markets rule, and losers in the economic game are … losers. If economics is the measure and broadly aggregate national well-being rather than local well-being the scale of address, then mapped poverty excites no interest except, perhaps, to warn folk away from the red-starred counties in the Enders map. But if one takes the Constitution as a moral declaration, a defining bedrock presupposition, then harm results to the nation at large in its ethical failure to promote the general welfare. From this perspective, the SAIPE maps identify a moral injury to some and should imply distress for all.

Consequently, we have known for a long time the deleterious effects of poverty on communities at large. "The [questionable] moral condition of the poor," the physician Andrew Buchanan argued in the 1830s, "is in great measure the *necessary consequence of the privations*, to which they are subject."[11] To blame people for what were then called moral failures—crime, illness, dissolute behavior, drunkenness, homelessness, unemployment, and so on—without indicting the conditions that drove them to those extremes was not only inappropriate but also just plain unethical. It was unfair. For Buchanan and other nineteenth-century reformers, poverty resulted more from a general social failure than a simple failure of individual character and will.

It was not lost on Buchanan and his contemporaries that systemic poverty decreased regional and national tax-based revenues while making greater demands on society at large for the care of the indigent (widows and orphans, for example) and social ne'er-do-wells (those in prisons and workhouses). The moral failure to ensure care resulted in an economic liability that over time, they argued, would be greater than the costs of needed support.

We know today that poverty's harm is not only moral and economic but in some cases mortal. The lower the income bracket, the higher the rate of mortality.[12] Average life spans decline with decreases in income. This holds demonstrably at every level from the urban to the national. Since a landmark study published in 1998,[13] for example, Scotland has tracked the inverse relationship between poverty and mortality (fig. 5.4). In 2012, for example, the "European age-standardized death rate was three times higher in the most deprived areas."[14]

The same relationship has been shown to hold elsewhere. That means a county map of life expectancy, or of early mortality, will correlate nicely with a map of SAIPE

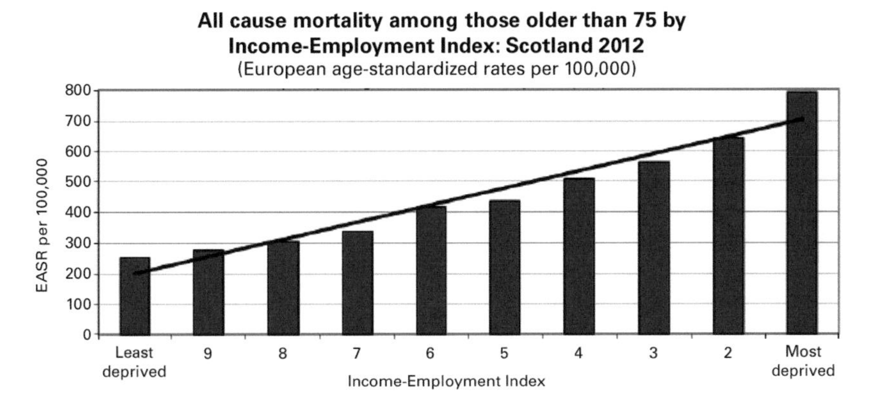

Figure 5.4

A representation of the straight-line relationship between poverty (unemployment) and mortality using Scottish federal data. Reprinted with permission.

poverty by county. A 2016 study described a strong correlation between poverty and rates of a range of cancers in the United States.[15] Not only were certain cancers more common among the poor, but they were diagnosed later and resulted in generally worse long-term outcomes (i.e., lower five-year survival rates). Similar corollaries can be found for mortality from cardiac disease, complications from diabetes, and so on.

Thus the Enders and SAIPE website poverty maps are at least potentially weighty documents, implying much even if in the end they say too little on their own. They can be read, like the redlined maps of the 1930s (fig. 4.1), as a way of identifying areas where investment should be shunned by opportunity seekers. Or, of course, they can be seen, at least in theory, as a call to action for those seeking a more perfect union.

Journalists and Writers: Poverty

Traditionally it has been the task of journalists and writers to particularize the statistical and transform the objective into a subject of moral indignation if not actual distress. Typically they do this by highlighting the effect of poverty on individuals. In the 1930s, the writer James Agee and photographer Walker Evans famously documented the lives of southern tenant farmers and sharecroppers whose lives were so restricted by structural poverty as to make any discussion of "buying power" a fantastic irrelevancy.[16] In the 1950s, CBS broadcaster Edward R. Murrow described US structural poverty and its effects as a "harvest of shame."[17] In that tradition, MSNBC's 2015 feature on the "geography of poverty" told the same tale, again.[18]

Agee and Evans's reports (and those of their successors) presented a kind of "morally indignant anthropology," condemning poverty and its effect as dehumanizing moral injuries.[19] The lives of the rural poor they described were "so continuously and entirely consumed into the effort merely and barely to sustain itself; so profoundly deprived and harmed and atrophied in the courses of that effort, that it can be called life at all only by biological courtesy."[20] This was, the authors argued, a moral wrong and thus an unconscionable national blight. In denying the humanity of others, they insisted, the landowners and office holders who profited from the poor lost claim to their own humanity as well.

Systemic poverty and extreme income inequality also present a moral injury in the original sense of an insult to the nation itself. "We must make our choice," Supreme Court Justice Louis Brandeis warned. "We may have democracy, or we may have wealth concentrated in the hands of a few. But we can't have both."[21] Democracy demands an engaged and vibrant electorate capable of understanding the issues of the day and then participating in the political life of their communities and their nation. Poverty most typically breeds illiteracy and ill health, not social commitment and knowledge. The poorest tend to be those least likely to participate actively in public debate and discourse. From this perspective, the poverty reported in the Enders and SAIPE-based maps presents a danger not only to the economics of the nation but also to the political well-being of the nation at large.

The argument against the reflexive acceptance of systemic poverty increases when its effects—increased mortality and decreased social engagement—are compared with

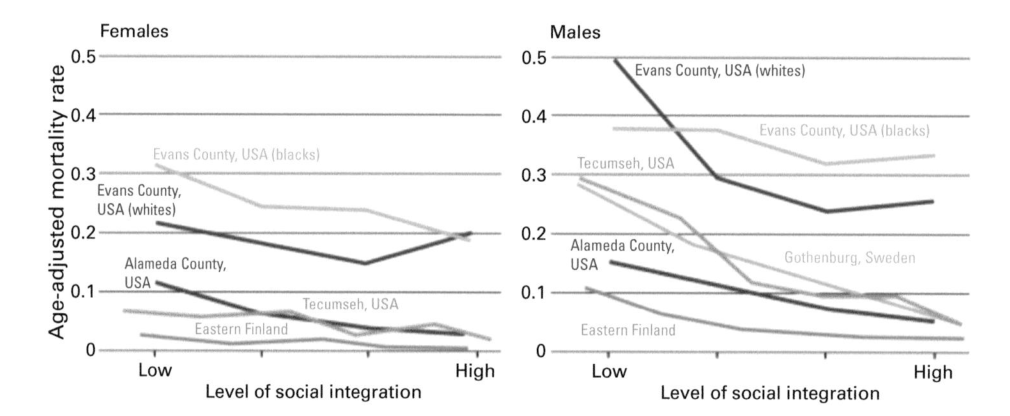

Figure 5.5
These graphs from a study published by the World Health Organization correlate social integration and mortality for three US counties and several in Europe. World Health Organization.

the reality in other countries. In a study of the social determinants of health, the World Health Organization compared levels of mortality and social engagement in several US cities and several European nations.[22] The trend lines shown in the study's graphs are stark. They too correlated higher mortality (a result of poverty) and levels of social engagement. The message, implicit but precise, was that it doesn't have to be this way in, say, Evans County, Georgia. It's not in the wealthier Alameda, California, for example; in Gothenburg, Sweden; or in eastern Finland. It's not inevitable but a result of choices we make politically in the nation.

Childhood Poverty

Others argue a similar message focused on specific populations. Jonathan Kozol, for example, has reported for twenty-five years on the effect of structural poverty on poor, typically African American children and their families living in America's inner cities. "The poorest children in America," as Kozol called his subjects, exist in a state of sustained deprivation with few real educational opportunities, at best minimal health care, and, of course, no real buying power at all.[23] The poverty Kozol describes, like Enders's "starred" poverty, persists over time and despite the sometimes heroic effort of parents to improve their and their children's status.[24]

"Buying power" is transposed in Kozol's work from a general economic conclusion into a specific catalog of goods necessary for children if they are to thrive. Children without buying power live in a constant state of stress and distress resulting in a greater likelihood of long-term illness and failure. Kozol might have hammered home the point by mapping "children in poverty" using SAIPE poverty estimates for all children in each county in the nation (fig. 5.6). The website's map calculator does this for two categories of childhood poverty: the poverty of *all* children under eighteen years old, and that of children between five and seventeen.

Figure 5.6 looks more or less the same as previous SAIPE maps but is, on closer inspection, very different. The dark-red counties with the most childhood poverty *begin* at 40 percent of the under-eighteen population and then expand to include those impoverished counties in which more than 67 percent of the youth are seriously poor. The next, lighter-red category describes counties in which roughly one-third or more of all children live in want. The divisor separating have from have-not counties in this map is 18.2 percent of the national population of children under eighteen living in the United States.

The map is an abstraction whose specific outcomes Kozol describes in excruciating detail: children who cannot go to school because of a lack of proper clothes;

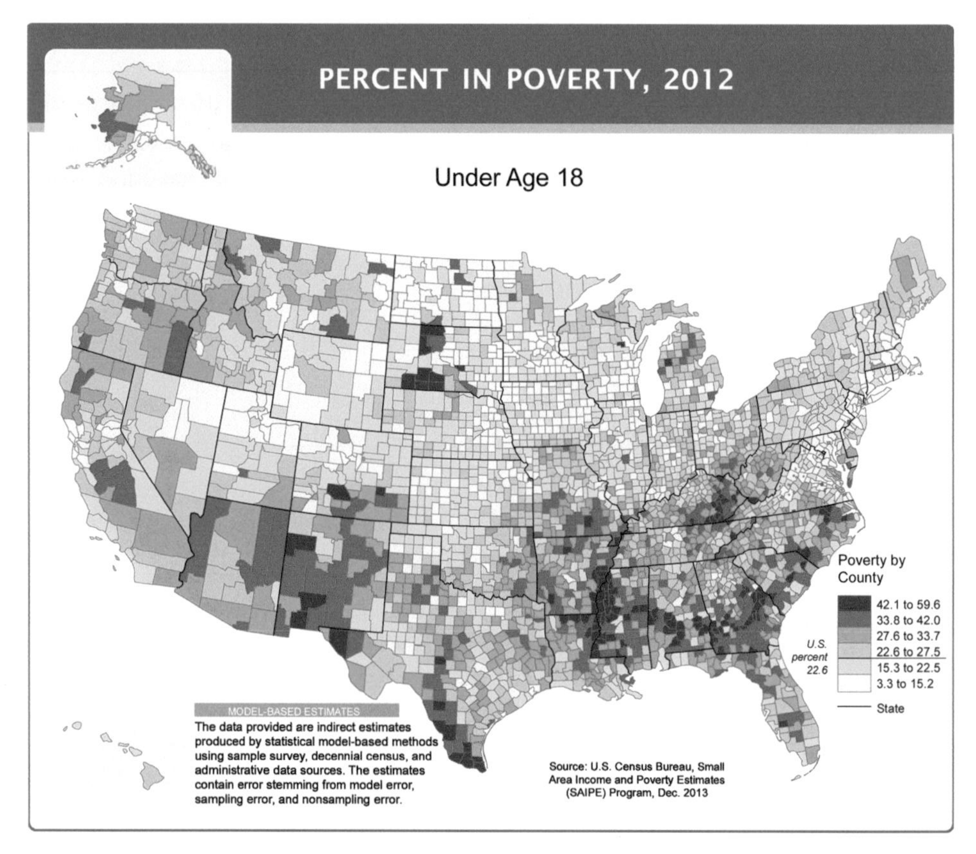

Figure 5.6
A map generated on the SAIPE website presenting county-level poverty affecting all children under eighteen years.

who are ill but whose families are so poor they cannot afford adequate health care. Distressed parents wish opportunities for children who will not receive them. In his books, and thus implicit in the map, are children who go hungry. Those like Kozol and others who moralize about this sad state do so on the basis of a virtue ethic in which dehumanizing poverty is not simply consequentially disastrous but morally unacceptable.

If, like Kozol, you believe that "the lives of children are the conscience of a nation"[25] (because children are our and our nation's future), then the SAIPE-generated map presents a conscientious moral injury that will adversely affect future generations. Children raised in the map's dark counties are physically harmed by the poverty they experience. "Their brain activity is less organized ... less well developed and less systematic."[26] They will be less likely to excel in school and be more prone to various illnesses. As a result, their potential to serve as thoughtful democratic participants will be diminished. As a people, the nation's collective future is thus harmed by the long-term effects of the poverty posted in the maps.

As virtue ethicists (believing in declarations of democracy, general welfare, and a more perfect union), we should therefore insist on structural changes that might change the map. As consequentialists we should be concerned about the long-term effect of a class of citizens who lack the potential to participate fully in the nation. As economists arguing consequentially, we can say that the cost of generations of poor creates a financial barrier to hopes for broader progress. The long-term cost of child poverty in the United States in 2016 was estimated at $700 billion, about 4 percent of the GDP.[27] As deontologists—well, it depends on which set of rules we choose to espouse.

Poverty as Contagion

This is not a new and radical riff, an unprecedented call for moral care. In the nineteenth century, as Christopher Hamlin writes, "concepts of liberty were often defined in terms of health: one could only be free to act if one were fit to act."[28] A poverty that bred ill health denied the impoverished person's equality of opportunity and thus his or her equal and full participation in society. Consequentially, those limits affected the lives of all. As John Ferriar, a nineteenth-century physician in Manchester, England, put it, "The safety of the rich is intimately connected with the welfare of the poor. ... Minute and constant attention to their wants is no less an act of self-preservation than of virtue."[29] Ferriar wrote during a time of ferocious epidemics[30] in which the overcrowded homes of the ill-fed poor were perceived (correctly) as being reservoirs for diseases that spread across class barriers to the enclaves of the well-to-do.[31] Nor was it lost on either Ferriar or his contemporaries that structural poverty provided a fertile field for social malcontents advocating radical social change.

Addressing the living conditions of the poor was therefore necessary if the well-to-do were to be spared devastating epidemics and the popularization of polarizing, revolutionary politics.[32] Here the moral imperative was not to community or humanity but to a kind of enlightened self-interest. Perhaps less virtuous, but for many more compelling, the motive for reformers was as much the preservation of the political status quo and an improving economy as it was civic solidarity and communal responsibility.

Income Inequality: Health and Disease

Today it is not poverty per se but income inequality—the distances between light-blue and dark-red counties—that is described as the most critical causal factor causing ill health, promoting transmittable disease, and reducing active membership among some citizen groups.[33] "The big idea," wrote the editors of the *British Medical Journal*, "is that what matters in determining mortality and health in a society is less the overall wealth of that society and more how evenly wealth is distributed."[34]

If we are morally obliged to promote population health (a critical criterion contributing to "general welfare"), then we are ethically obliged to address the problem of severe imbalances in wealth's distribution. "Low income predisposes people to material and social deprivation," wrote Juha Mikkonen and Dennis Rafael in 2014.[35] "The greater the deprivation, the less likely individuals and families are able to afford the basic prerequisites of health, such as food, clothing, and housing." The greater the comparative deprivation, the greater the distress experienced. The result, as Ferriar argued in his day, is that "disorders of marginalization will incubate and then be redistributed back down [or up] the urban hierarchy."[36]

"Poverty takes many tolls," the physician Peter J. Hotez wrote in 2012, "but in the United States, one of the most tragic has been its tight link with a group of infections known as the neglected tropical diseases [e.g., cysticercosis, toxocariasis, leishmaniasis] which we normally think of as confined to developing countries."[37] Their recent spread into the United States followed the fault lines of national poverty, Hotez wrote, across "the Gulf states of Louisiana, Mississippi and Alabama, where poverty rates are near 20 percent" and in pockets of extreme poverty "as high as in some sub-Saharan African countries."

Tuberculosis: Los Angeles

Hidden in maps of county and certainly state poverty are the divisions, sometimes, extreme, occurring within individual metropolitan regions. Beginning in 2007, Los Angeles's densely populated and extremely impoverished Skid Row district (an area too small to be seen on either the Enders or the SAIPE maps) was "ground zero for the city's largest tuberculosis outbreak in a decade."[38] There more than 7,000 Los Angelenos were exposed to a new and infectious bacterial strain incubated among the Row's homeless and near homeless.

Within a fifty-block radius (fig. 5.7), homelessness, poor nutrition, poor sanitation, and a lack of affordable health care created a veritable petri dish inviting pathogens

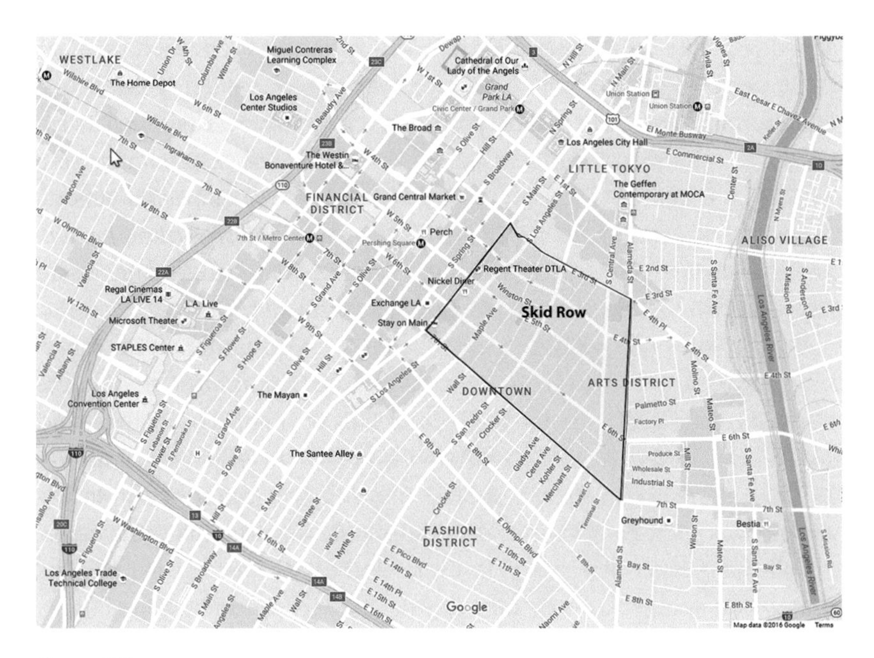

Figure 5.7
The Skid Row district of Los Angeles, where a new form of tuberculosis incubated among the poor. Google Maps.

to evolve and then proliferate.[39] While alarming, the outbreak was hardly surprising. "We've had outbreaks of other diseases before because of the poor quality of life in the area, so this is not a shock to me," a local police officer told reporters.[40] From the bacterium's point of view, Skid Row was a perfect environment not only for civil unrest and crime but for microbial colonization and diffusion.

Income Inequality and Democracy

Thus poverty and, more specifically, income inequality are consequential, the result injurious. "Perhaps the most important effect," wrote Richard G. Wilkinson, "is the reduction of goodwill and cooperation among the public at large."[41] Here again is moral injury in its original sense: an injury to the nation at large. Implicit in maps of relative county poverty is the alienating moral stress and distress amid a lack of education and opportunity that result in a diminished sense of citizenship and nationhood.

For those who choose to see things in economic rather than clinical, ethical, or moral terms, the whole can be reframed as a costly problem. "Inequality turns a large proportion of the population from net contributors to a society's economic welfare into net burdens on it."[42] In the polite economic language of modern sociologists: "The social and economic structure creates problems which impose cost burdens on the whole society, particularly on the public sector." To take but one example: Approximately $34.5 billion was spent in 2013 on uncompensated care of uninsured persons presenting at hospital emergency rooms.[43] Stabilizing if not curative treatment was required by law and its costs were borne primarily by the hospitals themselves. Those costs, of course, were then passed on to the greater public through higher service prices.

Other correlates, at once economic and social, include the relative rate of violent crimes.[44] Ching-Chi Hsieh and M. D. Pugh, for example, reviewed thirty-four different studies positively correlating income inequality and acts of homicide, robbery, and nonhomicidal violence.[45] More recently, Kate Pickett and Richard Wilkinson positively correlated with low income both general homicide rates and, separately, the percentage of births to adolescents.[46] The costs of both the crimes and their aftermath (the necessity of courts, policing, penitentiaries, etc.) and adolescent births (child care, medical and social support) add to other costs that poverty demands of society at large.

It is not simply that poverty decreases life expectancy, increasing mortality among the impoverished in a starred, red county. It is more precisely *relative* poverty that increases mortality among people living in red-colored counties compared to those in wealthier, blue-colored counties. Figure 5.8 correlates "all cause mortality" with "household Gini" (an inequality measure) and poverty.[47] If our morality insists on life as a precious thing to be nurtured and protected, and on our nation as the engine of a common democratic good, then we have an unacceptable result, a moral as well as economic injury to both the nation and the person.

Scale

The Enders and SAIPE-related maps of relative national poverty are about America. We may make that poverty disappear if we change the resolution and scale of the study. There are lots of ways to show this. Think, for example, internationally: Average per capita personal income in the United States in 2008 was $26,964,[48] whereas in Bangladesh in 2012 it was US $1,940 a year.[49] The relative poverty afflicting an average 15.2 percent of Americans in 2012 in this context is less important, except in extreme locations. It positively palls before the extreme poverty affecting 80 percent of the population of Chad and Liberia.

Figure 5.9 maps, as a definition of poverty, the percentage of a nation's population living on less than $1 a day. Based on statistics given in *The World Factbook* (published

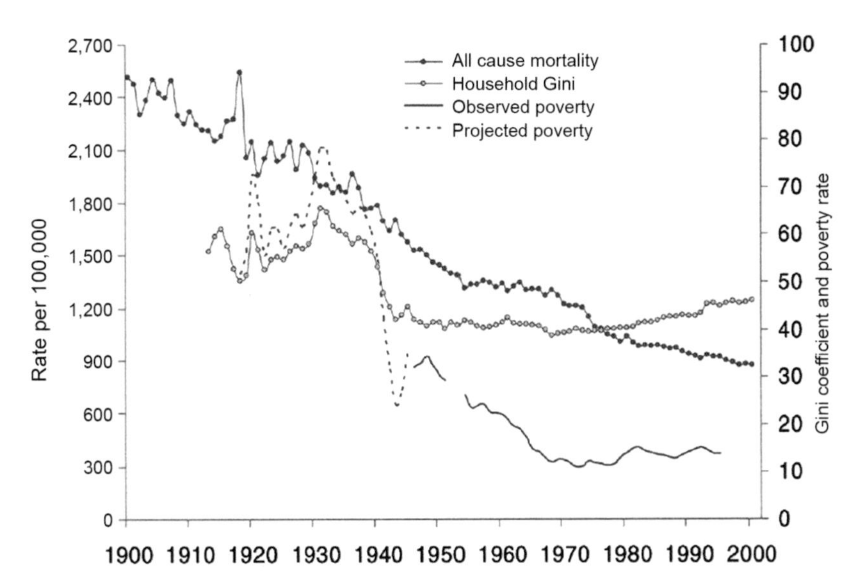

Figure 5.8

Income inequality, poverty, and mortality rise and fall together. Courtesy John Lynch.

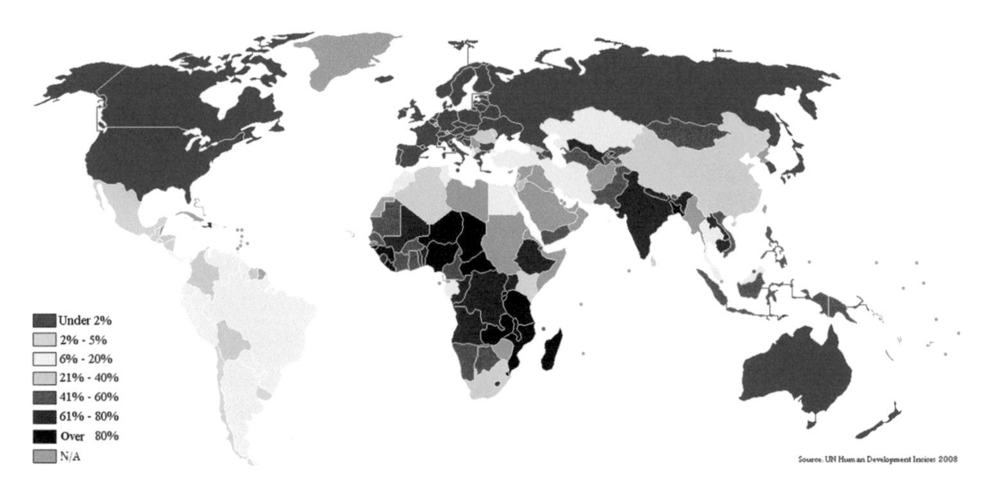

Figure 5.9

This map of persons living below national poverty lines is based on data from the CIA's *World Factbook*. "Measuring Poverty," Wikipedia.

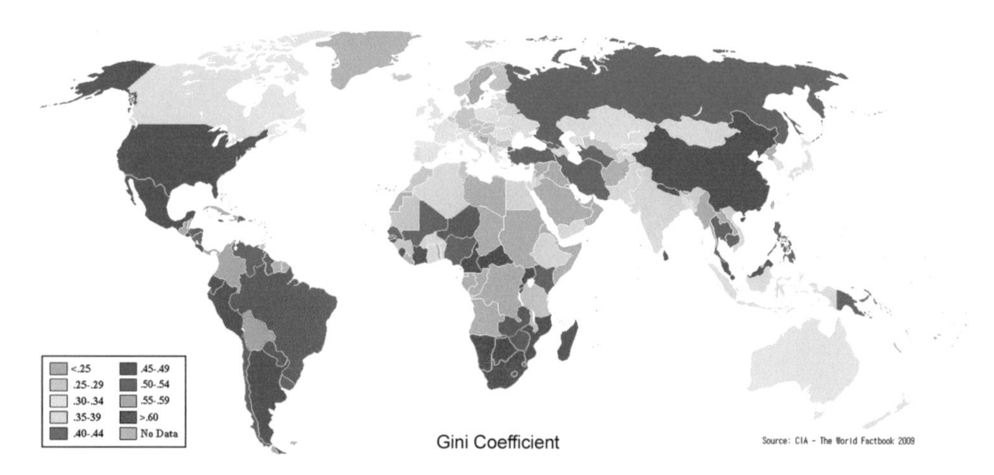

Figure 5.10
Using World Bank data, M. Tracy Hunter created a Gini index to map relative world inequality among world nations. Wikimedia Commons.

by the CIA), the United States, China, and Russia are all a healthy dark blue, because those governments report (accurately or not) that less than 2 percent of their total population is that poor. It's hard to ignore the idea of a poverty so extreme that a significant percentage of a population exists on less than $1 a day.[50]

If one is interested in global income inequality as a distinct, precisely calculated thing, the Gini index constructs a frequency distribution in which total equality is given as 1 and total inequality is 100. M. Tracy Hunter created a map of the world based on a set of Gini index calculations for each country using World Bank data (fig. 5.10).[51]

Who cares? Americans may argue a sense of responsibility to the poorest in their nation if they take seriously the idea of a nation dedicated to life, liberty, and the pursuit of happiness for all. Because the United States is a signatory to the 1948 *United Nations Universal Declaration of Human Rights*, at the least we should probably care as a nation about the extreme poverty of the dark-brown and red countries in the Gini map.

But if the scale of the nation seems an abstraction, its counties a geography we do not truly know, then the mapped world exists at an even greater remove, and the lives and deaths of distant persons are of little real moment for most of us who live elsewhere and in relative comfort. Pictures of starving children may give us a moment of moral unease, but it is brief. Chad, Brunei, and Bangladesh are not our problems. Catastrophic events—an epidemic,[52] earthquake, tsunami, or revolutionary war—may temporarily engage our sympathies, but otherwise let the kids collect for UNICEF on

Halloween. Simply put: the relation between "them" and "us" outside of a shared humanity seems hard to conceive. Harder still to muster is a sense of responsibility for the dire straits governing the lives of people living far from our homes or even our nation.

Conclusion

Deontologists might say that as long as our nation follows international rules set by agencies like the United Nations, then we are not enjoined to rectify the inequalities of the world. Nor, nationally, are we required to eliminate inequality if it is seen as a natural outcome of an equitable economic climate. Consequentialists might insist that the real issue is poverty's effects, the economic and social costs of structural, systemic inequality. Virtue ethicists, for their part, might argue that good people care for others, and poverty anywhere is about not caring about others. Humanitarianism should be the guiding ethical rule.

The maps and their demographic datasets engage none of these postures. They are "objective," and it is because they are "objective" that we instinctively trust them. Implicit in their construction is an "everything else being equal" caution, which absolves it from pairing the mapped data with contextual data. In their objectivity, however, they are stripped of the kind of obvious relevancies that might compel us to engage their arguments, let alone act on them. That is where the journalists and writers come in. But in their attention to detailed specifics, the general landscape of poverty—economic, moral, and practical—and its root causes are often lost.

At best the result is a kind of moral unease without an imperative to act. If the maps are seen as a general argument whose specifics can be unpacked in a context in which collective responsibility is demonstrable, then the issues become much clearer. As the next chapter makes clear, this is not hard to do. It is simply that we rarely choose to do it.

6 An Educational Example

All of this becomes applicably exigent when ethical suppositions based on moral definitions (justice as equality, for example) are codified in laws that set standards of required practice. Their violation becomes a matter of distress—a distance between declared belief and observed reality—and, to the extent codified ethical injunctions are violated, legal judgment. This sense of violation, and consequent demands for redress, lay at the heart of the legal challenge first advanced in 1993 by a coalition of New York City parents and educators. They described the chronic underfunding of inner-city New York public schools compared to other area schools as a violation of moral definitions of equality enunciated in American laws. To make the case, they created the Campaign for Fiscal Equity (CFE) which launched what became a decade-long court battle.[1]

In effect, their suit claimed that demonstrable underfunding of inner-city schools unfairly denied poorer students opportunities available to those living in wealthier areas of metropolitan New York.[2] If all students are equal and some are denied what others receive, then this inequality is unjust and must be remedied. Second, because the students adversely affected were largely African American, Haitian, and Latino, CFE proponents argued further the alleged inequalities violated Title VI of the 1975 Civil Rights Act.[3] So the argument was twofold: first, that some New York City schools were unfairly and thus illegally underfunded relative to other area schools; and second, that there was a racial bias underlying the observed inequalities adversely impacting some students

If successful, the legal challenge would require both redress and a prohibition of the practices inhibiting equal opportunity in education. The US Constitution's Fourteenth Amendment defines all citizens as equal, irrespective of color, removing race as a rationale for systemic inequalities. The CFE case thus became a constitutional justice case, and it was justice under the law (justice being a moral good in which fairness among claimants reigns) the CFE claimants argued was denied by the realities of unequal school-funding practices.

New York State Supreme Court Justice Leland DeGrasse found in 1995 that persistently inequitable funding levels did exist in a manner that denied inner-city New York students a legally mandated, roughly equal opportunity for a "sound basic education."[4] The nation's legal code, and the moral declarations underlying it, thus was distressingly breached. The judgment was appealed and in 2006 upheld in a final, presumably definitive decision resulting in the promise of major changes in funding. The effect of changes as a result of those problems has been, at best, partial.

The situation described in CFE court documents was hardly unique. Before Justice DeGrasse's 2006 ruling, nearly twenty other legal challenges had been brought elsewhere by coalitions similarly arguing against inequalities adversely affecting nonwhite students attending inner-city primary and secondary public schools.[5] What made the CFE case so important was that its locus was New York City, a symbol of America's energy, diversity, and, as a premier "global city," America's place in the world.

The case was thus from the start a heady mix of the economic, ethical, moral, legal, political, and social. In all its parts, it was profoundly geographic. New York City's impoverished schools existed in what Saskia Sassen has described as a "ring of poverty that runs through northern Manhattan, the South Bronx, and much of northern Brooklyn."[6] Outside lie progressively wealthier communities with far better funded schools. W. J. Wilson described the residents of the poverty zone as people who, like Agee and Evans's sharecroppers, lived with little hope of betterment.[7] Poor education in poor communities meant, experts said, urban poverty without end.[8]Thus the CFE school challenge targeted the effect of systemic poverty on an education system that effectively denied children from poor families the tools they needed to advance out of poverty in the future.

Geographer and multiterm elected Vancouver school trustee Ken Denike and I built a simple graph to track funding differences over a ten-year period between poorer inner-city and wealthier suburban school districts.[9] Our graph compared trend lines of funding per pupil from 1986 to 1987, published by Jonathan Kozol,[10] with data available a decade later from the New York School Department when the CFE case was first argued in court.

Figure 6.1 clearly shows not only that New York City schools received less funding per pupil but that the inequalities persisted across a decade in which schools in wealthy suburban municipalities—Manhasset, Jericho, and Great Neck—consistently received more funding per student per year (in some cases double) than those in Levittown, Mount Vernon, Roosevelt, and New York City. To this we added a "change" line that showed while funding improved for all students across this decade (a defense claim in the CFE legal case), increases were smaller in the poorer school districts than in

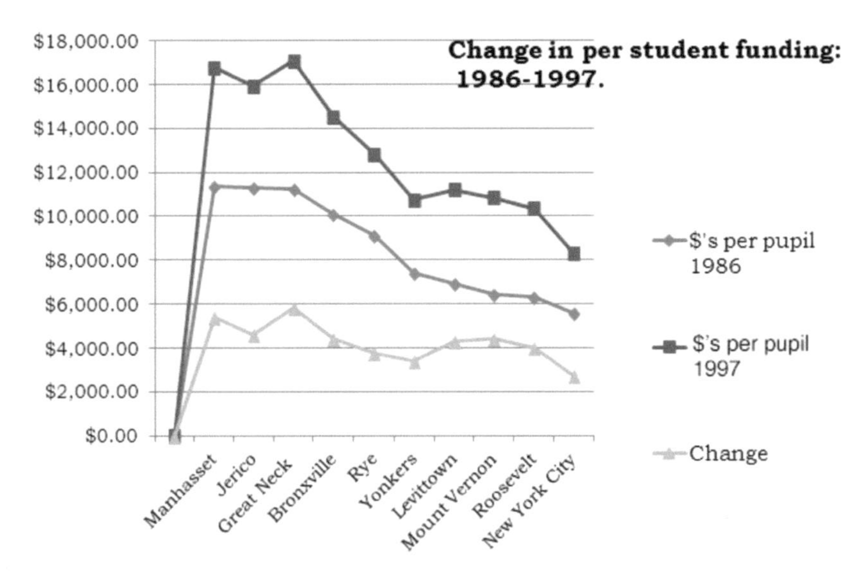

Figure 6.1
Monies spent per student per year were significantly lower from 1986 to 1997 when wealthier suburbs were compared with school funding in New York City. By author.

the wealthier. Funding disparities were persistent and real. But were they actionable, violating moral declarations of equality and justice for all? Was this truly distressful or injurious?

Geographies

Nobody claimed local politicians or school trustees were rabid racists maliciously or self-consciously shortchanging poor students. Most proclaimed themselves distressed by the challenge that funding disparities presented. The problem was, they said, not intentional but the consequential result of a system in which local school financing was (and in many areas still is) based, in large part, on revenues from local property taxes. Poorer school districts received fewer monies because the value of local properties was less and therefore there was less tax money for schools than in school districts with expensive homes owned by wealthier citizens. Here was, by the way, a demonstrable effect of the 1930s redlining of neighborhoods (fig. 4.1) carried into the present.

State educational monies were dispersed primarily on the basis of the number of students in a school rather than on the needs of individual schools or school districts. That funding formula insisted on an equality defined as monies per number of students in a school irrespective of individual need or local circumstance. Equal means equal, irrespective of need. State educational subsidies were largely per-capital, money per student, irrespective of the specific needs of students in local schools.

We sought to place these facts in a landscape in which relative poverty or at least inequality could be seen. Figure 6.2 mapped the percentage of children in free lunch programs (a SAIPE category) in area school districts as a way of showing the broad relation between poverty and school funding. The map served two functions. First, it was an obvious and pertinent statement of relative poverty among schoolchildren in various area school districts. Second, assuming that child poverty (fig.5.5 is a function of familial poverty, mapping the free lunch program in school districts would roughly reflect school funding based on household incomes. What the map did not show, but in retrospect should have, was that the poorest schools with the greatest number of students in the free lunch program also had the largest number of nonwhite students. The best-funded schools, mostly in Westchester and Nassau counties, had not only the lowest enrollments in the federal lunch program but also the fewest nonwhite children. The worst-funded schools in New York City had almost total participation in the need-based free lunch program and almost no white students. All of this was what the CFE suit had argued.

The long-term result was demonstrable. Public records made clear that most students from the well-funded, overwhelmingly white schools (where few students required free lunches) graduated high school and went on to college or university. Those studying in the less well funded schools with high lunch program enrollments were less likely to graduate and, if they did, were less likely to go on to higher education. A New York Bar Association brief stated the end result in its description of city school graduation rates: "Since the late 1980s, approximately 30% of the approximately 60,000 students who entered ninth grade each year do not receive any type of diploma."[11]

As late as 2012, the high school dropout rate in poorer New York City schools, mostly with large African American or Latino student populations, was 20 percent, and of those students who did graduate, only 18 percent received a full regent's diploma. Other graduates received lesser certifications. Among those who did graduate from the poorest city schools, most still needed some remedial education before they could seek advanced job training. Here was a moral injury, one in which the failure to ethically embrace an ideal of equality had an injurious effect.

The reasons for this were made clear in court documents. Funding per student was lower in school districts in poorer neighborhoods. Teachers in those neighborhoods were paid less because their schools received lower tax-based revenues per student. As a result, poorer schools had a higher percentage of inexperienced teachers as experienced

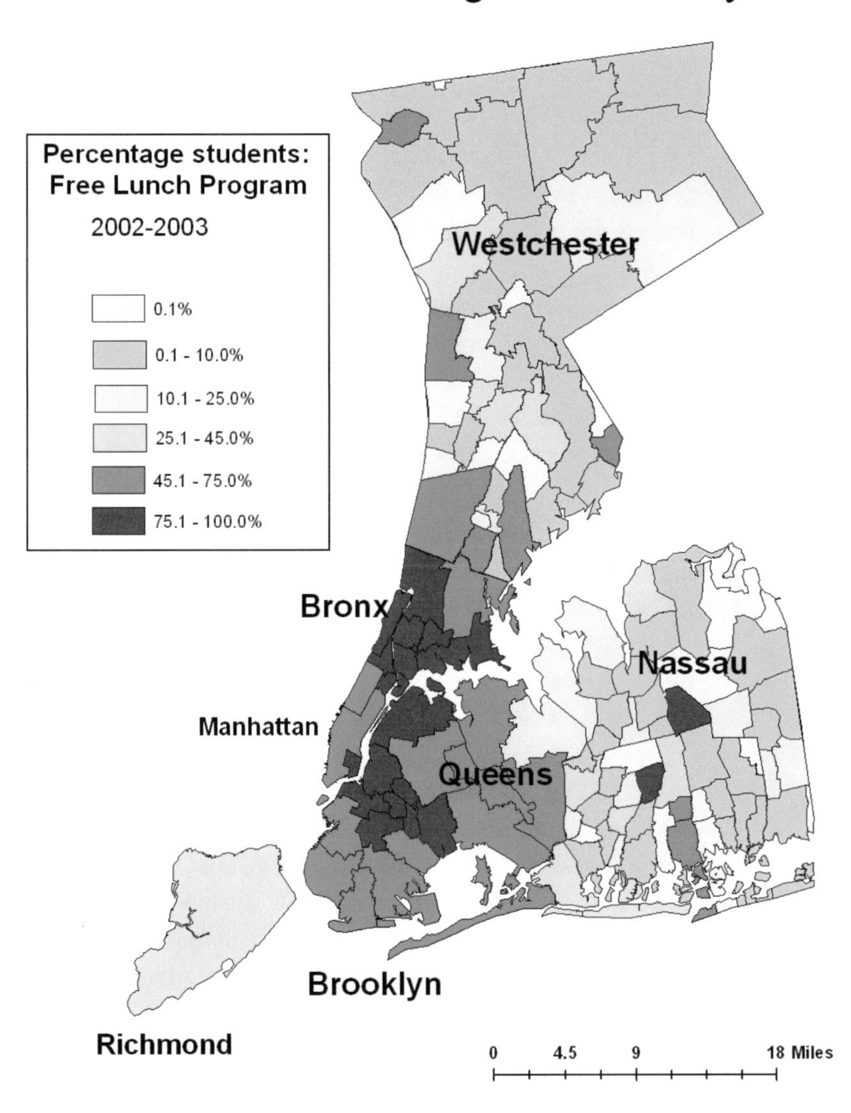

Figure 6.2
Choropleth map of New York City school districts based on the percentage of students participating in free lunch programs, one element of the SAIPE-calculated general poverty index.

teachers gravitated to better-funded schools elsewhere. Teachers in poorer schools had larger classes because there wasn't enough money for additional teachers.

Those larger classes led by inexperienced teachers met in overcrowded classrooms housed in school buildings in disrepair. Because the schools as well as the students were poor, classrooms lacked a range of resources and educational programs common in affluent suburban New York school districts like Great Neck, Jericho, and Manhasset. And despite a higher percentage of immigrant students in the poorest school districts, desperately needed ESL training was beyond the budgets of many schools with populations requiring it.

"Everyone wants to think of education as an equalizer—the place where upward mobility gets started," said Greg J. Duncan, an economist at the University of California, Irvine.[12] "But on virtually every measure we have, the gaps between high- and low-income kids are widening. It's very disheartening." The resulting gap in turn predicted a pattern of decreased relative future earnings and projected lower lifetime earnings for those without high school degrees.

The result has been a large and growing population of "disconnected youth" without careers, jobs (beyond the always precarious, low paid, and part-time), or real hope for personal betterment.[13] These young adults are not surprisingly concentrated in city districts where poverty was most evident in our map of free lunch programs, the school districts with the lowest funding per student.

The Community Service Society of New York, in association with the United Way of New York City, mapped first poverty and then the resulting percentage of disconnected youth (those neither attending school nor working) in 2000 and again in 2005 (fig. 6.3). The construction of a class of disconnected, disenfranchised young adults resulting largely from the failure of the educational system, was, Justice DeGrasse wrote in his court opinion, an injurious assault on democracy itself. Society suffers when generations of students are denied an "opportunity for a meaningful high school education, one which prepares [children] to function productively as civic participants."[14] Individuals who lack the tools for civil participation cannot serve as full members of a participatory democratic society (and economy). And so if democracy is a declared moral value, and if it requires an educated and engaged citizenry, then democracy itself is damaged by the funding inequalities evidenced in the maps.

This moral injury in its original sense—an injury to society—was a modern version of the "liberty" arguments advanced by reformers in the nineteenth-century British health-care debates. There, as recounted in chapter 5, the argument had been that health was a requirement if people were to be free to work as equal (taxpaying) citizens. In this case, the argument was that because the government failed to provide young

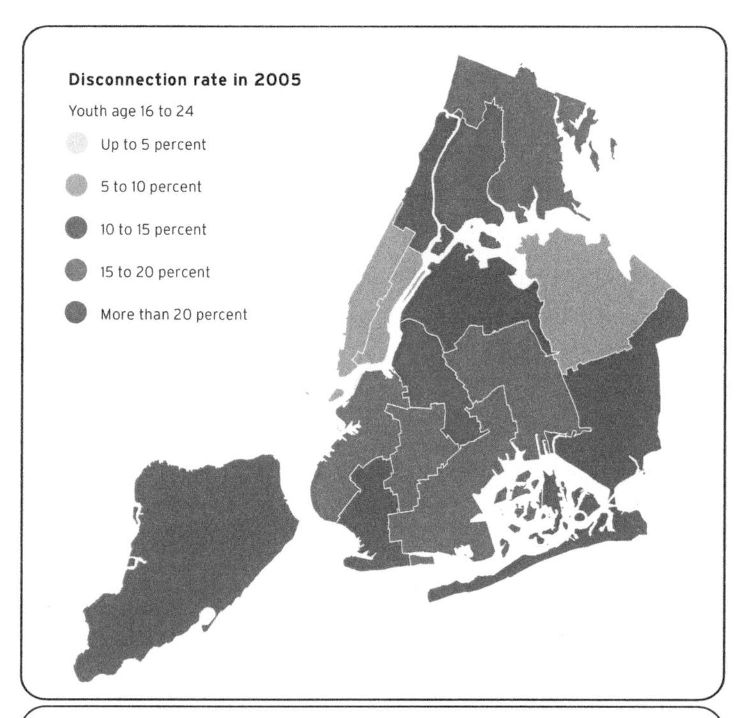

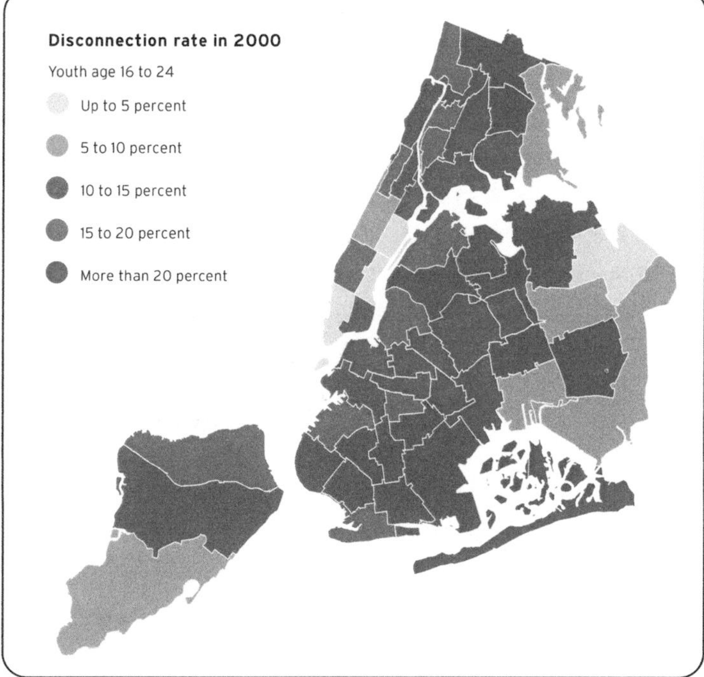

Figure 6.3

Maps of New York City's "disconnected youth"—those not in school and out of work—correlate with poverty rates and school lunch program rates in New York City. Courtesy Community Service Society of New York and United Way of New York City.

people in New York's impoverished public schools an adequate education, they were similarly denied equal opportunities and thus equal liberties.

Others described the so-called prosperity gap between rich and poor student education funding as economically ruinous rather than morally untenable and dangerous to the national weal. The "yawning educational achievement gap between the poorest and wealthiest children in America" costs the United States trillions of dollars each year in lost productivity and social services, one study reported.[15]

In 2015, the United States ranked twenty-eighth among thirty-three nations in math and science scores (behind Poland and Slovenia), in large part because of the failure to ensure suitable educational opportunities for all its children. Were the situation addressed, the cost of improved educational funding would be more than offset by a predicted increase in US gross domestic product of an estimated 6.7 percent and thus a cumulative increase of $10.6 trillion by 2050. Again, and not for the last time, what seemed morally appropriate and thus ethically dictated could be redefined as economically advantageous.

Results

The New York school controversy presented an embarrassment of riches. Its focus was the largest school system in North America, with more than 1.1 million students in a complex mix of more than 1,700 charter, public, private, and religious schools. The New York school budget in 2012 was $24.8 billion. In addition to the court transcripts that detailed the CFE case, available data included a wealth of annual reports—state and federal—on education, income, health, and so on.

The New York State Education Department, for example, made a host of statistics on student performance available to the public. Almost any educational measure (dropout rates per school, graduation rates, scores on standardized education tests, etc.) could be summed to show an inverse correlation between local poverty and student performance.

Ken Denike and I summarized the general problem in a graph that seemed to distill evidence from all the maps that we drew, or considered drawing, and all the statistics we reviewed. Figure 6.4 charts the complex realities documented by several agencies. For convenience, we used Kozol's data from 1986 to 1987 of dollars per student (fig. 6.1) for the varying school jurisdictions. The chart grouped school districts by dollars provided per student into three categories: high (group 1), medium (group 2), and low (group 3). To this we added the number of students in each of the areas for which we had funding data. We did not include a bar or line that would correlate the

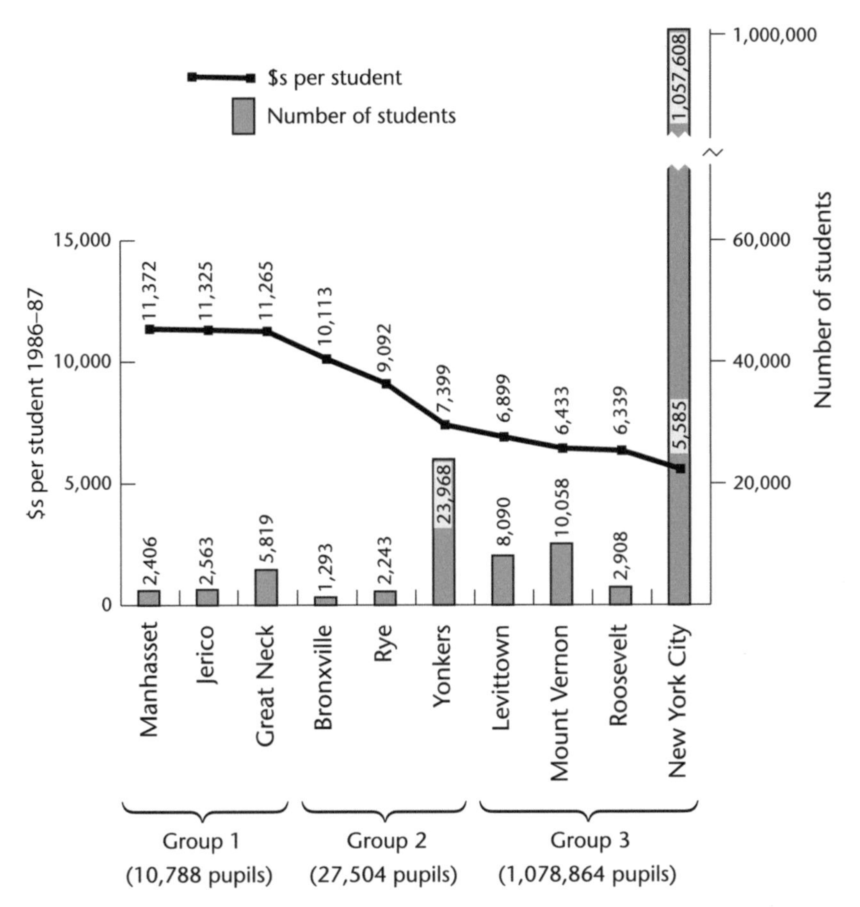

Figure 6.4
Using Jonathan Kozol's figures, this chart organizes student populations by dollars per student and population. By author.

general data with student ethnicity. It seemed so obvious we thought it unnecessary to do so.

By 2016, partially in response to changes made by the successful court challenge, things had improved somewhat. In a study for the Social Science Research Council's "Measure of America," Kristen Lewis and Sarah Burd-Sharps found a 24 percent increase in on-time (i.e., in four years) graduation rates in New York City schools between 2005 and 2016.[16] Despite that improvement, racial disparities reflecting economic barriers remained. While 85 percent of all Asian students and 82 percent of all white students graduated on time, the same could be said for just 65.4 percent of black students and

Table 6.1
Best and worst four-year graduation rates in New York City (*N*=59). Lowest figures are in the poorest school districts.

Ranking	Community	District	Percent 4-yr. graduation	Neighborhoods
Highest				
1	Manhattan	Districts 1, 2	95.1	Battery Park City, Greenwich Village, Soho
3	Queens	District 11	92.2	Douglaston, Little Neck
4	Queens	District 6	91.0	Forest Hills, Regent Park
5	Staten Island	District 3	89.0	Tottenville, Great Kills, Annandale
Lowest				
55	Bronx	District 4	63.4	Concourse, Highbridge, Mount Eden
56	Bronx	Districts 3, 6	61.4	Belmont, Crotona Park East, East Tremont
58	Brooklyn	District 16	61.4	Brownsville, Ocean Hill
59	Brooklyn	District 5	60.9	Morris Heights, Fordham South, Mount Hope

Source: Lewis and Burd-Sharps 2016, 4.

64 percent of Latino students who lived in the most-impoverished, least well serviced school districts. The number dropped to 40 percent for students with special needs, including "English language learners" who needed language training. Comparison of schools in the city, irrespective of greater distance from the suburban communities, made clear that students in poorer neighborhoods continued to be hugely disadvantaged compared to those in wealthier neighborhoods.

Table 6.1 presents the highest and lowest on-time (four-year) graduation rates for New York City public schools. Lowest figures are in the poorest school districts.

Racial Segregation

The geographies of school funding disparity exist along clear racial and economic divides, poor black and Latino communities on the one hand, richer white communities on the other.[17] The result has been what the sociologist Jeremy E. Fiel described as a kind of racial "resegregation."[18] While the intentional segregation of citizens, including students, is prohibited by law, economic disparities create divisions whose result is segregation, what Jonathan Kozol in 2005 called a shameful "restoration of apartheid." Simply, poorer schools are mostly black or Latino, while other (usually better-funded) schools are mostly white. The result is not maliciously racist but instead a consequence of the poverty considered in chapter 5. Regressive economic funding policies have traditionally advantaged the children of the well-to-do over those struggling unsuccessfully to overcome the barrier that systemic poverty presents. In most large cities, persons of color are, on average, poorer than white neighbors. Living in formerly redlined neighborhoods, they pay less property tax because they own fewer properties, and those they do own are relatively less expensive. And, tracking back, the poverty of those neighborhoods results from a history of poor educational opportunity and regressive policies affecting nonwhite populations over generations.

Limits

A problem this spatial, and one with such a wealth of available data (economic, geographic, and social), provided material for a series of charts, graphs, and maps in which we might have correlated race and ethnicity, poverty and race, family income and school monies with school performance (dropout rates, graduation rates, postsecondary attendance). To these we might have added consequential outcomes including resulting crime rates (higher in poorer communities), health status (Kozol writes about asthma epidemics in poor neighborhoods), health insurance disparities (the poor were less likely to have health insurance), mortality rates, unemployment statistics, and so on. We could have created an atlas. We faced, however, what was for us an insurmountable problem.

To accommodate its huge student population, New York has approximately 417 high schools of various types: charter, city, private, religious, and technical. Assessing outcome and performance data across this institutional mix would have been extremely difficult. As Canadians, we lacked the local knowledge required to navigate the labyrinth of New York's local complexities. Moreover, posting individual school performance, or any other scholastic measure, onto New York's dense geographies typically resulted in a map too dense to be read easily. To include high schools' performance or nonperformance as extracted towers (each school's height reflecting a performance attribute) resulted in what looked like a map of New York's skyline (fig. 6.5).

Another, less complex example was needed. Unfortunately, examples abound. It is still common in the United States to have school financing "that ties school budgets to the value of local property wealth" in a manner that concentrates educational dollars "within affluent school districts, and ensure[s] that low-income students are kept

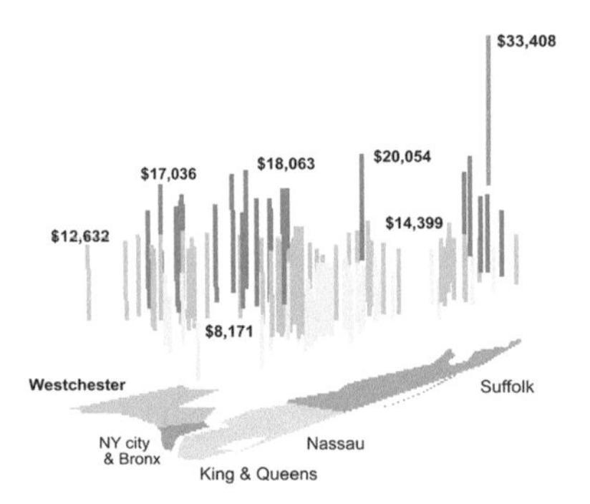

Figure 6.5
This map of New York education funding based on school catchments looks like a map of the city itself, confusing in its profusion of high-rises. Each column stands for per capita income at a single school. By author.

on the outside."[19] A national map of school funding (or rather, underfunding) looks almost exactly like the maps of SAIPE poverty presented in chapter 5. The only difference is that, in those maps, the metric is scaled to school districts rather than counties.

Buffalo, New York

Pondering all of this, I was in my hometown of Buffalo, New York, when the local newspaper ran a front-page story on "failing schools." "Some Buffalo high schools are set up to succeed," wrote Sandra Tan. "Others aren't."[20] Six of the city's fifteen public high schools had graduation rates under 40 percent. As they had been in New York City, the "failing schools" were those with the highest percentages of students for whom English was at best a second language; the greatest number of students with disabilities; and, of course, the highest percentage of students living in poverty. Here, too, lower property tax valuations meant less per capita financial support for the schools. It thus was perhaps inevitable that the poorest schools with the lowest graduation rates persistently reported the lowest student scores on standardized English and math tests and higher dropout rates.

The result, one high school principal told Tan, was that the principal and her staff "work 20 times harder to mitigate the extreme disparities that exist from school to school without the resources her school needs." The worst-performing high schools were, in Tan's words, "the last stop on the dropout train." They were the last stop because the best public high schools had admission criteria and tests that effectively barred most of the poorest students from transferring to them. Poor students who didn't score well on entrance examples (because of educational limits) had nowhere else to go.

The New York State Education Department makes available a database detailing graduation and dropout rates for all New York State high schools.[21] In addition, *U.S. News and World Report* provides an annual edition scoring all US high schools based on both demographics and performance criteria (like graduation rates).[22] Those data served in the construction of the insert in figure 6.6. The green bars post the percentage of college-bound graduates of area high schools, and the red bars post the dropout rates. Both are presented in a landscape whose surface reflects relative poverty in census districts.

The map and its insert emphasize the degree to which local poverty affects both dropout and graduation rates, with areas of higher poverty clearly grounding the worst outcomes. Both describe a striking but not surprising urban-suburban divide in which less-affluent inner-city schools sited in poorer areas have far higher dropout rates and lower graduation rates than their more affluent suburban counterparts. The one exception is the tall green tower of City Honors, sitting on a central patch of census-defined poverty, a magnet high school for the city's brightest students who, irrespective of home address, can pass its admissions test.

A simple graph based on the mapped data underscores the general relationship between poverty and performance. In figure 6.7 census-defined poverty and school dropout rates are correlated for the high schools mapped in the previous figures. Dropout rather than graduation rates were used because graduation rates are complicated by the welter of different degrees issued by area schools. They range from the statewide Regents diploma to local certifications. Dropouts who quit school without earning any degree or certification are a clearer indication of performance. These are the "disconnected" of the future, as New York's United Way would call them, once-students with insufficient skills (in language, math, or anything else salable) to become engaged as positive, adult community members.

Were this a book about educational opportunities offered and withheld, the Buffalo case would be just one of a number of more or less similar cases demonstrating the effect on student performance of persistent poverty and racial inequality argued in the CFE court case. In 2016, a National Public Radio Education Team partnered with *Education Week* to present a national portrait of school funding disparities (fig. 6.8).[23] Because most US public schools receive 45 percent of their funding from local monies (usually property tax revenues), 45 percent from state resources, and 10 percent from federal disbursements, the problem nationally was the same as it had been in New York City and Buffalo.

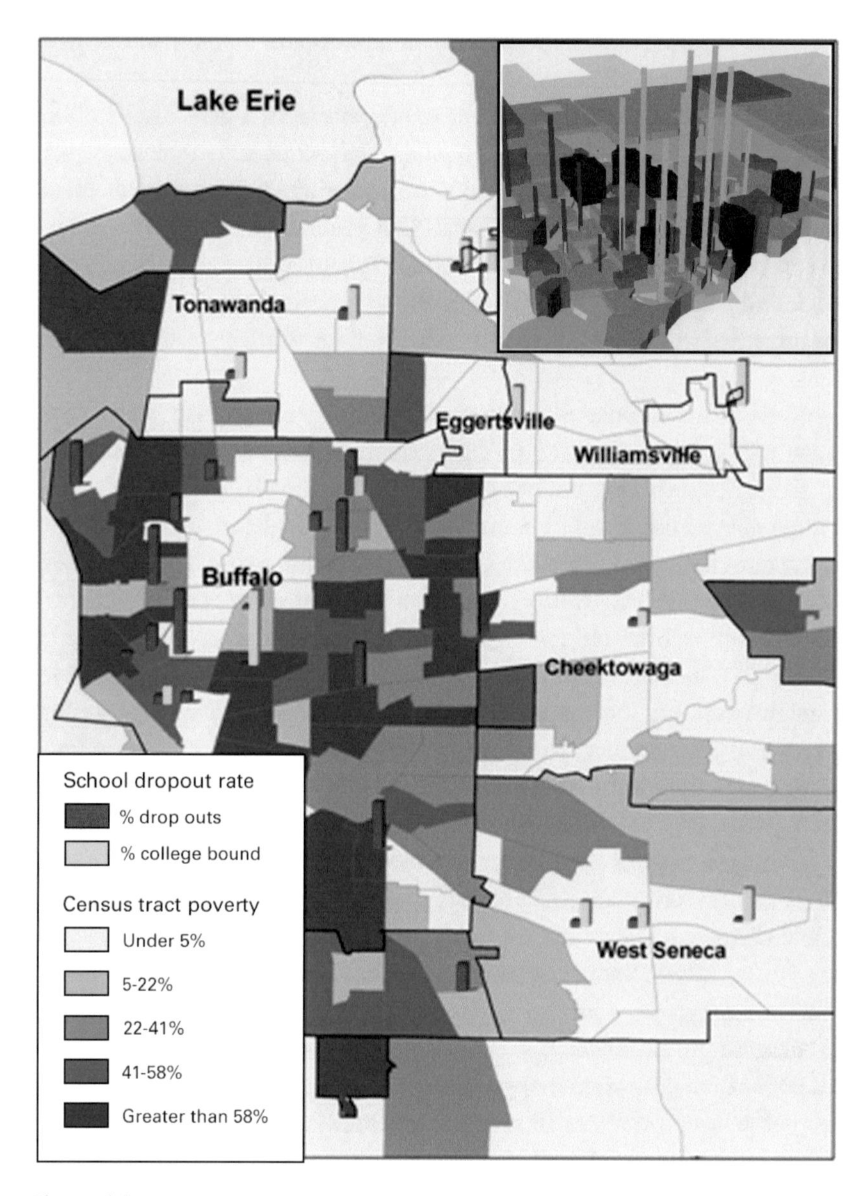

Figure 6.6
High school dropout rates for greater Buffalo, New York, on a landscape of relative poverty. "Failing" high schools are those in or near the areas of greatest poverty.

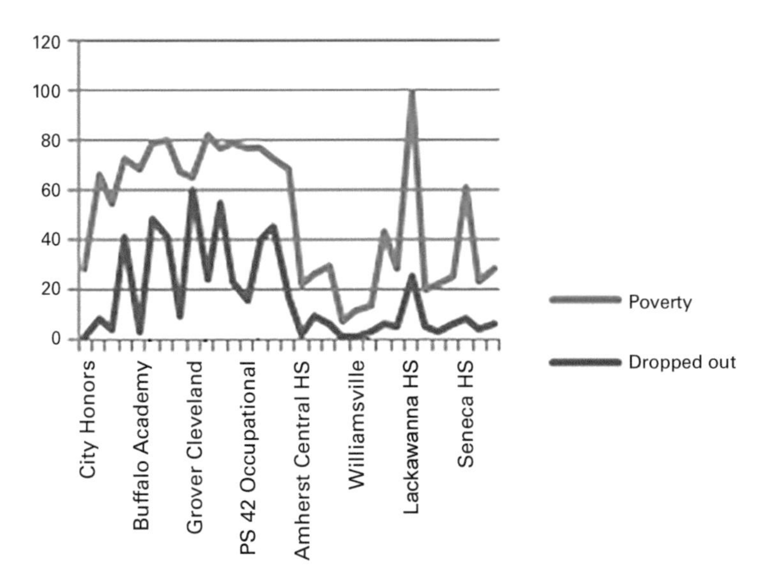

Figure 6.7
Graph of data from the previous map showing the correlation between poverty rates and dropout rates for students at Buffalo city and suburban high schools.

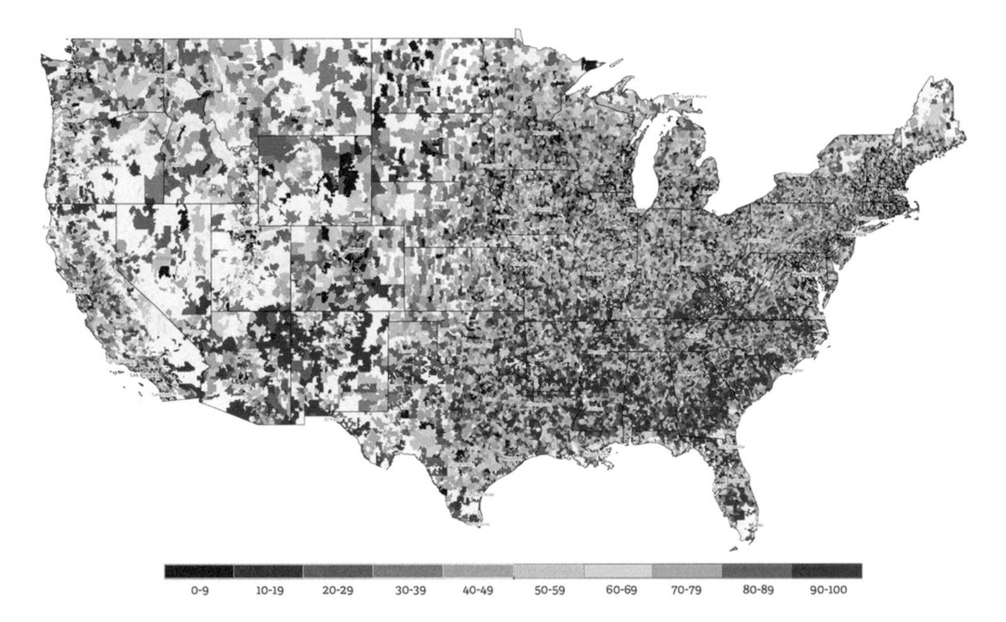

Figure 6.8
The National Public Radio Education Team mapped the differences in per student funding across the nation's school districts. The disparities reflected the ongoing realities of disparities raised in the CFE court case. Courtesy National Public Radio.

The NPR/*Education Week* story also included, as an example, a focus on schools in the Chicago area where money per student ranged from $9,794 in an inner-city school to $28,639 in an affluent suburban school. Similar disparities—and consequentially similar performance results (higher dropout rates, larger classes, fewer resources)—could be found across the country. Buffalo, where child poverty rates in 2013 (51 percent) were the third highest among the nation's seventy-five largest cities, remains an extreme case.[24] Broken down by ethnicity, that dismal reality included 16.6 percent of all Caucasian students, 39.9 percent of African American students, and 46.1 percent of enrolled Latino students. Alas, that reality is hidden in the NPR map, its scale too small to permit the local to be seen.

The poverty of have-not school districts across the nation signifies a range of woes that reach far beyond educational opportunities offered or withheld. In Buffalo, for example, race and poverty correlate with a range of health disparities affecting student performance in poor communities. At D'Youville Porter (Elementary) School, to take only one example, air pollution resulting in respiratory problems was so common that "instruction at the school includes reading, writing and, for some pupils, how to use an inhaler."[25] Jonathan Kozol reported similar respiratory problems in New York City's poorest schools.

Perhaps more alarming, lead poisoning was similarly epidemic in Buffalo's inner city, a toxicity that can result in lifelong neurological deficits.[26] The source, while environmental, was far greater in poorer neighborhoods where the money to replace lead-based house paints with new paint was often unavailable. The health problems that begin in elementary school have a cumulative effect on student abilities in high school and beyond.

Little of this can be blamed, as some Buffalonians suggested to me, on the influx of new immigrant families whose children "burdened" or "taxed" the system. Canadian studies have found not only that schools with strong immigrant populations recorded fewer behavioral problems, but also that significant immigrant populations often earned better scores in local schools than the general, nonimmigrant student population.[27] In Canada, however, tax-generated education funds are typically distributed by local school boards on the basis of the needs of students in their respective schools. Those with high immigrant populations needing ESL training or other special resources are thus more likely to receive them. Teachers with adequate resources can offer lessons tailored to multiple learning styles and paces in poorer, more immigrant-based communities.[28] In the same vein, Canada teachers often negotiate maximum classroom sizes in their contract talks with the government.

"Distressed Communities"

In recent years, academics have come to recognize that the issues of crime, education, employment, health, and housing are not separate but interrelated. As a result, they have begun to talk generally about "distressed communities" that lack the resources to provide equal opportunities in education, employment, and health. A study by the Economic Innovation Group (EIG) employed a series of seven indices, including percentage of the population over twenty-five years without a high school degree, median income, unemployment, poverty rate, and percentage change in jobs over time.[29] Not surprisingly, the mapped data appeared similar to the maps of SAIPE poverty in 2008 (figs. 5.1, 5.2, 5.6).[30] The extreme specificity of its resolution, distress by zip code, makes it even harder to read.

The study ordered cities based on the cumulative effect of the variables being studied. In figure 6.9, the now familiar map type of relative wealth and poverty is included as an insert to a map of the most distressed US cities. In it colored circles, whose size is based on population, present poverty's challenges in a way hard to perceive in zip code, county, or school district maps. The result makes bold the effects of poverty at the finer resolution.

At every scale or resolution, the point should be clear. The maps of poverty are maps of educational failure (one index) leading to unemployment (another index) and health problems. Poverty becomes the general category in which specific inequalities have adverse long-term consequences that limit individual opportunities and question the notion of a nation seeking "a more perfect union" for all. The government collects poverty-defining data to identify the disadvantaged areas of the nation requiring communal assistance. Help, however, is rarely forthcoming. In areas where the focus is education, Buffalo can expect little assistance from suburban Amherst, just as the Bronx can expect no help from its wealthier neighbors in Long Island. The ideas of national cohesion and regional cooperation are in this case just ideas, an ethical injunction rarely implemented.

Moral Stress, Distress, and Injury

There is certainly moral injury lodged in this congress of maps, charts, and tables and the realities they together present. The students whose education is limited by school poverty are injured when their opportunities for economic and social advancement are stymied. Their health is endangered by the poverty that diminishes their medical care as well as their educational opportunities. As one result, the likelihood of unemployment

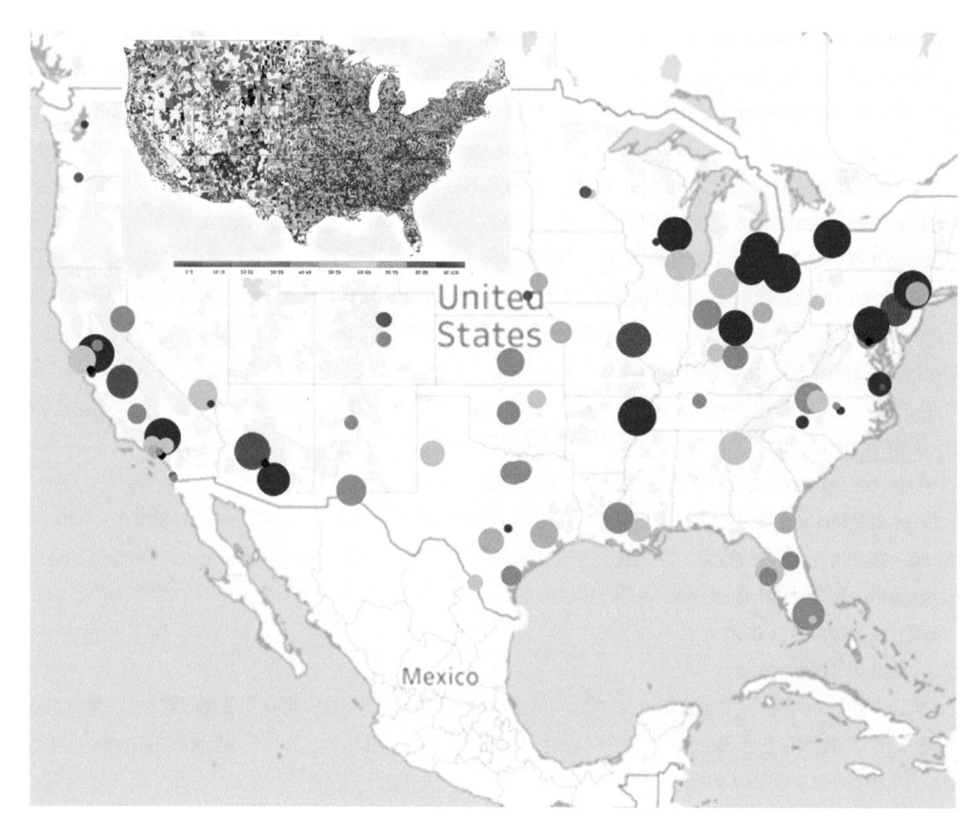

Figure 6.9
This map of "distressed cities" based on seven separate indicators locates and particularizes data in the national map of distressed regions by zip code. Courtesy EIG Group.

increases, and that of a prosperous future for those distressed is diminished. "Distressed communities" are the economically disastrous and at best ethically distasteful result (if we believe our moral declarations, then we should do more).

The nation is adversely affected by the many long-term effects of income inequality and systemic poverty adversely affecting education and thus collective futures. As Justice DeGrasse argued, the core ideal of American participatory democracy is injured through the creation of classes of disaffected, disconnected, and disenfranchised citizens without the education or the opportunity to fully engage in civil discussions and debates (remember fig. 6.3). The cost of even minimally maintaining those disenfranchised populations (from the criminal court system to the health needs that result and are treated pro bono in hospital emergency rooms) is vast.

Professionals who work in the education and health systems of distressed cities are morally stressed, and often distressed, to the extent they believe in their respective missions. Teachers cannot provide their students with the education they need, and physicians cannot provide patients with the treatment they require. Entering the system with ideals, young professionals (teachers, doctors, social workers, etc.) find those ideals impossible to realize. As a result, some leave their chosen fields or seek better-paying, less stressful opportunities among wealthier populations. "People think education is the means forward," one New York State Board of Regents members said to me. "But no matter what we spend, it doesn't matter. When it's about poverty in general, no single specific will help."

Supply-Chain Ethics

Mapping the correlates of poverty, its effects, and school performance (or health outcomes or anything else) creates a chain of evidence. Poverty leads to ill health and underfunded schools and thus to a failure of education and opportunity. The results are pervasive and create a kind of supply-chain ethics. Morally we declare our belief in human life and its worth. Because we believe that, we believe in the equality of all persons, and as a consequence, we believe all deserve an equal opportunity to thrive. Because we believe in those things, justice demands we treat each other fairly. Because we believe in fairness and justice, we insist on ethical programs that ensure an environment in which all should have the same opportunity to thrive. Each step in that chain of opportunity can be mapped in its relation to others within the morals that promote participatory democracy, which is our essential political covenant. And when the chain is broken, we see that, too.

It was this "supply-chain ethics" that lay at the heart of the 2015 US Supreme Court decision known as "Inclusive Communities."[31] In a five-to-four decision, the justices upheld and broadened the central thesis of the Fair Housing Act, passed in the week after Martin Luther King Jr.'s assassination on April 4, 1968. In that judgment, the justices declared that even where discrimination is not the intent, policies that result in discrimination are illegal under a doctrine of "disparate impact."

To simplify the legalities, the Supreme Court thus ruled generally what Justice DeGrasse had argued specifically. The law sets ethical standards on the basis of moral suppositions (equality irrespective of race, e.g.) requiring specific actions and outcomes. Whatever the intent, when those ethical standards are violated, the result is unacceptable under the law. If we believe in equality of opportunity as a moral good, and freedom to prosper as a civil birthright, then programs that deny their enaction are wrong. As the justices put it, policies that "otherwise make unavailable" to some communities necessities that are freely available to others are or should be considered illegal in a nation whose moral presuppositions include ideals of fairness, freedom, and justice.[32]

As cartographers, graphic artists, reporters, and statisticians, we usually ignore the ethical supply chain that carries the links of cause and effect to individual outcomes or specific circumstances. We are hired to assess school performance. Our job is to document hospital room admissions. Professional ethics require nothing more than the completion of those tasks. If the data are not maliciously tampered with, the result is deemed "objective," and we have done our jobs.

We are trained as professionals to ignore the consequential in favor of "the objective standpoint that constitutes the condition of good scholarship."[33] That permits and indeed demands a kind of tunnel vision that looks solely at the narrow outcome, not at its context or its potential effect. And so we collect, analyze, and map (chart or graph) the rate of educational dropouts, the location of students with lead poisoning, the poverty rates of communities, and so on; but unless we are ordered to do so, we never link one dataset to another. The result is at best only half the tale.

We may be disengaged, but that does not mean we are not affected. As citizens, we live with the policies our analyses advance. By *not* looking to the roots of school failure (or disease rates, etc.), we become complicit in the continuance of conditions that promote the things we chart, describe, or map. We thus promote through our inaction and perhaps willful blindness the uncivil society we then bemoan, the ethical violations of the morals we reflexively pronounce as good citizens.

The result is moral stress. Certainly in the mapping it was for me. I grew up in Buffalo and remember its economic and racial divides. I remember the 1960s, when the suburban schools were favored and city schools generally despised as, in the main, dead-end locations. Buffalonians I talked to in recent years blamed their schools' poor performance on the parents of impoverished children, teachers "not doing their jobs," or the school principals ... anybody and anything but a funding system that enshrined inequalities and racial disparities evident from the red-lined 1930s into the present day. I blamed myself. I left Buffalo as a teenager and never looked back.

The point is not simply to lament the means by which we come to accept, as I was trained to do, inequality as normal. It is not enough to bemoan the piecemeal manner in which the studies we engage offer at best partial truths obscuring the motive causes of our distress. Instead the point is to insist on an understanding that "objectivity" is necessarily limited and *always* bounded by our choices. We all are trained to advance small truths that tell big lies. Ethically, the result is a set of false truths that are no truth at all. As the US Supreme Court argued, "intentions" do not matter when the results are disastrous. When that happens, our communal moral declarations are violated, and we are all complicit.

7 Mapping Justice as Transportation

It is no surprise that the effective end of US racial segregation began on December 1, 1955, with Rosa Louise McCauley Parks's arrest for refusing city bus driver James F. Blake's order to yield her seat to a white passenger in Montgomery, Alabama. Rosa Parks was not the first to refuse to accept the segregation of the public transit system. It was not her name but that of Aurelia Browder on the seminal 1956 Supreme Court decision ruling state policies of public segregation federally unconstitutional.[1] But it was the face of young Rosa Parks, whom the US Congress would later call "the mother of the freedom movement,"[2] that focused the nation and the world on the systemic inequities of the then-accepted racial segregation of public facilities in the United States. It was her arrest and its attendant publicity that made the 381-day boycott of segregated Montgomery public transit services, then legal under Alabama laws, so powerful an act of protest.

The year before, the US Supreme Court had declared, in *Brown v. Board of Education*,[3] that the old rule of "separate but equal"—promulgated in an 1896 Supreme Court case[4]—violated the Constitution's Fourteenth Amendment. As it had been for Homer Plessy in the earlier case, and as it would be for the Campaign for Fiscal Equity (CFE) petitioners in New York City a century later, the argument was ethical: in a society declaring all persons equal, justice requires equality of access and opportunity. With these two 1950s Supreme Court rulings—one in education and the other in public transportation—justice in the United States was redefined.

In moral philosophy, justice trumps all other moral and political objectives. John Rawls called it the first virtue, one insisting on fair and equitable relations between all, and thus equality *for* all.[5] To deny equality is to accept that certain individuals in society will not be as free as others to act according to their best interests. Equality denied attacks the very notion of justice in its refusal of equal individual freedoms as a moral mainstay of society. When that occurs, the dignity of the person is violated,

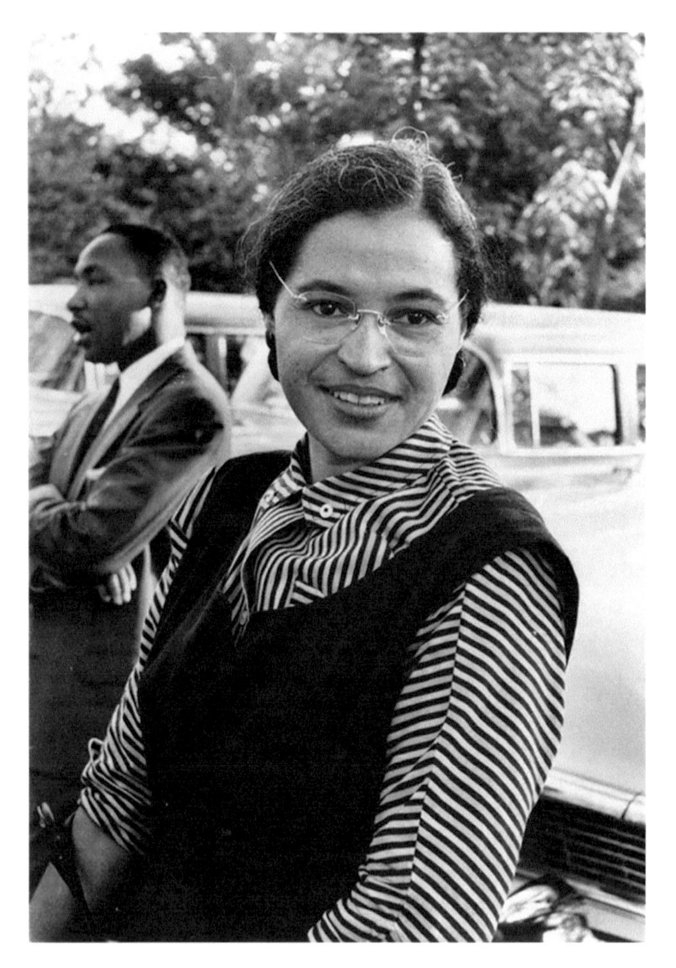

Figure 7.1
"The first lady of civil rights," Rosa Parks's refusal to yield her seat on a Montgomery bus highlighted both racial segregation and the critical place of transportation as an essential element of public life. Wikipedia.

along with the notion of full membership in the community and country in which he or she lives.[6]

What made Rosa Parks's protest so powerful was that public transportation was assumed to be an essential freedom without which a citizen's life is necessarily restricted. Citizens need to be able to travel the city in its many parts if they are to participate in its commercial and social activities. When transportation is restricted, so is the citizen. "Urban life is bound up with and predicated on transportation," Klaus

Schafer and Elliott Sclar wrote in 1980.[7] "The quality of human life depends on the amount of access we have to one another." Segregation ensured that equal access was restricted for some. And for individuals who cannot drive (or, if they can, cannot afford an automobile), it is public transit that either permits or inhibits independent access in modern urban communities.

It is in this sense that local and regional transportation is a critical constituent of what Harvey Miller described as "the individual's [essential] freedom to participate in activities in the environment."[8] One cannot be an equal citizen, free to participate, if one cannot get to city hall, the concert hall, or an employer's office. This belief in equality irrespective of individual differences led the United Nations, in its Convention on the Rights of Persons with Disabilities, to condemn the "attitudinal and environmental barriers" that hinder the "full and effective participation in society on an equal basis" of persons with mobility limits.[9]

So Rosa Park's protest, and the protests of others, exemplified an ethical attempt to right a moral wrong within the segregated United States, where equal justice and equal freedom were withheld from persons of color. Yes, she broke state law and violated the rules of the transit company. But they, in turn, violated a greater moral supposition. The result was certainly distress for her (the arrest), the driver (forced to follow the rules), and the nation at large (she broke the law, but was it a bad law?). The fundamental issue was America's image of itself and its allegiance to stated moral ideals.

Network Access

Transportation experts rarely talk about equality and freedom, about morals and their enaction. Mostly they talk about access, "one of those common terms that everyone uses until faced with the problem of defining and measuring it."[10] I use the term here in its most pedestrian definition: universal access means the freedom to go anywhere served by the transportation network. Limited access restricts a traveler's opportunity range. Inequalities occur when some people are denied access available to others.

Access is different from, but related to, the idea of "accessibility," the ease with which different elements of a transit system can be entered. A transit system may have great access to the city at large—its many lines and modes linked nicely together. But that matters little if the individual stops or stations are individually inaccessible. Where either access (a limited system) or accessibility (entry to the system at its nodes) is restricted, the accessible space of the city and its potential are diminished. Traveling urbanites must instead drive their own cars, pay for taxis, hire a private driver, or just stay home. Systems that provide universal access and accessibility are by this definition equitable, while those in which access and accessibility are limited can be described as less inequitable. Justice and its attendant freedom hang in the balance.

Transportation as Circulation Networks

For many years, urban transit systems have been understood as networks linking places within a city or metropolitan region. At another scale, air and rail services (or buses) link the city at large to the region and then the nation in which it is embedded. Experts talk about network "circulation." Just as humans are sustained by the circulatory system of the blood, so the circulatory transportation network sustains the urban body.

It was this idea that made the cover of the June 30, 2008, issue of the *New Yorker* so intuitively correct (fig. 7.2). In the cover illustration, New York City is anthropomorphized, simultaneously restrained and sustained by the bridges and transit lines that link its varying parts, one to the other, and the whole to the greater world. In the last

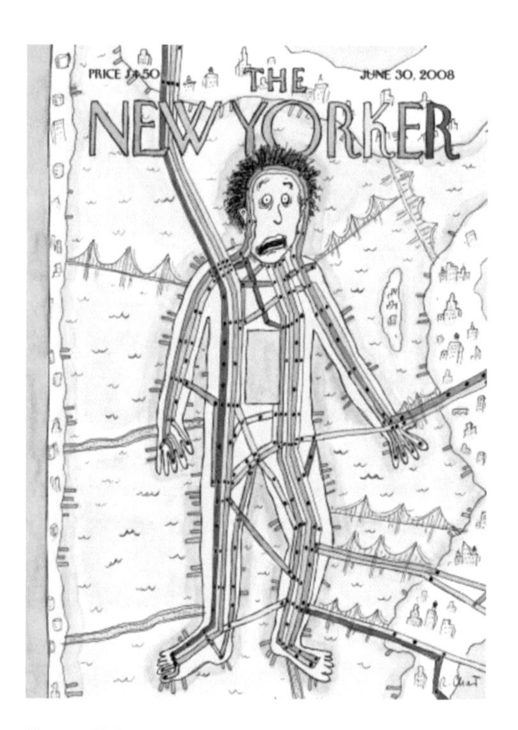

Figure 7.2
This *New Yorker* cover presents New York City as a body whose circulatory system comprises the rail and subway lines that run through its body. They, in turn, join the city to the greater world, across bridges that are also transit carriers. Courtesy the *New Yorker*.

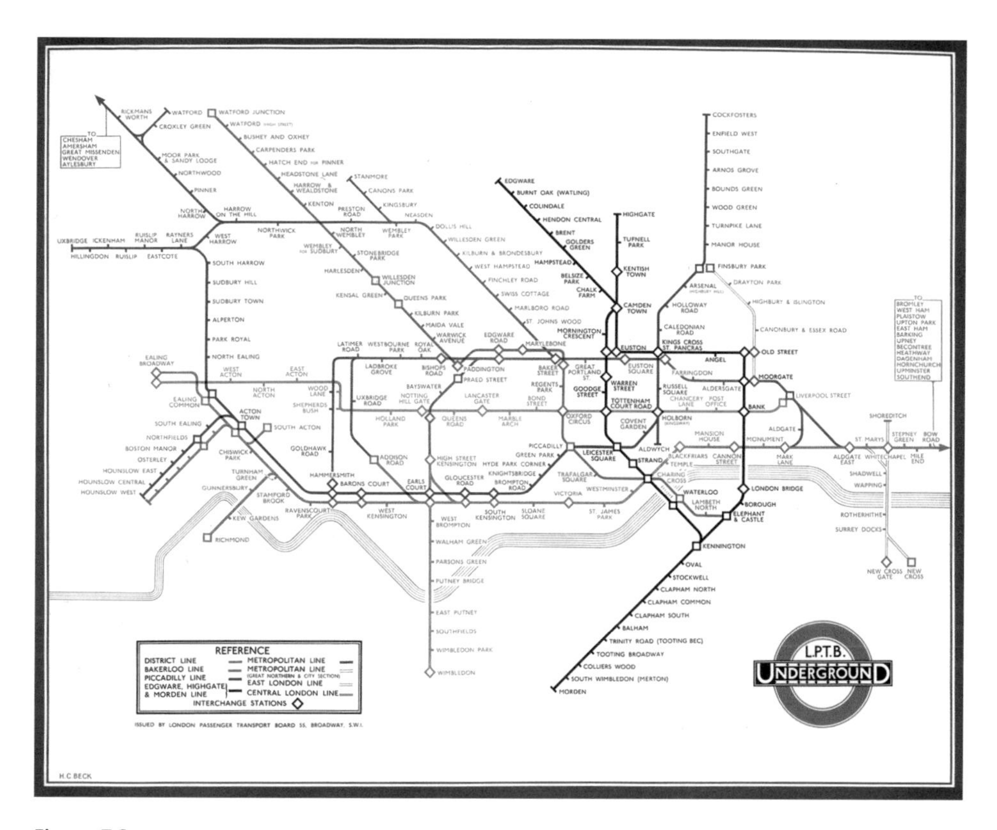

Figure 7.3

The original 1933 version of the London Underground map designed by Harry Beck, a map whose features have been widely copied for use by transit systems around the world. Courtesy London Transport Museum.

century, *circulation* was used as both noun and verb in describing the flow of electricity across a building's wiring and, by analogy, the electrified city. The idea of urban circuitry across a connected urban network powered perhaps the most famous and certainly the most emulated of all transportation maps, Harry Beck's 1931 map of the London Underground (fig. 7.3).

First published in 1933, Beck's spare, color-coded geometry posted the idea of a subway system as universally accessible urban circuitry.[11] Indeed, in 1933, Beck made another map of the London Underground using electric circuitry symbols in response to kidding from coworkers that his transit map "merely adopted one of the electrical circuits."[12] Just as electric circuitry ensures a free flow of all electrons in a wiring system, or in the human circulatory system blood cells move through the individual body, so transportation circuitry ensures the equal movement of all persons in and through the city.

For more than eighty years, Beck's map and its successors have served as "a magic guide to a hitherto totally bewildering city," wrote Ken Garland in *Mr. Beck's Map*.[13] "Before them [i.e., Londoners] was an orderly simulacrum for a disorderly, disjointed accumulation of urban villages, only barely discernible from one another on the ground, yet possessed with all the pride and exclusiveness of true communities." The mapping of the underground made those true communities part of one greater entity. In a real way, the Underground *is* London, its imaging a map of the city whose accessibility at every point is the presumed right and indeed the birthright of all Londoners.

The system has expanded since Beck's day. New stops and new lines have added to its reach; ridership has grown exponentially. At the end of the first decade of the current century, Transport for London supported 124.6 million passenger trips along its twelve, color-coded lines, each trip beginning and ending at one of the Underground's 333 stations. Some stops connect travelers to the national rail system and thus provide access to the nation at large. Heathrow Airport and Paddington Station connect travelers to the Continent and the greater world.

All of this is true for many Londoners and most visitors, but not in full measure for me in 2001, 2009, 2012, or 2014. Because I was hobbled by arthritis and walking with a cane, the high, narrow steps leading into and out of many stations, and the long corridors joining different lines at shared stops, were not mere impediments or minor inconveniences but barriers limiting my travels. If I can't safely navigate the stairs and walkways, then I can't get *to* the Underground's trains. And even when I can, on a good day, the effort typically is exhausting and sometimes dangerous if, when I am tired, my balance wavers.

Nor am I alone. Struggling mothers wheeling baby carriages can be found waiting at a station entrance until a passerby offers to help lift the carriage down to or up from platform level. At many stops, persons in electric scooters and wheelchairs are simply out of luck, as are those with other challenges that make even slow progress so dangerous and taxing they prefer to stay home.

If equality of access is an essential freedom, as civil rights activists (and signatories to the UN Convention on the Rights of Persons with Disabilities) proclaim, then the lack of accessibility to the London Underground presents a freedom denied, an injustice that isolates the mobility-limited user in and from the city.

The average Londoner experiences something like this during the occasional transit worker strike. "It's difficult to explain what a nightmare London can be without the

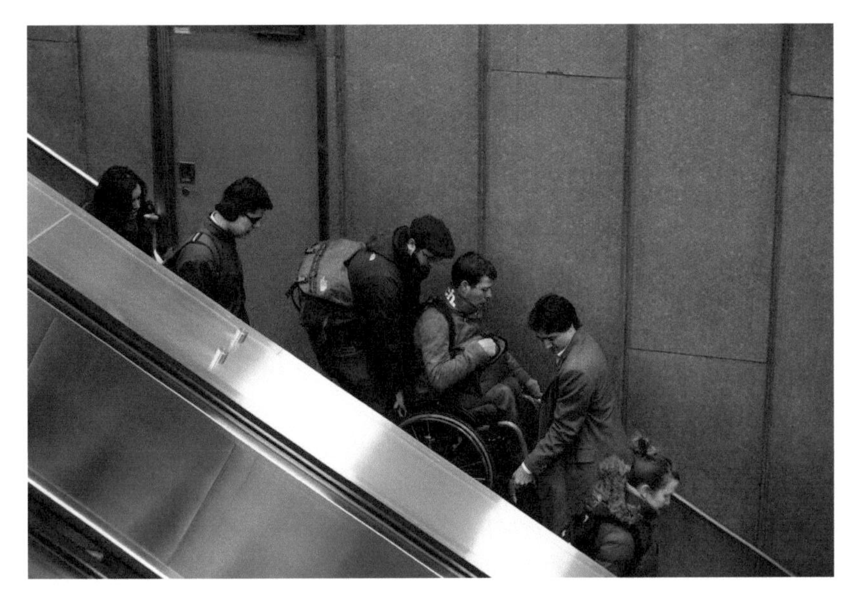

Figure 7.4
In 2016 Canadian Prime Minister Justin Trudeau was photographed helping to carry a wheelchair user down an inoperable escalator at a subway station in Montreal. Adam Scotti, official photographer for the Prime Minister.

Tube," wrote Jennifer Quinn in a 2014 obituary for Bob Crow, the longtime leader of Britain's National Union of Rail, Maritime, and Transport Workers. "Londoners sometimes just choose to stay home during a strike, rather than face the hassle of trying to get around a huge city with chaos on public transportation, which nearly 50 per cent of commuters use to get to work."[14] Those who cannot navigate the Underground's above-ground entrances and lower-level walkways know that "nightmare" on a waking, daily basis. Many simply give up the game and, as do Londoners during a labor action, just stay home.

I use London here as an example of the general problem that exists for mobility-restricted travelers in many cities. In the United States, Boston's MBTA and the New York City Subway have few elevators or lifts permitting mobility-limited entrance to the system. In other cities like Toronto, older streetcars have steps too steep for all but the aggressively able. The resulting inaccessibility also excludes people riding scooters or traveling in wheelchairs from using public transportation.[15] Even where there are elevators from the street to an underground or elevated transit station (or lifts on buses), they are often nonfunctioning. A 2009 survey of the Chicago elevated transit system found that more than 40 percent of the elevators that in theory provided accessibility in fact were inoperative.[16] So, too, were supposedly accessible doors and turnstiles.

In New York City, only 92 of the 425 stations—21 percent of the total—are wheelchair accessible. Of course, that assumes the elevators at those stations are working and, on an average day, 25 of the elevators at those 92 stations are out of service for a median time of four hours. That means, in effect, that at most 22 percent of the 21 percent of accessible stations can be accessed by persons with mobility deficits.[17] "I often wheel off a train only to discover that the sole elevator to ground level is out of service," Sasha Blair-Goldensohn wrote in the *New York Times*. The options are then to try another accessible station, often stops away, or hope folk will help carry him and his chair up the steps.

In a 2008 survey of US citizens over sixty-five, more than 20 percent of respondents reported staying home because of the limits of local transit systems.[18] Melanie Rapino and Thomas Cook call this a kind of spatial entrapment measured by a progressive reduction in accessible space or the necessary addition of travel time to get from one place to another.[19] For her part, Carol Thomas calls passenger exclusions on the basis of accessibility barriers an "impairment effect" that produces what Rob Imrie and Clair Edwards described as "disabled spaces," areas of the city that become off-limits to those with restricted mobility.[20] In 2002 Alison Porter named the result "transit disability," a state defined by system barriers rather than a person's physical capacities.[21]

For those in the disability movement, it has long been doctrinal that the problem is not solely this or that person's potentially limiting characteristics but society's refusal to accommodate individual differences.[22] The movement began in the 1970s in Great Britain, due in large part to the efforts of members of the Union of the Physically Impaired against Segregation (UPIAS).[23] Since then, the definition that has become generally accepted is, as the United Nations Convention on the Rights of Persons with Disabilities declared, that "disability results from the interaction between persons with impairments and ... barriers that hinder their full and effective participation in society on an equal basis with others."[24]

Racial segregation created an unjust limitation on personal freedoms based on a person's pigmentation, making it a "disability." Social segregation resulting from the systemic exclusion of persons on the basis of their physical or sensory characteristics similarly imposes inequitable and thus unjust limitations on the promised freedoms of affected persons to interact equally in and with the city.[25] That sense of exclusion, of diminished citizenship, constitutes the very essence of moral stress and distress: an attack on one's sense of self as equal based on a fundamental failure of justice's fairness ideal.

The London Transit Map

None of this is evident in maps of the modern Underground freely distributed in folding, pocket-sized editions by Transport for London at Tube stations and at the concierge's desk in most hotels (fig. 7.5). These maps, and those on the system's web pages, promise a justly equitable, universally accessible travel network of fourteen train lines in a wholly integrated network linked, at forty-five different transit stations, to national and international marine and rail transit systems.

What a map! The inheritors of Mr. Beck's vision have done him proud. In its current version, there are a total of 376 line segments, each connecting at least two of the 333 transit stations, one to the other. Some of those stations permit access to two or more different lines. Even where a station accesses only one line, however, it will of necessity connect to at least one other station, and from there another until it reaches a junction where a traveler can switch to a different transit line again.

Enter anywhere, the map promises, go everywhere. The diameter of the system, its length at its farthest two points, is forty-nine stations, stretching from the Piccadilly Line's Heathrow Terminal stations at the system's extreme southwest to the Upminster station on the District Line at the extreme northwest.

The mapped network is embedded in an economic landscape of nine concentric oval zones, each lightly shaded and numbered consecutively in the map. Zone 1 is the city center (Parliament, Westminster Abbey, etc.); zone 9 is the exurban periphery. Costs increase as a traveler crosses from one zone into another. Across this economic surface, the map promises equitable access for all who can pay the cost of the trip. Poverty aside, the map presents a promise of equality and universality in a London available in its many parts to all city residents and visitors.

John Pickles would call this an over-coded territory, one whose signs and symbols promise an organized, thoroughly accessible, hierarchical environment.[26] It is over-coded because the actuality may be experienced as chaotic and complex. Some, for example, Bieke Cattoor and Chris Perkins, think it *has* to be that way.[27] The result permits a kind of visual argument whose form and grammar are intuitively understood. The result screams, "Here is a system, accessibly open and well connected in its many parts."

The heart of the map is the moral declaration that underpins the complex realities proposed in its construction. Wherever you want to go, there's a Tube stop ready for you nearby. "There is general agreement that everybody deserves 'equity of opportunity.'"[28] That is what the map promises, and after all, that moral declaration is asserted not only in the United Nations Convention on the Rights of Persons with Disabilities

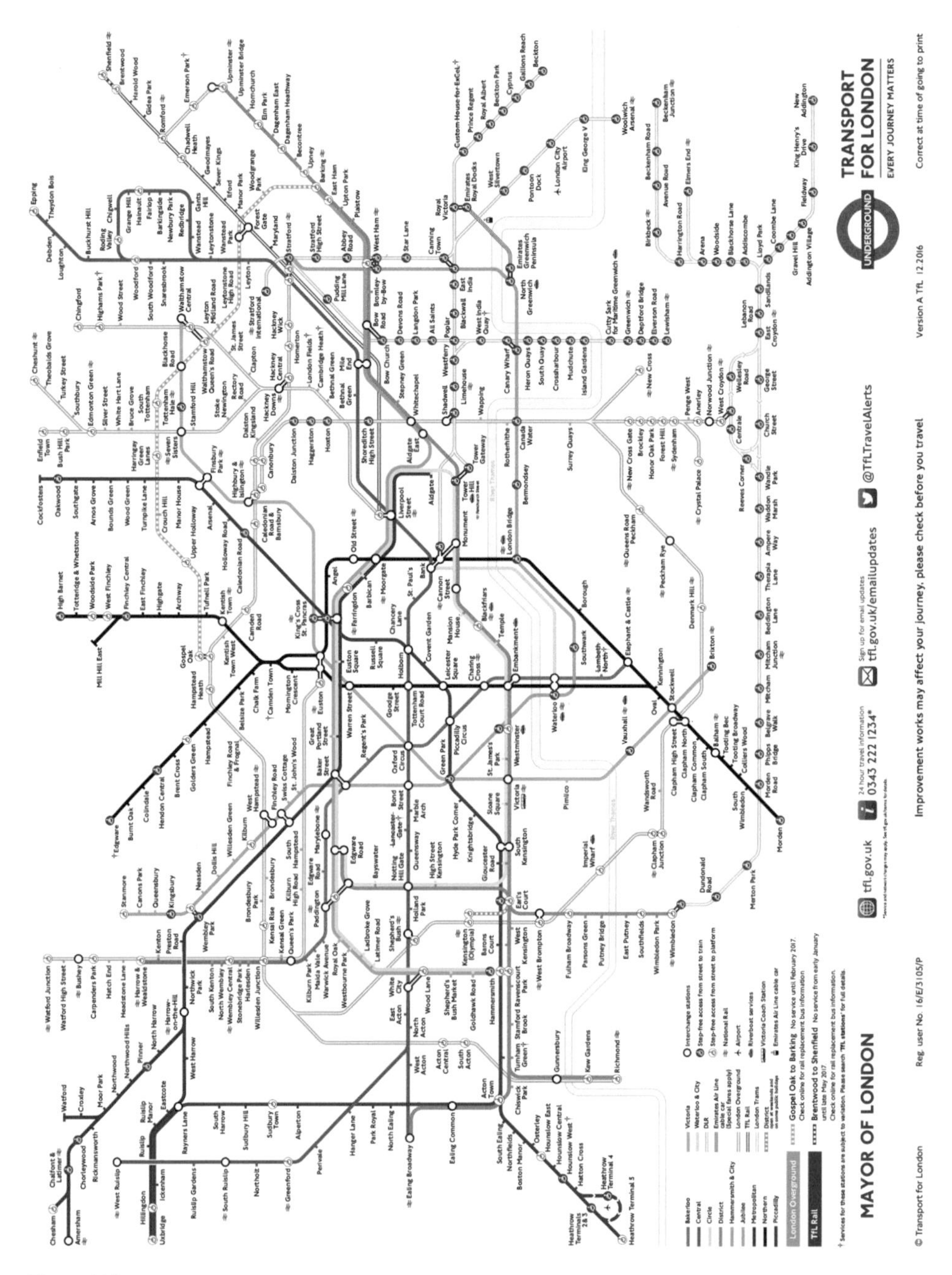

Figure 7.5

The official map of Transport for London promises a fully integrated, accessible opportunity for travel by all Londoners everywhere. Courtesy Transport for London.

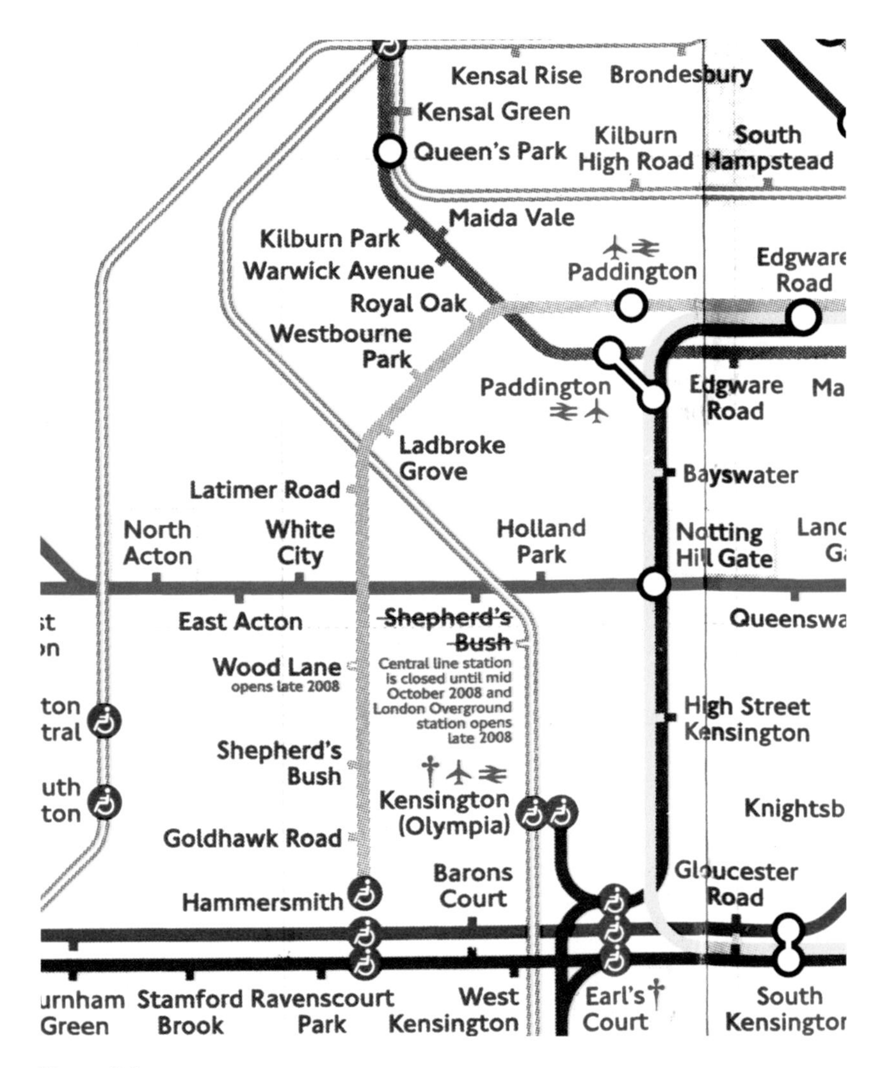

Figure 7.6

This detail from the Transport for London map shows the presence of "special access" stations, symbolized by a stick figure in a wheelchair, promising system accessibility at a minority of stations.

but also in Britain's Equality Act 2010[29] and, separately, Britain's 1995 Disability Discrimination Act, which was replaced by another, similar act in 2010.[30]

As if to emphasize these fine sentiments, across the mapped surface one finds 104 "special access" stations whose elevators provide accessibility for those with mobility restrictions. In the map, these appear as value-added locations. But for the mobility-restricted traveler who can enter (or leave) the system *only* at a "special access" station, 229 of the total 333 Underground stations are, in fact, *in*accessible. That drastically reduces the opportunity surface for the mobility-limited user. Inaccessibility, in other words, denies access in a way hidden by the map.

The number of stations between the Heathrow Airport terminals to the map's southwest, for example, and the Central Line's Epping station to the northeast shrinks by approximately 75 percent to ten accessible stations from the forty-one mapped for nonrestricted users. Access to the National Rail system at forty-five Underground connections available to the normal user was reduced by 29 percent to thirty-two "special access" rail connections. That meant slightly more than 71 percent of all National Rail connections in the city are *in*accessible, off-limits to the "special access" traveler.

To chart *that* reality, I made a map reflecting a mobility-limited opportunity surface that included *only* wheelchair-accessible "special access" stations (assuming all elevators were in fact working) and the links between them. The accessible city shown in figure 7.7 is radically diminished. Points of entry are severely restricted; so, too, are potential destinations. Even if one lives near a "special access" station, there is no reason to enter it unless the destination sought is near another station that is similarly accessible. As a result, whole lines are erased from the mobility-limited map as, one by one, inaccessible stations and their links are removed. The Metropolitan line north of Paddington Station and the District Line south of Earl's Court are gone. There is no point of entry or exit. The Circle Line that rings the inner city virtually vanishes, as well. Only the stops at Westminster, Bank/Monument, Liverpool Street, and St. Pancras remain. Where did the lines go? You can't ask Britain's most famous fictional detective, Sherlock Holmes, because there is no stop at Baker Street, where his office is now a museum.

Also removed from the map are most of the not necessarily accessible Underground stations linking the London Underground to the National Rail system. The standard map's symbols promising National Rail access are retained but moved off-center from their original locations. They float instead as symbols of promises withheld in the empty space of the mobility-restricted map, symbols not of connectivity but of inaccessibility.

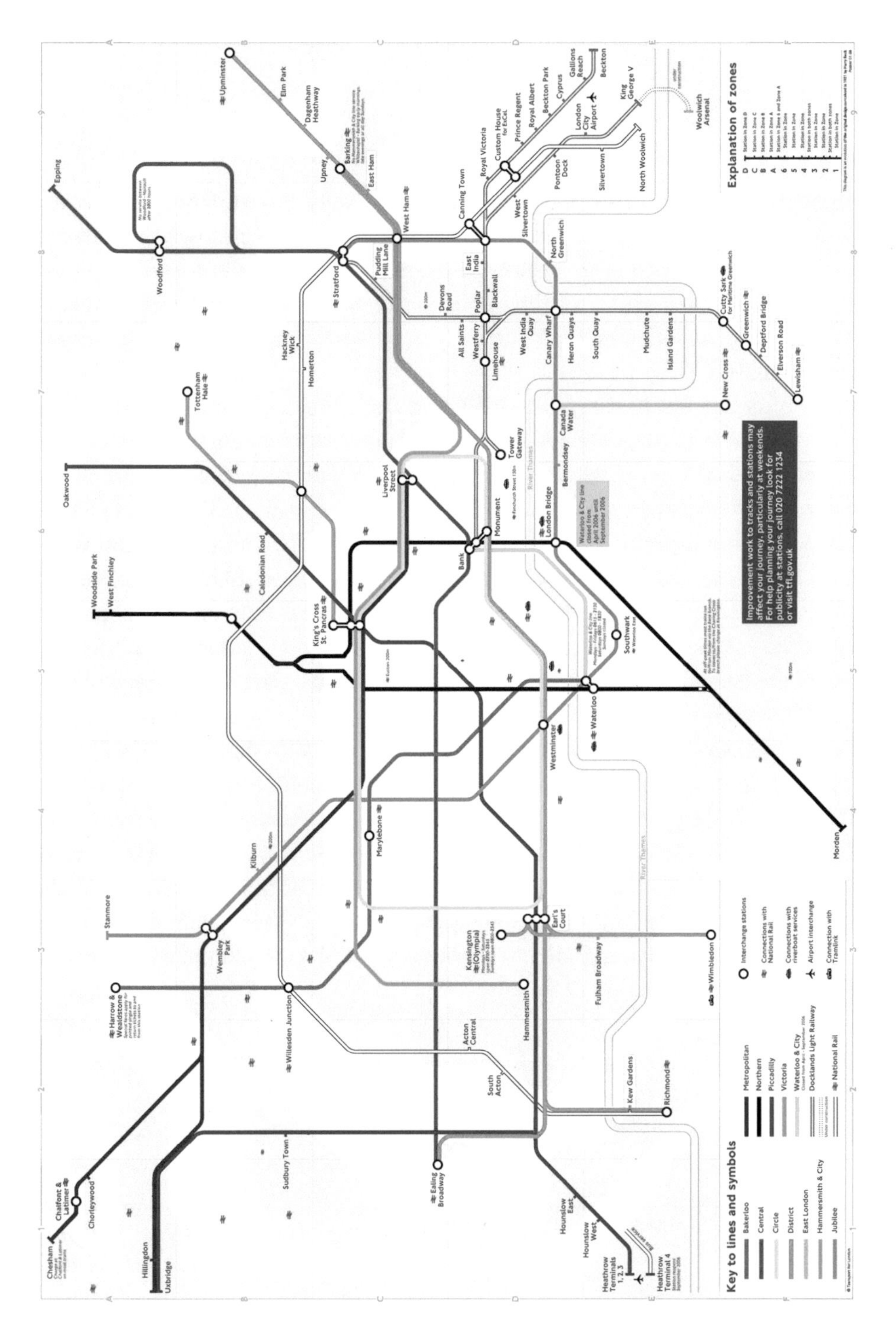

Figure 7.7

The author's map reconfigures the standard London transit map to reflect its reality to the mobility-limited traveler. Only stops accessible to wheelchair users, and the links between them, are included in this map.

Calculations

The mobility-restricted map is startling in its bareness, its opportunity surface drastically diminished. Its argument can be distilled into a set of quantitative descriptors teasing out the numeracy of exclusion. To do this, I asked for help from three transportation geographers: the University of British Columbia's Ken Denike; Simon Fraser University's Warren Gill; and Ray Torchinsky, who, for a time, taught transportation geography at SFU.

To quantify the effects of mobility limits, we first defined a direct connection as a single network link joining any two stations. Distances between any two stations were then considered additively, with an optimal shortest path described, in turn, as the fewest number of network links required to go from any *a* to any *b*. In considering the relative location and potential importance of different stops, and thus of regional differences in the city, we divided stations into two groups: inner stations in the central city (zone 1), and outer stations in the increasingly peripheral economic areas (zones 5 and 6). Zone 1 is the center of government—Metropolitan and National—and the area in which one finds London's most famous tourist sites, including the Houses of Parliament and Westminster Abbey.

The simplest measure of relative accessibility is the percent of stations open to potential travelers. Table 7.1 concludes that, overall, access for mobility-limited travelers was available at only 31 percent of all London's Underground transit stations during our study period. In the critical central area of the city, however, the percentage dropped to 15.5 percent, reflecting an uneven geographic distribution of "special access" stations. To state our findings declaratively: mobility-limited travelers were barred from more than 70 percent of the Underground network overall, and more than 85 percent of the network stations in the center of the city.

Table 7.1
Transit access: The number of accessible stations

	Number of Accessible Nodes		
	Total Number of Nodes	Number of "Special Access" Nodes	%
Full Network	333	104	31.23
Central Area	58	9	15.52
Outer Area	275	95	34.55

"Special access" Tube stations are distributed unevenly across the city with paucity in the dense central area compared to outlying suburban regions.

Table 7.2
Trips between accessible nodes

	All Possible Trips	Possible Accessible Trips	% Possible Accessible Trips
Within Central Area	3,306	72	2.18
Within Outer Area	75,350	8,930	11.85
Between Outer-Central	31,900	1,710	5.36
All Trips	11,0556	10,712	9.69

Of the total number of possible trips available to average London Underground travelers, approximately 92 percent are inaccessible to travelers requiring lifts and other access advantages.

Table 7.3
Trips between nearby stations (accessible nodes and nodes within one link of an accessible node)

	All Possible Trips	Possible Accessible Trips	% Possible Accessible Trips
Within Central Area	3,306	702	21.23
Within Outer Area	75,350	29,412	39.03
Between Outer-Central	31,900	9,288	29.16
All Trips	110,556	39,402	35.64

Even where access is defined by the "nearness" index of a station, the opportunity surface available to the mobility-restricted traveler is severely diminished.

An even greater reduction in travel opportunity was described by calculating the number of "seamless trips" available to the mobility-restricted Londoner. These are trips that do not require the inclusion of alternate travel modes (bus, ferry, taxi, etc.).[31] Table 7.2 concludes that fewer than 10 percent of all seamless trip possibilities (9.69 percent) available to the normal user were available to the mobility-restricted user overall. In the critical zone 1 at the core of the city, only 2.18 percent of possible trips can be accomplished seamlessly.

To better describe the effect of these reductions, we next calculated the number of trips between nearby stations available for the "special access" traveler (Table 7.3). For this we used one-link nodes as a measure of the coarseness or fineness of the urban network and thus of the travel opportunity space available to the mobility-restricted traveler. Simply, we used the number of nodes joining one link to another. If there was only one missing link, perhaps the mobility-restricted traveler could limp, crutch, or roll the distance. But where multiple stops were inaccessible, the likelihood of this was minimal.

Table 7.4
Mean nodal accessibility degradation index

	Average Links to Accessible Node	Percentile, Random Distribution
Full Network	1.40	97.7
Central Area	1.64	93.8
Outer Area	1.34	98.5

Mean nodal accessibility measuring expresses the average distance in links that must be traversed to reach a single accessible station from all other stations. For normal travelers, the average is 1.0.

These findings were again divided into those for the core city (zone 1) and then for the city at large. Using this one-link measure, we found that only 21 percent of trips within the central area and 29 percent of trips between the center and outer areas were available to mobility-limited travelers. For the normal traveler, of course, accessibility and thus access would be 100 percent.

Degradation

The reason why special access stations cluster along newer, outer segments of the network is simple. Older stations were built before concern for the mobility-restricted traveler was common. Newer stations built to serve the periphery are more likely to have elevators, escalators, and other mobility assists. To test for the degree of clustering exhibited by the distribution of accessible stations in London, we measured the average distance in transit links that must be traversed by mobility-limited users to reach a single accessible station from any other station (table 7.4). The resulting mean nodal accessibility degradation index (MNAD), developed by Torchinsky, is independent of both network size (number of nodes) and the relative number of accessible versus inaccessible stations. Using the cumulative frequency distribution for the full set of random iterations, we generated and analyzed a series of 100,000 random test distributions. The result is computationally similar to a first-order, nearest-neighbor statistic but differs in that nodes are separated into two subsets, and the distance measure is made from nodes in one subset (special access) to the nearest node in the other subset (all access).

The MNAD index can be interpreted as the average distance, in terms of network links, a mobility-restricted traveler needed to reach the nearest accessible node to his or her origin or destination. An index value of 1.40 meant a trip for mobility-limited travelers between any two rail stations in London would require, on average, at least three additional sequential rail links to get where they hoped to go. That is, there is the equivalent of a three-stop penalty for the mobility-restricted traveler compared to the normal traveler.

To test the conditional probability of the randomness of the distribution of accessible stations within the central and the outer areas, a second series of 100,000 random distributions forced the total number of accessible stations in the two areas to coincide with the observed number. The last column in table 7.4 presents the percentiles achieved in this simulation. The result again distinguishes, at a 95 percent confidence level, the diminished distribution of accessible central-city and out-area nodes available to the mobility-restricted user.

Other Travel Modes

Some say none of this truly limits mobility-restricted travelers' access to London. Those with sufficient monies may travel in taxis or drive personal cars. For those who cannot afford either or, like me, cannot drive (my low vision does not permit it), there are always buses. After all, Transport for London maintains a comprehensive and accessible bus network. At rush hour, the double-decker buses are typically overfull, and even if passengers can get onboard, those using canes and crutches are unlikely to find seats. Persons in wheelchairs may have to wait at an outdoor stop until a less crowded vehicle eventually arrives.

Even were occupancy unlimited, are city buses equivalent to the Underground? Is one travel mode equal to another? We compared travel times for the average Londoner with full access to the Underground to the travel time a mobility-restricted traveler would require accessing only "special access" transport services. To generate these two travel time profiles, we chose Heathrow Airport Terminal 3 as a destination and calculated travel times to it from all other Underground stations. Where the Underground was unavailable, bus travel was substituted and, in several cases, rail and marine ferry if they were shown to be the best accessible options.

Calculating relative travel times for all resulting origin–destination pairs was accomplished using Transport for London's online "journey planner." By 2014 the program we first used had been updated in a new online version.[32] The systems, old and new, both gave shortest-time travel options for all normal and separately mobility-restricted travelers. To generate comparisons, we entered the name of an Underground station in the "traveling from" box and entered Heathrow Terminal 3 in the "traveling to" box.

For all trips, we first queried the fastest travel option among all available transit modes for an average Londoner at 11:00 on a weekday morning. That start time is during a relatively slack transportation period, chosen to avoid comparisons during heavy commuting hours. Buses, if needed, are far slower during morning and evening rush hour commute times. Trip-planning parameters included "average" walking speed and a limit of ten minutes for pedestrian travel between stations or nodes (marine, rail). Then, using the "advanced options" button (now called "I need step-free access"), we calculated the same trip separately for mobility-restricted users unable to use escalators or stairs. Typically between four and six options were returned, all leaving within forty minutes of the 11 a.m. start time. These were averaged to give a recorded travel time (including waiting) between each of the 332 station locations and the airport station. Rolling or walking speed was self-assessed in the trip planner as "slow," and a maximum of four minutes pedestrian travel time was entered as a limit.

Not surprisingly, while most of the trips for the average traveler used the London Underground, those for mobility-limited Londoners relied primarily on bus and in some cases rail (mostly from Paddington Station). The number of steps required to get to Heathrow from anywhere in the city increased markedly (as the MNAD index predicted) for the mobility-restricted traveler.

On average (Table 7.5), it took the mobility-restricted transit user at least twice as long to get from any Underground location in London to Heathrow Airport. Columns 1 and 2 are the travel times for average and mobility-restricted users respectively. Column 3 is a simple ratio in which the first column is divided by the second. Thus a ratio of 1.5 presents a trip half again as long for the mobility-restricted user, a ratio of 2.0 means twice the travel time, and so on. The average time differential in this sample set of origin–destination pairs was 2.6:1. Calculations using the full set of travel times generated for all 332 transit stations to Heathrow Airport resulted in a system-wide travel time differential of a bit more than 2:1. Were the same test run during rush hour, when traffic flows slow markedly, the time difference would likely have been far greater. After all, the Tube's great advantage is that its trains run not simply underground but on tracks that avoid the gridlock of rush hour commuting.

But ...

A simple test of fairness and equality (and thus of justice) is this: Would the average person accept the restrictions that are placed on another? Would white bus passengers in Montgomery, Alabama, have accepted directions to sit only in the back of the bus and yield their seats to African American or Asian travelers? Would an Upper West Side Manhattan parent accept the condition of the schools that were the norm for students from, say, Harlem? Would Buffalonians who live in the suburbs of Amherst, Kenmore, or Williamsville accept for their children the school quality that existed in downtown Buffalo? If the answer is no, then the resulting inequality is clear. This kind of question (what if it were you?) lies at the heart of John Rawls's principle of

Table 7.5
"Special access" and normal user travel times to Heathrow Airport

From Tube Station	Normal Travel Time	Mobility-Limited Travel Time	Mobility-Limited "Penalty"
Acton Central	61	80	1.311
Aldergate East	53	114	2.151
Arnos Grove	72	140	1.944
Arsenal	60	125	2.083
Bank	58	112	1.931
Baker Street	40.3	106	2.63
Bethnal	65	133	2.046
Bond Street	48	109	2.271
Canonbury	71	135	1.901
Charing Cross	48	96	2.00
Edgware Rd.	42.3	103	2.44
Hackney Central	64	135	2.11
High Barnet	90	181	2.01
Hyde Park	47	85	1.81
Maida Vale	40	128	3.20
Marble Arch	46	123	2.674
Marylebone	39.2	112.3	2.865
Miles End	67	125	1.866
Monument	57	107	1.877
Newbury Park	83	157	1.892
Paddington	31	98	3.161
Perivale	56	113	2.018
Piccadilly Circus	42	113	2.69
Pimlico	54	106.5	1.972
Regents Park	44	118	2.682
Queens Park	44	108	2.455
Queensway	41	124	3.024

This table is a representative list of observed time differences between Heathrow Airport and London Underground stops.

justice "behind the veil," where one makes choices without knowing one's own precise circumstances.

Would the average Londoner accept without complaint a transportation system that required that he or she spend at least twice the travel time as his or her neighbor? Would he or she accept a system that largely barred him or her from travel on an Underground that was wholly accessible to that neighbor? The answer, based on the vociferous response to transit stoppages in the city, is no. The average Londoner would protest strongly, saying his or her access to the city and its opportunities—and thus freedoms—was being unfairly restricted.

Contemporary transportation researchers largely ignore these problems.[33] If you can't get there from here, they assume, another similar and more accessible "there" will somewhere be available. A clothier is a clothier, and if one won't do, then another will. Similarly, a doctor's office in one place is no different from one elsewhere. Issues of equality, freedom, and inclusiveness are thus avoided. This "place-based fallacy," as Harvey Miller called it, assumes not only that alternate locations will be more or less equally available, but also that they will be commensurable.[34] One church, doctor, or clothier is the same as any other. They aren't, however, not really. And where 70 percent of the network, including 80 percent of the urban core, is inaccessible, the reduction is simply too severe to suppose that easy alternatives exist.

The analyst's shrug seems to be based on the tendency, at least in the North American literature, to talk about access and accessibility in terms of automobile drivers who may have to drive a bit farther but are otherwise less obviously inconvenienced by mobility barriers.[35] Analysts whose models seek to "measure space-time accessibility benefits within transportation networks" typically take little account of needs of, and restrictions on, special user groups.[36] They simply assume the automobile is a universally accessible means of travel, the road system an equitable urban network. A small literature exists on travel barriers and opportunities for the sight limited, thanks to the work of the blind geographer Reginald Golledge, but this work is limited, largely experiential, and not system analytic.[37] The few who have attempted a general address of mobility limits have done so through theoretical computer models of such stunning complexity that their applicability remains untested.[38]

Discussion

In the standard mapping and in the professional's analytics, justice problems are buried in assumptions of normalcy. They assume we are all like electrons in the electrical grid, equally capable of transiting the system in all its parts. We are not, of course. The severe reductions resulting from limited accessibility present what the public health writer Barbara Starfield described, in another context, as a "vertical inequality" resulting when "people with greater needs are not provided with greater resources."[39]

Equality, equity, and freedoms acknowledged or denied are the result of both built and social environments that either promote or inhibit personal and professional opportunities.[40] Certainly the result is not simply distressful but also stressful for the mobility-limited Londoner. It was for me as I planned my travel in the city around the system and my own mobility limits. At the heart of that stress lie the moral declarations that are ignored, the ethical injunctions that are unmet. For me, the map became a kind of tease, if not a lie. More generally, the built environment reflects the social priorities of the society in which they are constructed, enacting the ethics of that society's moral vision. And here equality and freedom fell by the wayside in my struggles with city transit.

Maps and Mapmakers

The creators of the London Underground did not have equity and universality in mind when they built the first lines and their stations. They did not think about access for persons on crutches or in "basket chairs," the wheelchairs of old. Harry Beck did not think about these things when he first mapped the Underground as a kind of circuit board across which equally able Londoners might travel. The map that resulted deserves the overused descriptor "iconic."[41] In its clear, objective posting of transit lines dotted with transit stops, it has been the model for similar maps around the world.

The map (fig. 7.5) is "objective" in its mapping of Transport for London's Underground system, correctly relating the system's lines and nodes. Equally objective, however, is the map of London's Underground from the perspective of the mobility-restricted user (fig. 7.7). The first assumes a normal traveler with money to buy a ticket. The second takes accessibility as a critical determinant rather than a given and then refuses to include Underground stops and lines unavailable to mobility-restricted citizens.

Transport for London mapmakers might say, with a shrug, that this isn't their problem. They were hired to create a map of the transport network as it physically exists, not to critique its limits. They are functionaries doing what they're told. Thinking about equality, freedom, and justice is not included in their job descriptions. Nor is it the necessary brief of transport analysts and planners. They are, they could say, adding elevators where they can, when the money is available. It's an old system, after all, and things take time.

It is easy for functionaries to assert, as did one of the participants in the Regina workshop, that objectivity carries no ethical quotient, that morality is an ideal without a footprint. When as functionaries we take this position, we lose the opportunity to promote the moral values (equality, freedom, justice for all) that as citizens we purport to embrace. And that morality is clear in the laws and international agreements signed by Great Britain that promise equality of opportunity to persons of difference (I do not use the word *disabled*). We ignore our morality and its ethical injunctions until, perhaps, demands for redress make clear the limits of the work we have proudly produced. We ignore them until we sit in a wheelchair at a bus stop at rush hour or wait at the top of a Tube station we cannot access.

8 Ethics and Transplantation

Ethics become, in these examples, the standard by which the maps we craft, the statistics we generate, and the policies we promote on their basis serve to obscure or reflect the moral ideals we purport to embrace. Some will say, "It's just a map," or "they're just numbers," perhaps limited but certainly not malignant. But the consequences of the maps we choose to make, the statistics we self-consciously collect and arrange, directly affect lives, our own and those of our neighbors.

Consider graft organ transplantation in the United States, a subject introduced briefly in chapter 3. The ability to transplant a healthy organ from one body to another was one of the significant clinical advances of the last century. From the start, the problem has been that there have never been enough organ donors to provide what today is broadly advertised as the "gift of life" to those whose illnesses require a replacement kidney, heart, lung, or liver. We insist that the gift of an organ upon a person's death—and increasingly, for some organs while the donor lives (e.g., a kidney)—is a contribution to others that only the most churlish would refuse. We must, bioethicists and news commentators say, do more to increase the supply.[1]

The ethical ideal is beneficence, declaring as a moral good the active and selfless sharing of ourselves in a community of others like ourselves.[2] And so, as Nancy Scheper-Hughes wrote, we ethically promote organ donation while disparaging organ sales trafficking and the "organ tourism" that occurs when the rich of one nation seek organs from the poor of another country.[3] We insist that the commercial nature of such transfers not only is inherently inequitable—after all, the rich don't sell organs, only poor folks do—but violates the defined virtues of egalitarian sharing enacted (in theory) by graft organ donation in civil societies.

That said, organ transplantation is a quagmire of moral stress, distress, and perhaps injury. Joseph J. Fins describes the distress that results from overenthusiastic "hovering" organ collection representatives, waiting to "swoop in" to claim organs of those not yet quite deceased, "as if [they were] an entitlement."[4] Too often the families of critically ill patients are pressured to participate even when a patient's prognosis is uncertain and hope remains. The result is politely described as "premature harvesting."[5] All of this is made more complex by the clinical and moral problems concerning the criteria by which a body is declared deceased and thus, one might say, "organ ready." The result is what some call "justified killing,"[6] a willful termination of the still living for some greater good: "Although it may be perfectly ethical to remove vital organs for transplantation ... the reason it is ethical cannot be that we are convinced they are really dead."[7]

So there is the stress experienced by potential recipients waiting for life-prolonging donation, the distress of the family of the potential donor not yet dead, and that of organ transplant officials pressured to collect more viable organs. And then we have the moral distress of medical personnel like Fins who are engaged in a fragile patient's continuing, potentially at-risk care, as well as the distress experienced by those who see themselves as advocates for patients in need of new organs. Finally, there is the moral stress of the nation in which the national graft organ transplant system was created and is promoted today.

History: UNOS

In 1984 the US Congress passed the National Organ Transplantation Act (NOTA) "to create a national system in which an adequate supply of organs would be available on an equitable basis to patients through the nation."[8] The act defined transplantable graft organs as a national resource to be donated freely and distributed fairly among Americans, irrespective of a patient's income or social position. The moral principles underlying a national policy of organ donation were to be altruism and beneficence.[9]

Congress tasked the US Department of Health and Human Services (HHS) with the responsibility for organizing a national network for organ collection and distribution based on these moral suppositions. In its turn, HHS ordered a study on how best to structure a program that might enhance the supply of needed organs, improve the distribution of organs collected, and, of course, keep costs down.[10] "Equitable access to transplantation was a central issue," the report's authors insisted, arguing that a patient's financial status should not limit access to a transplant service.[11] That was as much practical policy as it was a moral declaration. If organs were to be donated "in a spirit of altruism and volunteerism and constitute a national resource to be used for the public good,"[12] then potential donors had to believe they, or their loved ones, were equally likely to be recipients if the need arose. If they were not, then they would be outside the community of equal giving and receiving. As a result, donations would presumably suffer.

The insistence that the system be equally accessible to all Americans reflected a justice provision declaring equality of treatment as a guiding national principle and thus, in theory, a principle of the systems it sets in place. The result was to be a model of the ethical application of this worthy moral stance. "No part of the health care system has done more to resolve questions of justice than transplantation," experts boasted in the 1990s.[13]

The NOTA-mandated HHS report resulted in the creation of the United Network for Organ Sharing (UNOS), which was charged with developing and overseeing a "national organ procurement and transplantation network" (OPTN). In the resulting system, UNOS organ procurement organizations (OPOs), typically located in or near transplant-performing hospitals, would be responsible for collecting and distributing graft organs across eleven national transplantation districts. The assumption was that "optimal quality as well as cost savings from economies of scale and experience could be realized through 'regionalization.'"[14] As one author cited in the 1986 HHS report put it: "By performing an economically efficient volume of procedures for any specialized hospital service, dollars can be saved with no loss in the quality of care provided."[15] So, from the start, the goal advanced a morality whose operational principle was cost efficiency.

Figure 8.1 shows a 2014 map of UNOS regions.[16] In this map, regional divisions are shaded in light, nonconfrontational colors in an equal-area, conical projection that seems, well, right. It is hard to see that Vermont is split into two parts, its eastern division set in Region 1, and the western part in New York State's Region 9. Nor does either the projection or its coloring raise questions about the inclusion of Hawaii in Region 6 rather than the more heavily populated Region 5. The map just feels correct, a fair division of the nation into parts (Northeast, Southwest, Pacific Northwest, etc.) that we intuitively understand.

Moral Geographies

Although organ donations are solicited from across the nation, the majority of procedures are performed at hospitals in major cities. Centralizing transplant procedures seemed to make pragmatic sense. Transplantation is a complex surgery, requiring specific expertise rarely available in smaller hospitals. Moreover, large urban populations are more likely to provide a quantity of immediately available viable organs. Because organs degrade outside the living body—when the transplanted heart, for example, is

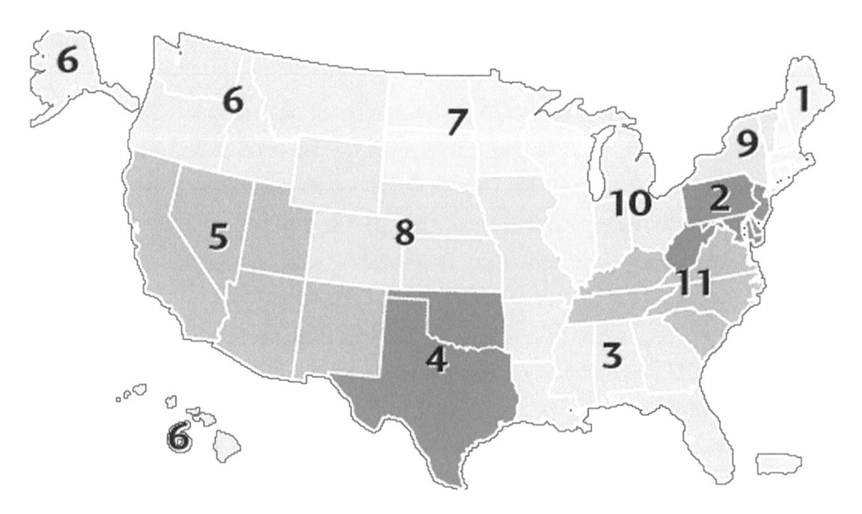

Figure 8.1
A map generated in 2014 by UNOS of its 11 districts within which donated organs are registered and then distributed. UNOS.

separated from its living host—speed of both collection and distribution is essential.[17] So the proximity of both donor and recipient to a transplant center is desirable; distance from a transplant center is a negative factor in choosing which needy patient will get the donated heart, lung, or other organ.

The result is "biased toward higher density areas," and the system's maximizing goals are "achieved by reducing the travel of the many as much as possible, while accepting greater travel for a few."[18] The unintended result, HHS Secretary Donna Shalala informed Congress in the mid-1990s, was a systemic failure of the "equable distribution" promised in law by NOTA. "In some areas of our nation, patients wait 5 times longer or more for an organ than in other areas. ... In the worst case, patients die in areas where waiting times are long while at the same time organs are being made available to less ill patients in areas with shorter waiting times."[19] Shalala proposed a series of changes designed to decrease observed spatial disparities.[20]

If, as she claimed, the system failed to meet the standards of equality of treatment ethically required by the legislation's justice ideal, then the failure was moral (all people were not equal), ethical (if equality is a standard, then it was not met), and geographic (discrimination was being practiced on the basis of location). Legally, Shalala was thus obliged to assert HHS oversight to ensure that the law's ideals were enacted. Consequentially, doing so would enhance the idea of a participatory community whose members give and receive equally, irrespective of location or personal circumstance.

UNOS launched a highly public campaign opposing Secretary Shalala's proposed changes. The result was a bitter battle over means, not ends. All agreed that graft organ transplantation was an important good and that organ donation was a beneficent act to be encouraged. Everyone agreed fairness was important, even if nobody was quite sure what fairness meant. "We have general principles," UNOS president Dr. Larry Hunsicker admitted, "but we don't yet know how we as a community want to measure the question of fairness."[21] The result was a problem in what David M. Smith calls "moral geography": "a rubric for empirical investigations into various aspects of spatial patterns and relations which invite a moral meaning."[22]

Modeling the Problem

I became involved in all of this after reading an article by Alan B. Pritsker, then the doyen of simulation modeling.[23] In 1998 he strongly defended the UNOS system as efficient, equitable, and, if not perfect, then so good it certainly did not require political interference. Not coincidentally, Pritsker had spent three years as a consultant for UNOS. I had, however, been researching issues of equity and fairness in organ distribution for Toronto's Hospital for Sick Children.[24]

In a letter to the editor, I suggested Pritsker's model largely ignored both spatial and socioeconomic disparities.[25] After all, as Robert Steinbrook put it, "Although the procurement system is national, patients' access to it is not. Patients must generally either have health insurance that will pay for transplantation or [must] be able to pay for it themselves."[26] In a nation with, at that time, more than 40 million persons who lacked health insurance, this seemed a serious deficiency if equality of care was a goal. Where was fairness if the uninsured poor (wherever they lived) were asked to be organ donors but could not afford to be recipients? Where was the justice in a system in which regionalization and urban concentration favored some over others?

Pritsker's condescending response led me to propose an article mapping the geographical inequalities Shalala had argued and Pritsker had dismissed. While his specialty was liver transplantation, and others had considered kidney transplantation, I chose to focus on hearts. Renal patients can live for years on dialysis, and for those who qualify medically, kidney transplantation is a nationally funded program in which questions of insurer or patient economics are dramatically lessened. Liver transplantation is complicated by that organ's remarkable ability to fully regenerate if it is partially damaged. Partial liver resections can be performed without unduly endangering the lives of living donors. But for cardiac patients there is no life-supporting, dialysis-like treatment, no regenerative partial graft. Moreover, the ischemic rate of degradation is more rapid for the heart than for either kidney or liver. Finally, the heart has a mythos that, in an article criticizing a well-known, well-established expert like Pritsker, offered polemical advantages.

Substantiating the geographic inequities that Shalala described proved relatively easy. Using publicly available UNOS data, I located all US hospitals performing heart transplants, added to a worksheet the number of heart transplants each performed in 1996. From UNOS I collected data on mean wait times (MWT) for potential recipients at each hospital. If the problem was regional geographical disparity, then the question was not simply the average or mean waiting time per hospital or region. Rather, the real measure would be cumulative waiting time across the UNOS regions. Where Shalala had found, to her dismay, a disparity of five to one between patients from different cities, this broader regional measure reported a disparity as great as ten to one between different UNOS regions.

Figure 8.2 summarizes the geographic imbalances. The disparity between regions is evidenced through an eccentric color ramp designed to emphasize the differences in patient waiting times among the different UNOS regions. Including the urban clustering of transplant-performing hospitals made clear the locational inequalities of service that presumably contributed to regional disparities. In a supposedly national program, more than eleven states had no program at all. In other states, where hospitals were listed as transplant service centers, few or no transplants had been performed during the study year. The number of organs per hospital in a city determined the size of the circles used to locate them on the map. Regional disparities certainly seemed to violate the ethical framework set out in enacting legislation.

Unconsidered in either UNOS's rebuke of Shalala's proposal or Pritsker's analysis was the need for patients from underserved cities and states to travel at their own expense to established urban transplant centers. Yes, persons from regions with few if any transplant services were getting transplants. But to do so, they first had to travel to other cities, states, and UNOS regions, where they might wait for months in hopes that an organ would become available. This "organ tourism" is rarely compensated by an insurer and requires patients seeking transplant organs to have not only health insurance but also sufficient monies to fund months of travel out of city and often out of state. Patients too poor to pay for that would not qualify as potential recipients and would thus from the start be off the UNOS list of transplant candidates.[27]

My close examination of these issues resulted in a series of journal articles, a doctoral dissertation, and, nine months after its defense, the publication of *Scarce Goods: Justice, Fairness, and Organ Transplantation*.[28] The data used in those studies became

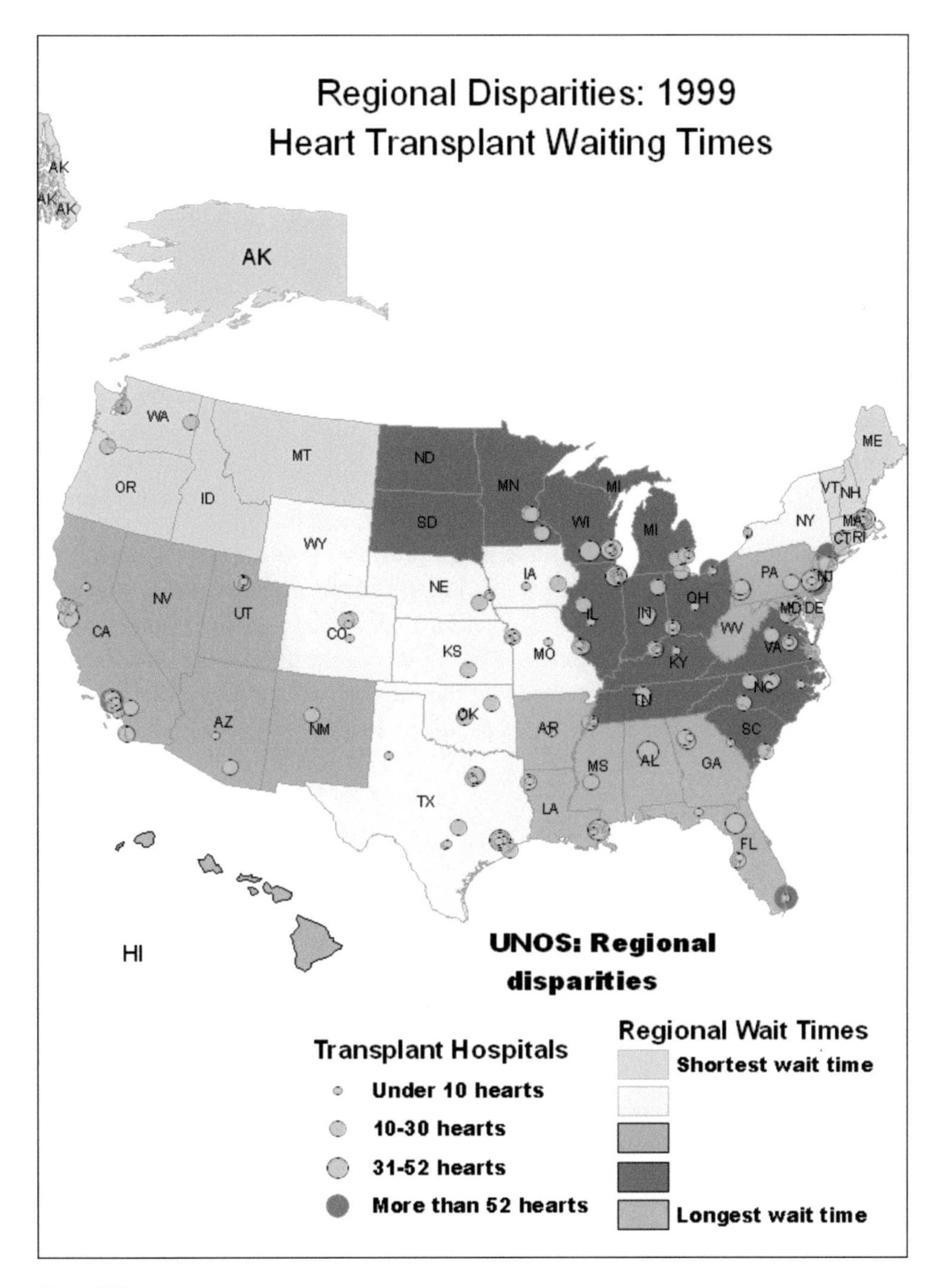

Figure 8.2
Mapped mean waiting times by UNOS region for people entering the heart transplant waiting list in 1996. Included are the locations of all hospitals performing heart transplants in 1998 and 1999. By author.

the basis for an undergraduate student laboratory exercise at the University of British Columbia. In Geography 381, "Spatial Analysis using GIS," which I cotaught with my friend Ken Denike, we asked students to locate new US hospitals to perform heart transplants. Students were required to justify their choices on the basis of geographical equity, efficiency, justice, or some combination of these criteria.

Not surprisingly, the choices depended on the criteria used. Students seeking maximum efficiencies (and profits) chose sites in major metropolitan areas near existing heart transplant centers. Others, seeking greater geographical equity, located their new centers in underserved western states and northern New England. The hope was that greater geographical equity would boost regional donor participation.

Several students suggested a North American program in which New England and Quebec would be joined into a single transplant region, and the underserved US Northwest would be partnered with Canadian prairie provinces (Alberta, Manitoba, and Saskatchewan). Alaska would be added to the British Columbia region. While this made good locational sense, it raised a series of jurisdictional problems. Not the least of these was the gulf between the US system of fee-for-service medicine and Canada's commitment to universal healthcare. Bridging that gap, whatever the efficiencies, made the result an exercise in political ethics as well as a moral philosophy lodged in the landscape.

The Regions Today

Look again at figure 8.1. There is, as one would expect, a New England region. Moreover, there is the Mid-Atlantic. But why is Illinois part of Region 7, hanging like an appendix, and not Region 10? Why isn't New Mexico joined to Texas rather than California and Arizona? In theory, regionalization promotes the efficient distribution of services. Do the regions in fact provide equitable national coverage, or as Donna Shalala argued in the 1990s, are they a template for spatial inequities?

Table 8.1 is based on UNOS data describing total heart transplants between 1988 and 2014 by region. In it regional differences in performance are manifest. The number of transplants per UNOS regional population between 1988 and 2014 ranged from a low of 117.7 per million in the Pacific Northwest to 238 per million in the Mid-Atlantic states of Region 2. At the least, it seemed obvious that the regional system appeared to create persistent population imbalances that affected the number of organs donated and thus the number of procedures performed.

Figure 8.3 attempts to maps these regional disparities. It shows the number of heart transplants performed across UNOS regions between 1988 and 2014. To this

Table 8.1
Heart transplants, 1988–2014

	Pop. (2000)	Pop. (2004)	Hearts Donated	Total Hearts Transplanted	Transplants per Mil. by Pop. (2004)
Region 1	13,922,517	14,263,833	2,199	2,207	154.726
Region 2	29,155,893	29,929,841	6,601	7,123	237.990
Region 3	38,602,965	36,807,686	8,729	7,323	198.953
Region 4	24,302,474	26,430,721	3,123	5,746	217.398
Region 5	45,052,752	48,315,730	9,350	9,199	190.393
Region 6	13,350,137	13,994,818	2,083	1,647	117.686
Region 7	24,099,491	24,999,667	5,048	5,273	210.923
Region 8	17,716,259	18,564,700	4,343	3,931	211.746
Region 9	18,976,457	19,316,116	2,855	3,511	181.765
Region 10	27,372,069	27,963,605	5,607	5,287	189.067
Region 11	28,870,892	30,529,315	6,867	6,189	202.723

Transplants per million is a coarse performance estimator that divides total transplants by 2004 population and then multiples by 1 million. Source: https://optn.transplant.hrsa.gov/data/view-data-reports/center-data/.

is added the number of donations in relation to the number of transplantations across the same period. In keeping with the UNOS map's light pastel color scheme, the variation in the number of heart transplants per region is presented similarly. The data are repeated a second time in bars that reflect the number of donations and heart transplants performed in each region. To distinguish my map from the official one, I used a different projection, one whose breadth contrasts with that of the UNOS conical equal-area projection.

The color scheme chosen at once acknowledges the presence of regional disparities and, in their pastel hues, mutes their importance. The addition of bars signifying the numbers of transplants per region clearly makes manifest the argument that equity is an unfulfilled promise. But neither the regional map nor the summary table (table 8.1) tells the real tale of geographic inequality that Secretary Shalala first argued unsuccessfully in the 1990s.

Regional mapping and statistics smooth the relevant data, rendering it invisible. Some states have organ procurement organizations but no transplant-performing hospitals at all. So organs donated in those states are shipped elsewhere in a region or to other regions. Figure 8.4 instead posts the number of transplants per state population. In the map, the raw number of transplants performed is signified by red bars located

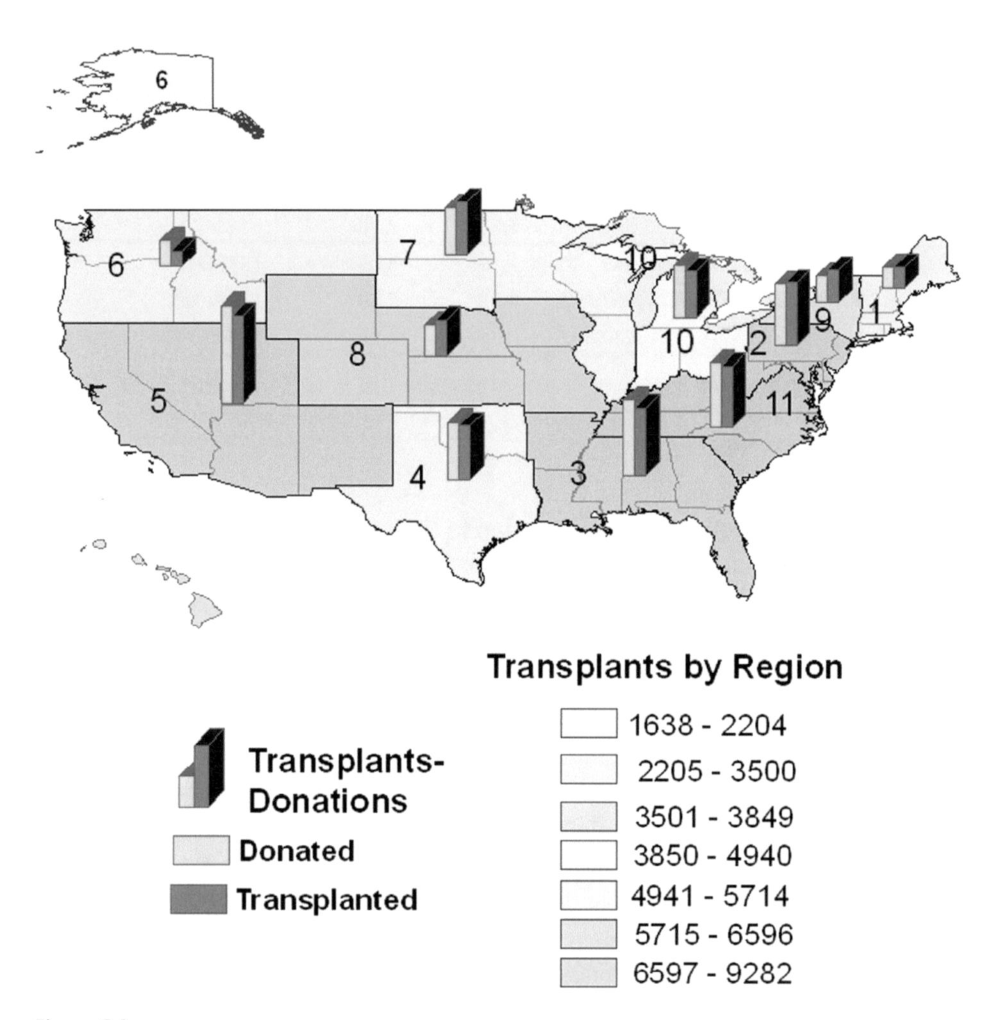

Figure 8.3
Regional heart transplant performance mapped using UNOS data from 1988 to 2014. By author.

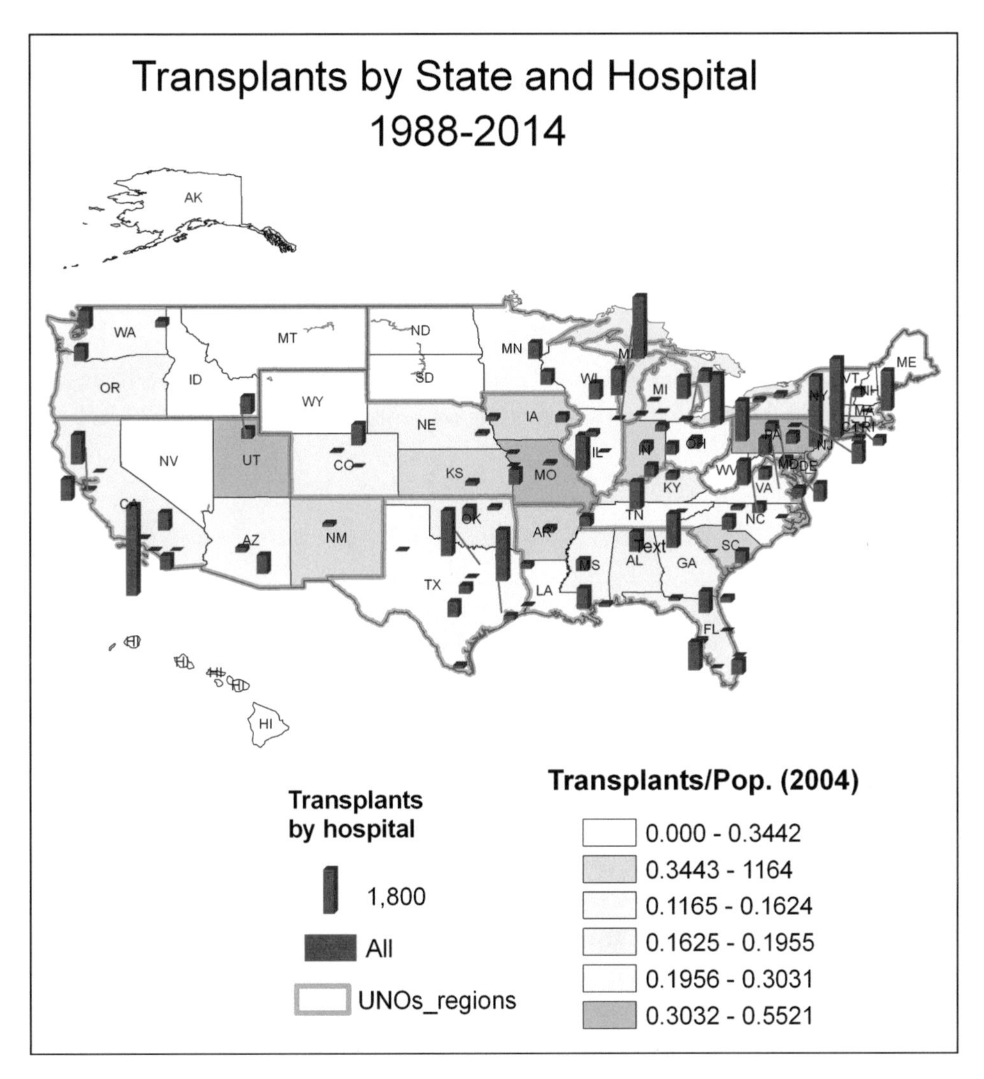

Figure 8.4

Cumulative number of heart transplants performed between 1988 and 2014 by state. The bars symbolize the number of transplants per city at all hospitals over the study period. By author.

in cities with transplant-performing hospitals. Where two or more hospitals perform transplants in a city, their numbers were combined. In coastal areas like Los Angeles, the bars are set slightly off-coast for ease of reading.

Because the data are based not on where patients live but on where transplants are performed, some states now show no heart transplants at all. It is not that nobody in Montana or Maine received a heart transplant but that no patients received a transplant in their home states. Moreover, we do not know if the person transplanted at Cedars-Sinai Medical Center in Los Angeles is Alaskan, Californian, Chinese, Hawaiian, Japanese, or Montanan. Nor do we know if a patient at the Cleveland Clinic in Ohio comes from Cleveland or Saudi Arabia. The US system permits some US organs to go to foreign nationals who can pay the cost (approximately $1 million) of heart transplantation.[29]

Socioeconomic Inequities

Clearly geographic inequalities were and are inherent in the US graft organ system of collection and distribution. They appear to be based on the relative distribution of populations in the varying UNOS regions and the concentration of transplant-performing centers in major cities. Some would say such inequalities are unavoidable, at least if maximum efficiencies at minimum cost is the standard. That said, as some of our students argued in Geography 381, changes in regional configurations might lessen existing disparities. There is, however, a more fundamental problem, briefly mentioned in chapter 3: UNOS transplant data include only patients accepted to the transplant waiting list. What about persons without health insurance or, like Denzel Washington's character in the movie *John Q.* (itself a careful case study of moral stress, distress, and injury),[30] whose insurers would not pay for a lifesaving heart transplant for his son? Those who do not have sufficient insurance and cannot afford a transplant, as well as the postoperative drugs and treatments a successful transplant requires for the rest of a patient's life, never make it onto the UNOS waiting list.

The UNOS system therefore is at best *only* as equitable as the national health-care system within which it is embedded. Poverty and wealth influence, where they do not determine, both the health of the person and the speed with which a patient may be added to the transplant waiting list. During the controversy over Shalala's "Final Rule" in 1999, for example, patients who earned more than $40,000 a year were twice as likely to be added to the waiting list for kidney transplantation as those who earned less than $10,000 a year.[31] And *that* procedure is universally funded by federal legislation.

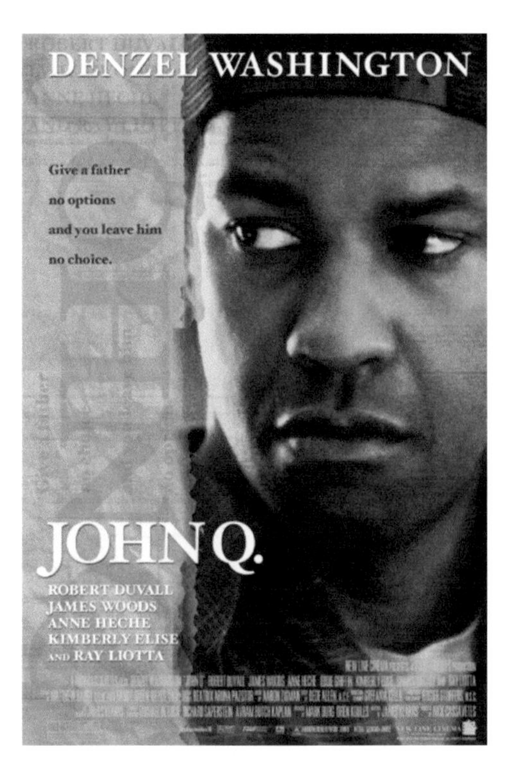

Figure 8.5
John Q. is the story of a father whose health insurance will not cover the desperately needed transplant procedure his son needs to survive.

More generally, for patients without health insurance, the likelihood of being accepted as a transplant candidate plummets. Think of the persons in Enders's starred purple and red counties (fig. 5.1), and those living in the poorest sections of Buffalo (fig. 6.6) or New York City (fig. 6.2). All would be accepted as organ donors, but many would not qualify as recipients because they lack health insurance or family resources. They would be … off the map. Figure 3.4 was an early attempt to calculate the effect of income and insurance on the transplantation patient pool, using the percentage of persons without health insurance as an indicator.

Ethnicity/Race

While UNOS is, in theory, color-blind, the Institute of Medicine, referenced earlier, acknowledged that "African Americans are less likely than white patients to be referred for [transplant] evaluation and are typically placed on waiting lists at a slower rate."[32] The reason, the report explained, was not race per se but "socioeconomic status" (SES). Poor persons who lack health insurance or the monies for private treatment are less likely to be listed as organ recipients. If those patients happen to be nonwhite, the result is simply an unintended consequence of economic realities. That assessment, however, ignores the inconvenient fact that "race is an antecedent and determinant of SES and racial differences in SES reflect, in part, the successful implementation of discriminatory policies" resulting in poverty.[33] We saw how this happens in the field of education in chapter 6.

Even where poverty is not an issue, persons of color are still less likely to be added to a transplant waiting list. In a stunning article in a national magazine, Vanessa Grubbs, an African American physician, reported that her partner's needed kidney transplant was delayed for years in a manner that made racial discrimination hard to dismiss.[34] Grubbs's partner was, like her, an African American professional with good health insurance, a solid income, no history of alcohol or drug abuse, and a strong social support network. He was carefully "compliant," taking all the medications he was prescribed. And yet he waited far longer than Caucasian patients in equal (or lesser) medical need. "Not once in my three years of training," wrote Dr. Grubbs, "did I hear a nephrologist [kidney specialist] talk about referring anyone from our mostly black [local] patient population for a kidney transplant."

For some, this was simply more proof of ongoing medical discrimination by white medical professionals treating African Americans. Here is the legacy of the Tuskegee syphilis project, in which poor blacks with syphilis were not treated with penicillin so that the study of disease effects could continue without interruption.[35] Here, too, is the story of Henrietta Lacks and her immortal HeLa cancer cells, recently retold by Rebecca Skloot.[36] Medicine has never been immune to patterns of general discrimination.

So it is perhaps not surprising that organ donation rates by African Americans were, throughout the 1990s, assumed to be lower than those of Caucasian citizens. To insist on a sense of altruism and beneficence in a context of historical racism and persistent socioeconomic bias is to ask a great deal. It is to presume communal solidarity for persons whose communal standing is limited. If persons believe themselves, their family, and their friends unlikely to receive organs, why should they donate? Would you?

When Dr. Grubbs and her partner asked about the delay in his organ receipt, they were told at least one reason was that African Americans organ donation rates are lower than those of Caucasian citizens. As a result, the likelihood of a precise organ match is similarly lessened. Nobody asked, apparently, if that was true.

Ethnicity and Race: Calculations

In 2014 the US Health and Human Services (HHS) website posted UNOS-collected data on the ethnicity/race of graft organ donors by regional organ procurement organization (OPO).[37] It also posted an ethnic/racial breakdown of graft organ recipients by transplant-performing hospital. Without patient addresses or at least postal codes, there was no way to know for sure where exactly patients came from: were they local residents or organ tourists from another city, state, or country? But the data did provide a means by which relative rates of organ donation and receipt by ethnicity/race could be calculated, if not, alas, accurately mapped.

Between 1988 and 2014, 75 percent of all heart transplant recipients were white. Of the remaining 25 percent, 15 percent were African American, 7 percent were Hispanic, and 2 percent were Asian American. The remaining 1 percent included foreign patients, Native Americans, or those whose ethnicity was unknown. Census figures for 2010 reported that approximately 72.4 percent of American citizens were white, 12.5 percent were African American, and 16.3 percent were Latino. Going solely by these figures, therefore, it would seem nationally that inequities, if any, most seriously affect the Latino community, whose members receive fewer than half as many transplants as one would expect based on a percentage of national population.

Those national figures are too coarse, however, to be definitive. What is the ratio of organs donated and transplants performed by ethnicity at finer scales with more precise resolution? I used the HHS data to create a new set of spreadsheets. The first included the total number of heart transplants performed since 1988 at each UNOS-listed hospital and the reported race of those donors. The second recorded the ethnicity of transplant recipients reported by the OPO collection agency in the catchment in which the hospital was located.

Buffalo, New York

Without better spatial data locating donors and recipients (their zip codes or home counties, e.g.), it was impossible to know the actual home city of an organ's donor or its recipient. Accurate mapping was therefore impossible. Instead I chose tables as the best medium to explore imbalances between organ donation and receipt by ethnicity/race. As a kind of proof of principle, and a way to check the thesis that persons of color are not donors, I calculated rates for three US cities.

I began with Buffalo, New York, where ethnicity and income were seen, in chapter 7, to influence quality of education and general health status among students. US

Table 8.2
Buffalo-area heart donors and recipients by ethnicity, 1988–2014

Buffalo	Total	% White	% Black	% Latino	% Asian	% Native
Population	261,310.00	50.40	38.60	10.50	3.20	1
Donations	277	82.67	13.60	2.89	0.36	0.07
Transplants	113	89	6	4	0	0

Looking at organ donations and heart transplants for Buffalo, New York, reveals a series of inconsistencies between rates of donation and heart transplantation by race.

Census Bureau web pages provided base information on the city's demographic profile.[38] Organ donations from 1988 to 2014 were reported through the Buffalo-based OPO, Upstate New York Transplant Services, whose catchment extends toward Cleveland in the west and Rochester, New York, to the east. Heart transplants were reported at three different Buffalo hospitals: Children's Hospital, Buffalo General Hospital, and the local VA hospital.

White citizens, who make up about half the population of metropolitan Buffalo, received 89 percent of all hearts transplanted between 1988 and 2014. African Americans, who make up 38 percent of the population, received just 6 percent. Latinos, who in 2012 made up almost 11 percent of the population, received 4 percent of all hearts transplanted at Buffalo's three heart-transplant-performing hospitals during the study years. These imbalances were not reflected in donation rates, however. African American organ donations were significantly greater than the percentage of transplants performed on members of those communities. Latino donations were lower than the relatively meager percentage of transplants performed on community members.

The percentages in table 8.2 do not precisely sum to zero. There are two reasons for this. First, some people report themselves as being of mixed heritage, and that category is not included in this table. Moreover, there are small groups—for example, Europeans or Pacific Islanders—whose members are not represented in this general summary but who were patients in area transplant hospitals. For the sake of clarity, those very small communities were ignored in this table.

New York and Los Angeles

Is Buffalo unique? Are the apparent imbalances between donation and transplantation by ethnicity/race a local anomaly? To consider that proposition, I generated donor and transplant profiles first for New York City (table 8.3) and then for Los Angeles

Table 8.3

New York–area heart donors and recipients by ethnicity, 1988–2014

New York County	Total	% White	% Black	% Latino	% Asian	% Pacific	% Native	% Mixed
Population	8.34 mil.	33.00	25.50	28.60	12.70	0.10	0.70	4.00
Donors	1,868	39.03	22.70	32.39	2.68	.00054	0.05	3.00
Transplants	3,112	62.08	17.71	14.46	4.72	0.10	0.06	0.87

This table uses US Census Bureau population data to anchor a comparison of donation and transplantation rates in the New York County area provided by UNOS reports, 1988–2014.

Table 8.4

Los Angeles heart donors and recipients by ethnicity, 1988–2014

Los Angeles	Total	% White	% Black	% Latino	% Asian	% Pacific	% Native	% Mixed
Population	9.82 mil.	27.79	9.60	47.74	13.50	0.27	0.19	0.26
Donations	4,279	52.61	7.92	35.38	2.99	0.23	0.40	0.30
Transplants	3,550	64.17	10.70	15.44	7.97	0.87	0.23	0.62

A third comparison of donation and transplantation rates, 1988–2014. Data for Los Angeles were taken from US Census Bureau and UNOS report data.

(table 8.4), both large, multiracial cities that are home to multiple transplant-performing hospitals and extremely active OPOs. In these tables, there were sufficient populations of Pacific Islanders ("Pacific"), primarily Hawaiians in Los Angeles, and First Nations communities ("Native") to warrant inclusion. In addition, the numbers of those reporting a mixed ethnicity were sufficiently large to include as well.

The startling statistic that the Caucasian population of New York City is under 35 percent of the metropolitan population of 8.34 million requires a word of explanation. US Census Bureau statisticians do not consider "Hispanic" or "Latino" a race but instead a cultural or at best ethnic classification. Thus persons who identify themselves "ethnically" as Latinos must also identify themselves with a race, most often "white." To clear up the confusion, the US Census Bureau statisticians created the category "white (not Hispanic or Latino)." The census data thus include two categories, "white" (44 percent of the New York population) and "white, not Hispanic or Latino" (about 33 percent of the population). Only by using the latter percentage did the ethnic profiles sum to 100 percent.

White (not Hispanic or Latino) New Yorkers donated 39 percent of all hearts transplanted since 1988 and received in return 62 percent of all hearts transplanted at New

York City hospitals. African American donations were significantly lower (22 percent of all donor hearts), but that figure well exceeded the percentage of heart transplants community members received (17.71 percent). Of the three major population divisions, Latinos were relatively generous, with 32.4 percent serving as active heart donors; but with the receipt of only 14.5 percent of hearts transplanted, Latinos far less well served than either African American or Caucasian neighbors.

The situation is even more imbalanced in Los Angeles. In table 8.4, US Census Bureau population data anchor a comparison of ethnic/racial donation and transplantation rates in the Los Angeles County area.[39] Again "white" as a census category represents 50.7 percent of the population but is severely reduced when "white (not Hispanic or Latino)" is used in its stead. And, again, only the lower figure permits the rest of the census profile to sum to near 100 percent. Even so, the numbers do not quite sum because of a small percentage of cases listed as ethnicity "unknown," likely reflecting nationalities not included in the questionnaire (Mongolian, Monrovian, Tibetan, etc.) or questionnaires not properly completed.

Unlike New York, where more transplants were performed than organs were received from donors, there was in Los Angeles a surplus of organs donated and presumably then dispatched to other transplant centers in Region 5. In Los Angeles, white Angelenos, representing 50 percent or less of the population (depending on the way "white" is categorized), received the majority of hearts, over 64 percent. Latinos, while representing more than 47 percent of the area population, received only 15.44 percent of the hearts transplanted during the study period. That was less than half the percentage of the organs they donated. In this case, white donations (52.6 percent) were lower than the percentage of organs received (64.2 percent), and African American Los Angelenos donated fewer organs (7.9 percent) than they received as a community (10.7 percent). Latino donations (35.4 percent of all donated hearts) were more than twice the percentage of transplants performed (15.4 percent).

If these cities are an example, then these tables at the least support the idea that ethnic and racial shortages of organs for persons of color are not simply the result of the communities' failure to donate. Moreover, these coarse comparisons insist that fundamental racial imbalances do indeed exist. Look again at figure 6.9, the Economic Innovation Group's map of distressed American cities. The most distressed are typically large cities with multiple organ transplant centers and significant percentages of nonwhite citizens. If the pattern holds in those places, then it certainly challenges the equity of the system and the self-confident insistence, quoted earlier, that "no part of the health care system has done more to resolve questions of justice than transplantation."

Does It Matter?

From the start, the US system of graft organ transplantation was based on two very different perspectives. The first was moral, advancing justice in an equitable system available to all citizens in need irrespective of a needy patient's ethnicity or finances. Ethically, altruism and beneficence were to be the motive force for donors, whose "gift of life" might be matched by a similar gift to them or their loved ones in need. The operative principle governing relations between donor and recipient groups was to be reciprocity among citizens, giving and getting as partners in a community and nation. The second was economic and thus focused on cost efficiencies, which financially, geographically, and socially distanced some Americans from the lifesaving care they needed. The first principle has long been trumpeted, but it is the second whose ethic has dominated.

Mortal and moral harm is done to those whose chances of receiving a graft organ are diminished or denied by dint of a combination of ethnicity, location, and poverty. As OPO members push aggressively for a donation when a loved one is injured, perhaps unto death, moral stress is suffered by the patient's families whose acquiescent participation is demanded. Should African American or Latino families ignore disparities for some greater good or deny donation because the likelihood of reciprocity is low? How must Dr. Grubbs and her partner have felt when told that his transplant was delayed time and again? How do we feel about a system so aggressively advertised and promoted that appears to fail in its legal promise of equality and justice?

UNOS officials might say their job is to collect and distribute graft organs as efficiently as possible. It may be that transplantation rates reflect inequalities built into the US system of health care and employment-based health insurance. It may be that socioeconomic disadvantage affects some groups more than others. None of that is the business of UNOS. If there is a problem, it is for Congress to fix. If the economics of race are an underlying issue in these disparities, UNOS cannot be held accountable. And if regionalization creates disparities, contemporary administrators might protest, those disparities exist in a system designed by experts decades ago. It's not their fault.

Similarly, the Institute of Medicine analysts of the 1990s might say they were not *asked* to look for economic, ethnic, or racial disparities in the UNOS data they were given to analyze. They were not told to consider patients who never made it to the transplant waiting list. The analysts did their job, which was not to unearth inequalities buried in a system that trumpets its moral virtues and ethical propriety. Had they been given that task, then perhaps their conclusions would have been different. They, too, did their job with the UNOS data they were given. The local hospital's shills for their transplant programs will point to the lives they have saved through transplants. If doing so requires an aggressive hand with the families of this or that patient, well, look at the good that results. It's ... their job.

Some might even say none of this really matters: Who cares if folks in less-populated states have to mortgage their farms and homes to travel to cities with transplant-performing hospitals? So what if the system is weighted toward the well-to-do and thus the white? The fine moral declarations enshrined in law are just ideals that in practice sometimes get lost. What is important, some might say, is that since 1988 UNOS has collected and distributed thousands of organs and has done so quite efficiently. Lives indeed have been saved as a result.

And really, if there were a problem, wouldn't bioethicists, the self-appointed guardians of medical ethics, be criticizing UNOS? Since 1988 scores of medical ethicists have engaged in an "at times almost scholastic" debate focused on the imbalance between organ donation and demand.[40] Some have argued for a market in organs with remuneration to donors, an idea that others (like me) have flatly rejected. Most have vocally criticized the organ tourism that takes the wealthy of one country (e.g., Israel) to another country whose poor become their organ providers (e.g., Turkey).[41]

Most bioethicists have been resolutely silent, however, on the American context in which the desperately ill may be required to travel at their own expense hundreds if not thousands of miles to enter transplant programs where the organs they eventually receive may come from donors who by dint of poverty (or race) had little hope of being recipients themselves. Bioethicists have similarly been generally silent on the possibility of systemic inequities and inequalities based on socioeconomic criteria, which, in turn, are heavily biased by ethnicity and race.

It is unlikely that the materials I present here will have much effect. The research is tentative and incomplete. Because publicly available data do not include donor or recipient home addresses, zip codes, or even counties, I can't say if the heart transplant recipient at Buffalo General Hospital is from Buffalo or Saudi Arabia. I can't say if the donor is from Buffalo, elsewhere in the OPO, or perhaps a surplus organ donor from ... Ontario. I can suggest strongly but not prove absolutely a consistent and precise correlation between ethnicity and income, on the one hand, and organ receipt, on the other. The data are suggestive but certainly not definitive. A series of tables comparing donation by race and transplant service in the most and then least distressed cities described in the EIG report (fig. 6.9) would be instructive, if still not definitive.

The clear harm is that we do not even ask about these things. We do not question the distance between the morals we espouse, the ethics that seek to implement them, and the inequities and imbalances these maps and tables appear to describe. Since

Secretary Shalala's Final Rule and the subsequent political firestorm it created, neither politicians nor researchers have been anxious to question the status quo. Until they do, we are left with that queasy feeling where everyone does his or her job while carefully ignoring the divide between, on one side, broadly shared moral definitions and their resulting ethical propositions and, on the other, their apparent failure in practice.

Clearly, the ethics of graft organ transplantation are enfolded in the greater issues of inequalities of income, education, and healthcare. *Of course* those differences are going to be reflected in transplantation rates. Education affects long-term income, which affects a person's health. Lack of education means less likelihood of anything but a precarious job, and that means a person is less likely, in the United States, to have comprehensive health insurance. None of this should be ignored, but in the ongoing discussion about graft organ supplies, it is almost never mentioned. The moral crime here is that UNOS officials and medical ethicists apparently accept a near-complete disconnect between morals and practice. They never argue our ideals as a rationale for changes in health care in the United States. Inequalities in organ transplantation thus become, in this reading, a symbol of a greater set of moral injuries and harms resulting from economic and social inequalities embedded in the practical realities of medicine and health care in the United States.

If we believe in equity and equality, in fairness and justice, then those must become the presuppositions against which we test the realities of our world. Should we ignore them and advance marketability or system efficiencies as our prime virtues, demoting fairness and justice as secondary concerns? That is one possibility, and one that seems to be the default choice. But in doing so, we abdicate any pretense of allegiance to the morality that we proclaim as governing the ethics of the programs we have created in a nation we insist is ethically robust and morally strong.

Imagine the effect if UNOS officials or Institute of Medicine analysts said, "Sure, there's a problem. But it is greater than our program." They then might of necessity become advocates for laws requiring insurers to pay the expenses of patients who need to travel to the urban centers where transplants are performed. They might insist that, for the law's moral posture to be fulfilled, the nation *must* make all transplantation, not just kidneys, a nationally funded trust. At the least, they could acknowledge and seek to correct the manner in which efficiencies of scale have trumped the declared virtues of equality, fairness, and justice.

Nor are any of us free of responsibility for the system as it exists or the changes that might be needed. We sign donor cards. We sanctimoniously promote our virtue by participating in the system as it exists today. News outlets annually lobby for readers and viewers to get with the program. Because the national graft organ system was legislated on the basis of a moral structure that we accept as defining (equality, justice, and fairness are American bywords we trumpet to the world), we could as citizens insist on reform *before* signing graft organ donor cards. At the least, we might acknowledge and protest the means by which some are denied and others are delayed in the provision of the "gift of life," whose promise is supposedly equality for all.

Or, like the statisticians who collect the data and the officials who administer the program, we can shrug and say that it's perhaps unfortunate but not our business. That is, we can do so until a friend or loved one urgently needs a graft organ whose receipt is delayed by ethnicity or denied on the basis of location, income, or simply "socio-economics." Until then, it's easier to ignore the moral promises we make and then in practice deny. Consequences be damned. Virtue ethics are something best left for the other guy.

III Moral Communities and Their Members

Members of a culture are members of a moral community who work to construct a shared reality and who act as though they were parties to an agreement to behave rationally within the terms of the realities they share.

—Richard Shweder, *True Ethnography*

9 The Ethics of Scale, the Scale of Distress

There is a scale to the ethics we propose as moral peoples, to the sense of responsibility we develop as persons. How could it be otherwise? We embrace, in theory, a set of moral definitions that define us as citizens whose governments craft laws based on them and then sign international covenants that promote their message. At least in theory, we believe in them not simply as citizens but as individuals because they seem to us, and others like us, honorable and right. An ethical perspective follows on those moral declarations that in theory are universal and thus everywhere applicable but in their actualization become particular.

"The existence of a hierarchy or system of rank," writes Princeton's Peter Singer, "is a near-universal human tendancy."[1] Our sense of obligation and the field of opportunities for ethical action based on moral definitions can be distinguished spatially, ranking close and far, familiar and foreign. Adam Haslett describes this as a spatial hierarchy by which we "attend to suffering and injustice. ... There are friends and family, whose suffering is ineluctable. There are people in the immediate communities, physical and virtual, that we live in whose troubles we see and talk about. And then there is the pain of distant others, people who live in places we've never been, news of whose suffering arrives through the media if it arrives at all."[2] And so with scale comes resolution, a degree of attention to the images we see in the world as we see it.

Philosophers call this practically preferential ethic the "morality of special relations," a sliding scale whose imperatives are greatest where the person is most intimately active, lessened as the degree of direct engagement diminishes.[3] Moral definitions don't change, but the imperative to their ethical enaction is more urgent the closer we are to home. Chris Kaposy addresses the issue in a different context: "For many of us, the most valuable aspects of our lives revolve around these relationships of intimacy—whether they derive from intense friendship, relationships with lovers, or from familial ties. Those who are not given this 'special relationship' status are owed [only] the baseline of ethical obligations that prevail among strangers."[4]

The closer we are geographically to those in need, the greater the familial and social ties that bind them to us, the more we are called on to help. And at the large scale of the personal, the more we are able to help. Our options for practical involvement decrease rapidly as we move from the local and personal to the national and then international. With distance, the seeming need to enact ethical engagement lessens. It is not that our moral presuppositions are spatially dependent but that our ability to act on them decreases with distance.

It's the ethical-moral equivalent of Waldo Tobler's First Law of Geography: "Everything is related to everything else, but near things are more related than distant things."[5] The result is a kind of distance decay affecting the urgency of our moral intuitions and the strength of their resulting ethical imperatives. The farther we are from home, the less clearly we see injustice or feel its force. We may feel a sense of pathos when a flood hits India, an earthquake decimates an area of Japan, or another hurricane ravages Haiti. Unless we are from India, or Japan, or Haiti, our response is minimal. We may note the human suffering that results from these disasters but will not see them as our problem or a call by us to supportive action. But when the flood happens in our city or the earthquake rocks our neighborhood or state, we are engaged immediately in our concern not only for ourselves but our neighbors.

When forced to confront the distance between thin principle and thickly complex realities at greater remove (for example, those starred counties on the Enders map), we may feel queasy, even a bit guilty. But that's as far as it goes when the object of our concern is ... away. Put another way, for most people, distress only becomes injury when it is personal.

Think back for a moment to figure 5.1 and its companions. We see the mapped poverty, but as middle-class (or better) US citizens, we do not easily equate it with our lives or world. The scale is too grand for association; the idea of nationhood and its responsibilities is too thin to spark active outrage and a concerted call for redress. Think back to the maps of New Orleans after Katrina. Like the NACIS members who presented at Map-Off, we prefer to see the city's flooding as a natural disaster rather than the result of years of inaction by governments we elected. Officials responsible for the state of the levees would say that they asked for monies to shore up the city's defenses but Congress refused their request in favor of other priorities. If you want to blame somebody, blame them. Congressional legislators might say they were elected on a platform of lower taxes and good business—and that, not a possible hurricane, was their mandate. But us? Well, not really our fault, and thus not our responsibility.

The Amahl, or Satya

This is why charities that seek financial contributions for the welfare of children in impoverished countries do so not with a global map of poverty, or one of global income inequality (figs. 5.8–5.9), but with an endless succession of sad-eyed children, their bellies distended, standing in front of dismal thatched huts with earthen floors. A voice gives the child's name (call him Amahl, or her Satya) and details his (or her) pitiful destitution. You can save Amahl, we are told—or others like him (or her)—for just pennies a day, a few dollars a week. Just a few hundred dollars a year. Help him (or her), and "your" child (who is illiterate and does not speak English) will write back! The relationship will be reciprocal, and the child not a stranger but an acquaintance, a person linked to you. The obligation to care will be based not on distantly thin moral definitions of human allegiance and solidarity, or on simple pity, but instead on an interpersonal relationship whose ethical obligations are as clear as they would be if Amahl or Satya lived next door. The realities of global inequality and poverty are thus scaled back to a personal point: Amahl, Satya, and you or me.

Signing up, you won't be signing up for the salvation of Amahl or Satya, of course. They are totems, symbols of the need of children across the dark-red regions of the maps of world poverty, the reddish sections of the map of inequality. Your child will be someone else, one of the many otherwise nameless children living in villages so small you'll never find them on any but the most local of maps. And so as the advertisements seek to personalize poverty in a way that requires we seek its reduction it simultaneously objectifies its young subjects who in the end are merely fungible, examples of a class of needy who are all nameless.

The advertisements seek to invoke and thus focus in the child a moral definition of human solidarity whose result is an injunction to care. A sense of ethical propriety, of moral righteousness, is what they're selling. If you don't contribute, then you feel guilty or at least queasy because you've abandoned human beneficence and solidarity, suppositions that you thought you held. The ideas and ideals that power these advertisements are lodged in the United Nations' charter and subsequent covenants our nations have signed which seem to promise to all a minimum of care, food, health, housing, and maybe education.[6] The advertisements invoke that ethic as a practical, personal proposition: If we are persons with a moral compass, then we will *want* to help, if only to confirm our own humanity (which is to say our status as moral persons). And if we want to help, who better to help than this needy child? If our nation can't do something, then, well, we individuals will.

This transposition of broad moral ideal to practical human context is what at another scale made Agee and Evans's writing about southern sharecroppers so powerful; Edward R. Murrow's "Harvest of Shame" so, well, shameful; and the work of Jonathan Kozol documenting the lives of poor inner-city schoolchildren in the United States so damning. The psychiatrist Robert Coles chose to argue the general from the perspective of the particular in his Pulitzer Prize–winning five-volume *Children of Crisis* (2003).[7] In the same vein, think of Andrea Elliott's and Ruth Fremson's "Invisible Child," which describes the life of Dasani, one of twenty-two thousand homeless children existing in New York City shelters.[8] This isn't the far side of the world but our own backyard.

But those descriptions of individual life are so particular that they are not easily generalized as a mandate to care. What do I in Canada care about the homeless children of New York City (or Austin, Texas)? I care a bit as a human being, but it's not my nation, city, or neighborhood. And even if it were, the idea of what are in effect third-world children living in first-world countries challenges us in ways most do not want to consider.

That is why television charities do not invoke the need of an Amahl in Harlem, a Satya in rural Mississippi, a Michelle-Jean in Buffalo, New York—or any of the more than 2.8 million American children living in households with incomes in 2012 of less than $2 a day.[9] To do so would be to challenge our sense of the nation as able, prosperous, and moral in its treatment of all its citizens. It would insist on an ethics of local and national action and redistribution, or at the least a consideration of the distance existing between the nation's moral ideals and its realities that we prefer to ignore. A Charity for America (not for Africa or the Sudan) would invoke an ethical judgment obliging us to demand programs at once costly in tax money and, perhaps more importantly, in their damage to our self-esteem. To focus on the nation's ongoing failure to embrace the morals we trumpet to others, the ethics we espouse to the world, would indict our own failure as citizens to insist on that long-promised more perfect union.

Most of us *do* care more about our immediate neighbors than about those who live on the far side of the nation or the world. The exception is those who are from those places, the new and first-generation citizens for whom the far side of the world was home. Still, for most, the spatial drop-off is steep. In western New York State, the high school dropout rate in Buffalo's poorest schools was … news. But the families of suburbanites in Amherst, Kenmore, and Williamsville outside Buffalo safely ignored the structural inequalities that are its root cause (fig. 6.7). They could tisk and stay gratefully uninvolved, ignoring the long-term effect of high school dropout rates and disaffected youths in their region. And, too, they could ignore the imbalances and inequalities that encourage white flight to the suburbs and penury in the inner cities of New York State and the nation.

When the gulf between our moral posture and ethical programs is pointed out, most of us become defensive and a bit ... queasy. This isn't the "avoidance problem" presented by Nancy Berlinger (described in chap. 1), in which a problem is simply ignored. Instead the source of the problem is scapegoated. If one forgets the reasons for those school failures—systemic poverty and funding formulas that ensure inequalities of education service—then one's responsibility for them diminishes in a defensive moment. Blame the parents who don't supervise their kids, who then drop out of school; blame the teachers charged with their failed education, or the reluctance of the kids themselves to learn. And, sure, suburban schools are better, but isn't that why people with children move to the suburbs? Too bad, Buffalo, or Rochester, or any large city with the same problem. We look after our own first. You inner-city folks should do the same.

In mapping the problem and not the context, the test results and not their rationale, we invite this type of response.

Global Scales

Consider *The State of the World Atlas* (fig. 9.1), now in its ninth edition.[10] First published in 1981—and quickly followed by its companion, *The War Atlas* (updated edition in 1991)[11]—*The State of the World Atlas* deploys a range of cartographic techniques to present a mass of data arguing that the state of the world is inequitable, unequal, violent, in trouble. Map after map posts key indicators and vital statistics of global life, its dangers, and its many inequalities.

One map presents nations like the United States that are major exporters of the weapons used in the active wars of the day. A map of the wars where the munitions are used ... that's on another page. There is a map of national military expenditures and, a few pages away, another detailing the inverse relation between military expenditures and monies spent on education and health. Flip forward to a map of life expectancy, and not surprisingly, it is lower in countries where poverty is a constant and war is simply business as usual.

The politics of the *Atlas* are antinuclear, antiwar, antipoverty, pro-equality, and aggressively humanist. It *invites* indignation, implicitly demanding that nations pretending to an ethics of moral responsibility to change policies, change rules, change the *maps*. It thus encourages, at least in theory, readers who live in the wealthy nations to lobby as citizens of those nations for a different and more equitable world.

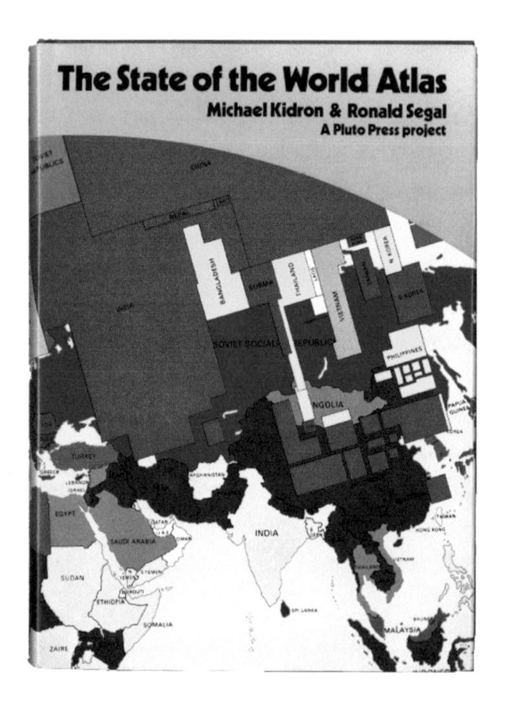

Figure 9.1
The State of the World Atlas has been, since its first printing, a persuasive mapped indictment of global inequalities. Penguin Books.

In more than thirty years and across nine editions, the *Atlas* has not provoked an international movement to disarmament, income equality among nations, or an international fight against poverty. At best, its maps confirm a liberal reader's view of the world as a dismal, sorry place (more than 700,000 copies of the *Atlas* have sold to date). We feel queasy in the face of the reality the *Atlas* presents, but we see no way to influence its arguments. The result for most readers is less a call to action than a sense of exhausted resignation, of general moral decay.

I may express solidarity with humanity everywhere, but in 2016 the world population was around 7.46 billion persons and expanding by 1.07 percent annually. It is impossible to conceive of that number of persons and even more impossible to think about having a personal responsibility to them all. The world is too vast and complex a place for most people to feel a personal presence and thus to sense an individual responsibility for its current state until and unless—as it did with the Ebola epidemic of 2013 to 2015—something from afar seems to threaten their own cities and homes.[12]

Look again at figures 5.8 and 5.9. Most people are drawn first to their own country—for me it is Canada—and then to one's native region (again, for me, North America). The eye then travels to other countries one knows, where one has lived, perhaps. I always look next at Ecuador and Guatemala, countries where I worked on health-care projects in my youth. Then the eye follows a general survey of the map's surface, the color ramp of its presentation, in which one sees the dark reds and bright oranges of poverty on continents whose countries we often do not know (Where *is* Chad?).

Unless one is contemplating moving to Bolivia or Haiti (an island almost too small to be seen at this worldly scale), the dismal realities lodged there, in the map, will be perceived as perhaps lamentable but personally inconsequential. Even if one knows where Chad or Haiti is located, their individuality is lost in the coloration. They are just one more small, red-colored polygon in an event class of mass poverty too vast to be internalized without going mad. And in the end, what do the realities of the poorest countries in the map have to do with me, in Canada? Well, look: We are pretty fine, thank you. The global scale smooths into invisibility our pockets of extreme poverty among rural First Nations, the local sites of want that exist in each and every Canadian city.

There are exceptions, of course. The death of more than 1,100 Bangladeshi workers in a 2013 factory collapse "turned a lens on poor conditions endured by workers and brought fresh focus to production practices used to create affordable goods."[13] Canadians were shocked to learn that Bangladeshi sweatshops with abysmal work conditions and low pay rates produced a popular Canadian clothing brand. Promises were made by the manufacturer to increase oversight of their offshore factories.

Sales did not suffer for long, however. Things soon returned to normal. In 2016 conditions in most factories still included forced overtime, unreasonable production targets, and unsanitary (and in some cases unsafe) work conditions.[14] Attempts by workers to organize into unions were met with ferocious resistance. Canadian consumers, however, were again mostly unconcerned. Progress, we were told, had been made. Things take time. Situations like this are complex. And after all, we were told, what seems to us to be a pittance of a wage might seem to a Bangladeshi munificent and life sustaining. In buying Bangladeshi clothes, we are actually supporting those workers and that nation's economy! That's the glory of global trade.

National Maps

Our sense of involvement and thus responsibility comes into only slightly sharper focus at the scale of the mapped nation. Here the injunctions are clearer, even if the sense of solidarity is no less liable to distance decay. I was born in the United States and have visited thirty-one of its fifty states. As a voter (I am both a Canadian and a US citizen), I have some say, albeit minor, in the nation's policies and thus some responsibility (at least as a virtue ethicist) for urging it toward ethical programs reflecting moral definitions that the nation in theory embraces and should thus promote. At the scale of the nation, I may lament but am not personally engaged with the poor of Mississippi, a state I only once briefly visited, or Tennessee, where I have never been. While I endorse, in a general way, the idea of a "war on poverty," its necessity remains an abstraction imaged in the maps and leavened by tales of want so local and specific as to be, for me, irrelevant. Higher taxes? Please, no.

In Canada it's much the same. I may lament the sorry health state of impoverished northern communities and endorse, in a general way, government plans for their improvement. But it's a long way from Toronto to a First Nation Cree community at the mouth of the Attawapiskat River on James Bay. I have read about their dire need, and I hope, in a general way, that things will improve, but it's hard to rally a sense of personal engagement. The average urbanite can muster at most a bit of queasiness, a sense of inchoate moral stress. We're Canadians, after all, and so are they. Somehow we should do better.

Resolution

Just as a world map obscures the variances existing in a country's map, so a state map smooths the often intense variations existing at the finer county resolution. Figure 9.2 shows a 2014 map imaging levels of SAIPE-calculated poverty in 2012 in the fifty states. The first panel (upper left) presents poverty as a general feature of state populations. Beside it is another map with a different color scheme that presents the SAIPE-calculated poverty of young people under eighteen years of age. Below these maps are others that present the same poverty among those aged five to seventeen, and finally, in the lower right, for children under five. Because most young children live with their families, one would expect their poverty to reflect that of the general state population. After all, few children are significant wage earners. And so in looking at the maps, we see commonalities more than differences.

Across the four map panels, the darker states, which are the poorest, are generally in the Southeast—Georgia, Louisiana, Mississippi, South Carolina, and Tennessee—and Southwest (Arizona and New Mexico). The richer states are in New England and the Midwest. A closer inspection shows that, map to map, there are shifts of one level of poverty on the color ramp, up or down, depending on the particular map's

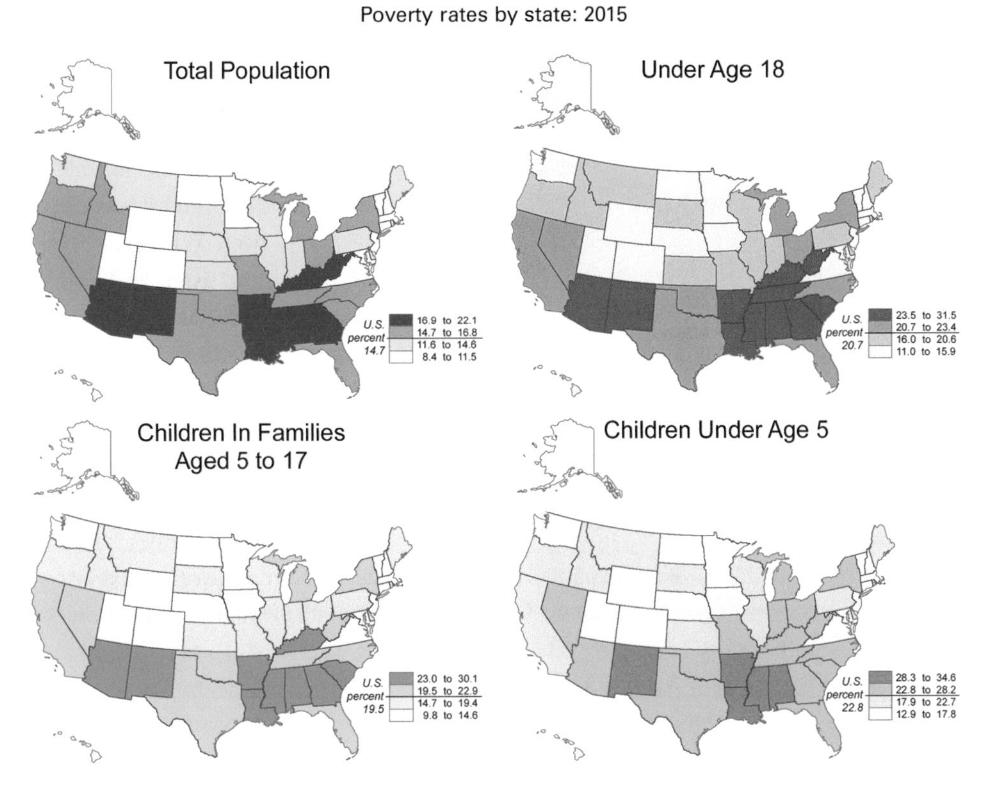

Figure 9.2

These US Census Bureau maps of SAIPE-defined state poverty compare poverty as a general population characteristic and its effect on underage children.

demographic focus. We see this in California, Idaho, Montana, Nevada, and Oregon. We do not know what causes these shifts, or what they mean, but the changes are not so visually radical that we who live elsewhere are likely to see them as critical testimonies that ethically require national policy initiatives.

In the four-panel page, we have a broad statement that childhood poverty is epidemic across the plane of US states, although uneven in its prevalence. Moreover, map to map, the poverty is worst among the youngest of citizens. But as we look at the maps, our eye is drawn first to the states colored so lightly they seem empty. What's the real scoop here? Are things really so good that you can color poverty in those states as … blank?

Look again, and a bit more closely, at this official, automatically generated map set. The earlier, SAIPE-generated maps of county-level poverty used as many as six divisions in their color ramping. The computerized map program at the state level on the SAIPE website employed four mapped divisions. County data on poverty (remember the Enders map [fig. 5.1]?) are smoothed at the state level. The quartile division smooths data again. A five- or six-division choropleth color ramp would emphasize differences that the map in figure 9.2 ignores or at least reduces. The result says poverty isn't so bad, not really. And where it is, well, the colors are somehow calming, a dark woodland green or a pale blue.

Consider the details in the legends of these 2014 maps based on 2012 SAIPE data. The dividing line between "have" (light color) and "have-not" (darker color) state populations has risen, in the upper-left map (total population), from 13.2 percent of all Americans in poverty (figs. 5.2–5.3) in 2008 to 15.9 percent of young people under eighteen. In the map beside it (under eighteen), the divisor increases to 22.6 percent. In the lower maps, left and right, the bar distinguishing have and have-not states rises yet again to 21.1 percent (children in families) and 25.6 percent (children under five) respectively.

For US citizens these are *our* Amahls, *our* Satyas. The number increases as the age of the children decreases to one in every four children under five years of age. And yet that abysmal conclusion is hidden, albeit in plain sight. The very solidity of the maps on the page, the blocks of states in their comforting familiarity, lulls us into acceptance.

Look again at the earlier maps of SAIPE-calculated poverty in US counties, and also at the starred orange and red counties in the Enders map (fig. 5.1). In those maps, poverty is real, persistent, and in some counties extreme. But the maps are so chaotic there is nothing to anchor the message; we see so many counties, it is hard to locate one's home and harder to see how, across a landscape so varied, anything could be done. Moreover, we have little idea what the maps mean for those living in red, and especially starred red, counties. Are the American Amahls and Satyas without food or clothing? Are they without healthcare? What about education? What do we *do* with the map and its data? Should we really get involved; should we care?

It's Not in the Map

None of this is just about maps or the means by which they are produced. Maps are just exhibits, ideas presented in two dimensions, and to think that this is about mapping is to ignore a map's real message. Nor is this about statistics as a methodology whose divisions transform rows of columned data into a graphically presentable numeric conclusion. The problem is not the algorithms used to generate the computer-generated SAIPE maps or the statistics of poverty on which they are based. The computer-generated map of child poverty is accurate, saying what it was created to say about poverty in youth in America. The statistics are firm and verified to high levels of statistical confidence. One can quibble with the automatically generated color ramps critique the number of divisions in the maps categorization. One can ask, with Enders (fig. 5.1), for a symbol that shows the areas of most-enduring long-term poverty in children. But those are the edges of the problem, not its heart.

The maps exemplify the manner in which the ethical supply chain is interrupted, the means by which a narrow focus and a general perspective permit us to feel at worst a bit queasy about our practical ethical disengagements. Just a tad of moral distress, perhaps.

The scale promises a context, geographic and political; the resolution determines the specificity of the material presented. But somewhere along the line, the rationale behind the collection of the data is lost. The stated *purpose* was to identify areas of the nation where citizens need but do not receive assistance so that with the nation's help they and theirs will have an equal chance in life. Data on impoverished children, our Amahls and Satyas, are collected to identify those who need but are not getting an equal chance to thrive, an equal opportunity to become the best citizens possible, the democratic participants we need. As we saw in chapter 5, that is *why* federal officials collect poverty-related data. The moral ideals of equality of opportunity and freedom are the motivating rationale behind the moral imperative to identify the needy so that we can then collectively help them. That moral call for ethical actions to ensure moral goals gets lost in the telling.

In the same vein, data on global income inequality or outright poverty ($1 a day is the measure) are perfectly presented in maps. The statistics of the Gini index, or any other index of inequality, are ably constructed. They are supposed to awaken us to humanitarian concerns, to the dreadful existence endured by others like us who live in a different place. But they don't, at least not often, and then not without damning text describing the short, dreary lives of those in the beleaguered regions of the map. Why?

One reason, I think, is that in mapping numbers, we are still seduced by the idea of their objective truth. That's just the way it is, as the demographer in Regina would say: numbers are just facts, and as such we can blissfully ignore the context of structural poverty that makes those numbers real. We lose the greater meaning when we retire to the safety of the broad numbers set alone, the objective fact without a context that gives depth and meaning to the abysmal portrait of millions of impoverished children whose futures are endangered. If numbers are just numbers, then consequentialists can rest easy. There is nothing truly consequential until those numbers are correlated with ill health, a lack of education, and social dysfunction.

The ethical injunction to aid and care is not wholly lost in the specificity of the numbers posted in this or that chart, map, or table. We know we *should* feel something. We know that poverty is more than a statistical conclusion based on census data collected and manipulated by statisticians. It has a human face, and in glimpsing it in the reports of writers who focus on the particular, we know that somehow our moral suppositions are violated, our ethical goals unmet. We know as well that structural poverty is costly economically, politically, and socially. Billions are lost in taxes not paid by the unemployed; billions more on the health of those who have no money to pay for insurance or health care. And, too, we know that a disenfranchised, semiliterate, unemployed population is unlikely to participate in the issues of the day, the participatory democracy we purport to value. So, like readers of *The State of the World Atlas*, we are left with a kind of moral exhaustion when confronting ethics we feel but can't quite see and do not know how to enact.

Professional Ethics

As professionals, we are trained to ignore our individual ethical sensibilities. We are trained as well to ignore the broader context. A focused research grant's subject does not invite a broader critique. An assignment to identify relative poverty in the United States (or Canada, or the United Kingdom, and so on) is not a brief to indict inequitable national tax structures that ensure poverty will be as constant a landscape element as mountains, lakes, and rivers. Like the cartographers at Map-Off or the fictional reporter in Raleigh, North Carolina, our task is specific, and if we don't like it, well, like the *Challenger* engineer Bob Ebeling, we just can find another job.

And so our ethics are in liege to those of our employer of the moment. Did Institute of Medicine researchers *ask* about individuals who never made it to the transplant list? Did they question the criteria by which some organ recipients may reflexively be disallowed because they can't afford postoperative care? Did they demand a clear breakdown of ethnic or racial divides at the level of local organ procurement organizations? To have done so would have raised fundamental questions that their employers (and certainly UNOS) did not ask them to address. As "professionals," the researchers were constrained even if, as people, they might have questioned the entire enterprise.

"As educators, but also as inhabitants of the world," wrote the geographer Jim Tyner in 2009, "we have a responsibility to act. ... To know that poverty exists, to know that infants and children are dying from malnutrition and inadequate health care and to do nothing ... is to participate in and perpetuate a culture of impunity."[15] Tyner argues a kind of ethical two-step. He takes as given that the ethics of the professional instructor are related to his or her being in the world and responsibility to it. He enjoins geographers and cartographers to teach these realities as a means to expose, if not personally combat, a "culture of impunity." The cartographers, geographers, and statisticians thus trained are enjoined to promote accurate public information as a way to identify the social ills their expertise enables them to document. Think of it as a fugue played on three keyboards: the first is professional (the cartographer and geographer); the second is expressive and instructive (the teacher); and the third, a muted-pedal addition, invokes the responsible citizen embedded in a culture and world of potentially reversible moral improprieties.

In the end, however, Tyner's clarion call rings hollow. Teaching is a good thing, but it's usually a safe thing. It puts the onus on the student to act in a way the teacher him- or herself need not. Moral indignation is the order of the day, a way to bleat at inequity without personally engaging its core realities in a substantial manner. The base notes of personal citizen engagement are largely absent in Tyner's call to ethics. As teachers, they do not need to organize student food drives or work in the homeless shelters of their cities. They need not tithe to charities. Their careers need not focus on the many ways we might combat economic and social inequalities in our neighborhoods, cities, provinces, or nation.

There are exceptions, of course, but most professional lecturers and researcher (and journalists) remain safely disengaged. If they did anything else, they would be activists and not lecturers or writers who in theory are supposed to be as objective as Peter Singer's universal observer. Here one may observe an inverse of Tobler's law at play: in general, the more distant the inequity, the more academics and other so-called experts trumpet their distress, calling for radical change.

North American bioethicists are outraged by the transplant tourism of Israelis seeking organs from poor countries in the Middle East, as well as by China's program of organ harvesting from criminals (many of those organs ending up in foreign transplant tourists). But to talk about organ transplantation inequities in the United States, to see the resegregation and ghettoization of the poor in inner-city Buffalo, Chicago, or New York ... no way. At least, not in a manner that would require them to actively involve themselves in seeking solutions.

In the same vein, federal statisticians calculating SAIPE poverty are enjoined to keep a professional distance from the realities their work implies. As citizens, they might feel a tad queasy about the data, but once the numbers are collected and computed, they need do no more as citizens or as moral persons. Certainly they are not called on to be activists. Perhaps one of the federal statisticians made a donation to a charity after his or her work was complete. But to take the maps as a clarion call would be to step beyond the professional role into one that is personal. "You want to do something," a supervisor would say, "run for office. Here we just do our jobs." Consequentially, ethics and their attendant morals end precisely there. Professionalism becomes in this way a retreat to the amoral, to personal disengagement.

Think Local, Act Global

The current cant enjoins us all to "think global, act local." But the global is exhausting, and its relation to the local unclear. It thus becomes a recipe for inaction or, rather, for actions that are largely symbolic, like driving the family SUV to the annual Earth Day celebration. "Think global" permits us to be vocal in our indignation at the inequities that exist in distant places while remaining largely agnostic about those in own neighborhoods, cities, and nations. Remember the redlined neighborhoods of the 1930s federal maps.

To "think local," on the other hand, to see at home what one may condemn abroad, is to require action by those who wish to see themselves as ethically engaged, moral citizens. To see in one's immediate environment a reflection of the world at large insists on addressing local consequences in a way that is more personal and perhaps immediate. Few people perceive the world in this way, however. And to be fair, it requires a perspective that professionals are trained to resist from their undergraduate years (it's about the data) to their own later careers ("Here's what I want from you").

Habits of the Heart

It is rare these days to find a moral philosopher or a practical ethicist talking about the nature of citizenship or the responsibility of citizens; the link between the person and the ideals of his or her community and nation. The very idea that as a people we might proclaim a moral platform whose suppositions are the basis of our ethical postures is eccentric if not radical. And yet it is in the distance between those morals and the ethical stance they promote that moral stress and distress exist for many. This is the perhaps inevitable conclusion of what Alexis de Tocqueville called the "habits of the heart" resulting from a moral perspective that leaves "the individual suspended in glorious, but terrifying isolation."[16] Published in two volumes (the first in 1835 and the second in 1840), Tocqueville's *Democracy in America* (*De La Démocratie en Amérique*) reported on the nature of the then-young American body politic. There he found the idea of freedom increasingly equated with individualism, "a calm and considered feeling which disposes each citizen to isolate himself from the mass of his fellows and withdraw into the circle of family and friends." As a result, the sense of responsible community and reciprocal solidarity was lost, except perhaps within a family and a small circle of friends. Thrown back on the local and individual, each person is thus locked "in the solitude of his own heart."[17]

Tocqueville perceived a conflicting set of moral suppositions at the heart of the American ethic. On the one hand was a belief that "each man learns to think and act on his own, not counting on the support of an outside power."[18] In this ethic of individualism, wealth, not moral rectitude or social service, became the defining standard by which worthiness was measured. At the same time, however, "The political dogma of this country is that the majority is always right." And so individuals beholden to no one were free only to the extent that the majority of their fellows gave permission to their beliefs and their practice.

The inevitable result was a "unity of disunity" that is not, as others have suggested,[19] the result of modernity but instead a thing deeply embedded in the American consciousness. The disconnect becomes dysfunctional because we are *not* alone, locked in our own solitudes; we are members of interlocking sets of communities, each active at varying scales and resolutions stretching from the home and its neighborhood to the city, state, and then the nation and world. American individualism thrived in its earliest incarnation *because* of a sense of active reciprocity, of solidarity (and thus equality) among peoples in its mostly rural, isolated villages and towns.

"Nothing struck me more forcibly," wrote Tocqueville, "than the general equality of condition among [those] peoples." That equality permitted individuals to act on an equal basis with neighbors in their shared community. It was, for Tocqueville, America's most defining characteristic. It is that prerequisite equality in the midst of constant interpersonal exchange that is challenged, map by map, statistic by statistic, across this book. We fail to the extent it is denied at the varying scales we promote as requiring our allegiance.

If equality and freedom are moral imperatives, their range must be actively local. From there it extends naturally and necessarily to the interlocking realities of governance and trade. Economies are linked, local to regional to national to global. Local factories serve national interests active in global economies in the kind of transnational mercantilism (today we call it globalism) that Adam Smith railed against in *The Wealth of Nations*.[20]

We have the ethical propositions that follow on a set of agreed-on moral suppositions. The form is clear: if we believe x is good, then we should, if we are ethical, do y. Conflicts are inevitable, and Hegel's tragic hero embodies the moral distress of us all, a fact of modern daily life. Sometimes it is extreme, sometimes a persistent, chronic discomfort, but it is always there, poised at the edge of the heart and mind. It is always there, its traces calling from the edges of the map.

10 It's ... Complex

In *Gorgias*, Socrates takes on the master rhetorician who boasts of his ability to convince others of whatever point of view he may be employed to promote irrespective of its effect or its merits.[1] For Plato, the result is mere trickery, a technique but not a *technê* whose goal is (or should be) real and thus actionable, shared knowledge about the world and our place in it. The rhetorician, while not mendacious, is nonetheless dangerous to the common weal because, as Plato puts it, "Nothing is worse for a human being than false belief," and by his own admission, Gorgias is as happy arguing logical but ultimately insupportable falsities as he would be those that are deeply held, firmly supported, and socially beneficial. The result, Plato concludes, perverts justice and damages the community at large through the promotion of half-truths that are ultimately false truths.

Plato thus bequeathed to Western thought a clear distinction between hard-won insight and mere stratagems of persuasion that masquerade as knowledge. Taken as a whole, the dialogues present a carefully planned argument for a kind of knowing in service of a kind of being in the world with others. From Plato comes the moral definition of truth as something greater than the individual argument. It is instead a presupposition, to return to the language introduced in chapter 1, that by his definition first serves the community at large rather than an individual or single group. It is not that the rhetorician lies but that he does not tell a truth whose ultimate aim is social. The charge against Gorgias is not sophistry but, worse, bad citizenry where an informed citizenry is a moral good for which we all should strive.

A second lesson of the dialogue is that truths are neither immutable nor self-evident but manufactured. Moreover, they have social consequences as we attempt to act ethically and honorably on their basis. Plato created, in effect, a consequential standard for the evaluation of arguments based not simply on (he said, she said) facticity but on their effect on society. When truths seem to conflict, when suppositions differ, then they must be evaluated by a communal, rather than an imperial (Singer's

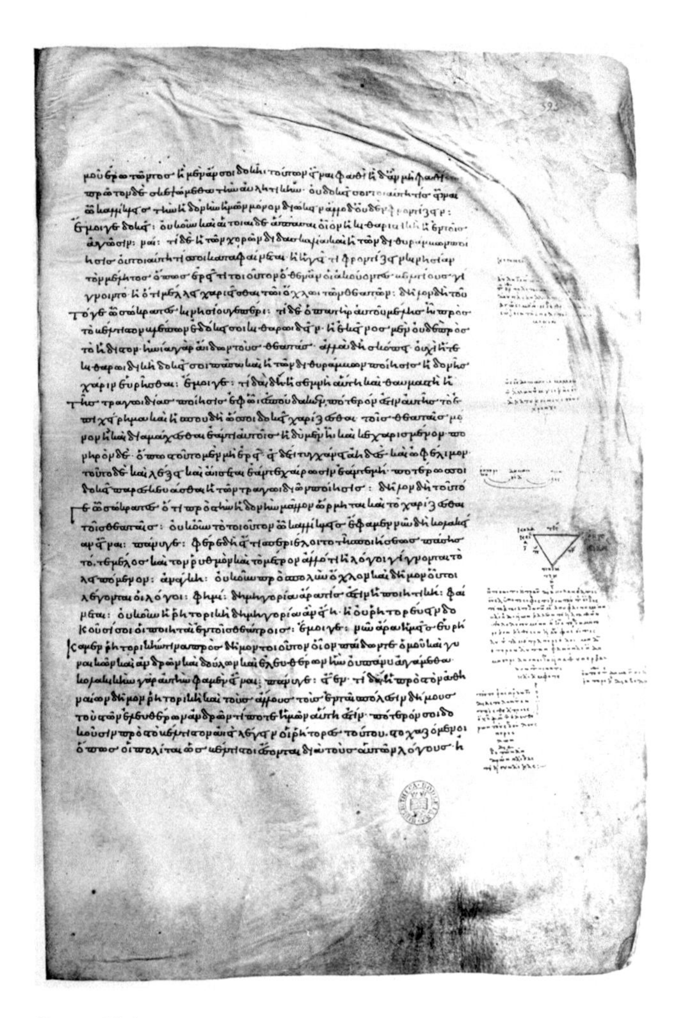

Figure 10.1
A page from a version of *Gorgias* produced in AD 895. Wikipedia.

objective observer) or idiosyncratic ("It's true because I say it is"), yardstick. There is nothing virtuous about the rhetorician; the real virtue is society's indulgence of his trade.

Mapping and statistics are techniques that, like the rhetorician's persuasive speech, can be used to advance almost any argument, any proposition. Daily journalists similarly have no fixed subject; few have a specific expertise beyond the ability to present in relatively clear language another person's point of view. It's been that way for a long time, and the rationale is that reporters who are not experts may more faithfully broadcast another's argument *because* they are not particularly informed. They are thus assumed to report without preconception or personal bias. Whether the reported statement is ethical or merely rhetorical is the speaker's responsibility, not the reporter's.[2]

Like the rhetorician, reporters are a persuasive lot whose task in theory is to promote only the smallest of truths (he said, she said). But there are a thousand ways in which any single story can be shaped. Young reporters learn them quickly (I certainly did) and learn, too, how to be persuasive. There is nothing wrong with that. Plato's dialogues were themselves masterpieces of rhetorical construction. But in them he advances as a moral bedrock "human thriving," and thus a socially grounded orientation, as the difference between his arguments and the self-promoting posture of those like Gorgias whose pride is grounded in ethical and moral vacuity. For today's journalists, that perspective is, if not foreign, then rarely argued and more rarely advanced.

In the last of his dialogues, *The Laws*, Plato insisted that disconnected information is meaningless when severed from a setting in which people work together to achieve broadly desired social ends. The problem with the literature reviewed in chapter 2 was that most writers tried and failed to find a distinct morality and subsequent ethic unique to cartography, geography, graphic arts, journalism, or statistics. The authors assumed their own uniqueness, their own solitudes, taking Peter Singer's objective world of disconnected, disinterested realities as real.

But as the examples of the past chapters demonstrate, any attempt to build an ethic in which independent, Olympian objectivity is the measure of success inevitably fails. "The truth of any statement, scientific or otherwise, which ultimately must rely on some anchoring, in order to avoid being completely arbitrary, is undecidable."[3] Data can't serve as the sole anchor of our ethical judgments, a thing outside us, because data are not independent. Data do not speak. Their voice is not real but apparent, like that of a ventriloquist's dummy. From the idea that sparks data's collection to the approved methodologies that guide their organization, data are an artifact of our ideas, the propellant of the propositions we seek to enact. Data do not speak through us; we speak through them. In charting, graphing, mapping, and writing, we define and refine a dataset's selective message. And so not simply as authors, cartographers, demographers, geographers, reporters, and statisticians, but more importantly as citizens, we are faced with a choice. We can be like Gorgias, arguing or at least analyzing whatever we are told to support or analyze. Or, like Plato, we can begin from the perspective of the shared moral good, one we then seek to define, refine, and defend as citizens through our work.

Rawlsian Geometry

"We should strive for a kind of moral geometry with all the rigor which this term connotes," John Rawls wrote in his *Theory of Justice*.[4] That geometry is inherent in the structure of the map is why maps serve so well as an evidentiary medium in this discourse. "They link the territory to what comes with it—which is to say all of the desires, needs, and aspirations humans bring to them."[5] It is those aspirations—ethical, moral, practical, professional, and scientific—that they express.

The Rawlsian geometry of a map's moral underpinning is based on the mapmaker's own beliefs and perspectives, his or her ethical propositions; his or her presuppositions dictate the result. Across a two-dimensional plane, maps reveal the results of our ethical choices in a landscape we understand as our own. Seen in this way, the map is the practical end point of an ethical supply chain that begins with a set of shared moral definitions and resulting injunctions that underlie propositions enacted in the construction of the mapped landscape. That underpinning expands from the map itself to the news stories that employ it or the journal articles that use it, not simply illustratively but substantially. But when that moral basis is that of the employer or speaker, not the mapmaker, he or she is often faced with an ethical disconnect. The work is his or hers, but its bias is not. Ethical and sometimes moral distress is the inevitable result.

This is not just about the map, or mapping. Maps serve here primarily as a medium for the exploration of the ethics and moralities that we embed in their construction. Charts and tables are others, as those used in previous chapters demonstrate. Nor does it matter overmuch if the maps, tables, or charts are being used by demographers, journalists, researchers, or statisticians. It is simply that in the mapping one can see more easily, and more dramatically, the limits of the methodologies by which we fashion ethical arguments and moral definitions.

For the deontologist, rules are preeminent. Those rules are designed to ensure a kind of social performance whose goals presumably reflect a particular moral perspective. When the result seems unethical or, worse, immoral, our role becomes that of a Gorgias or, at worst, simple drudges whose labors we would disavow if we could. The issue is not simply the efficacy of the rules—the way schools are funded; the way subways are constructed—but the manner in which they promote social outcomes that we seek either to embrace or to reject.

Understanding Ethics

And so we come to the central insight of the American pragmatism advanced in the nineteenth century by the mathematician Charles Sanders Peirce. Its fundamental premise was that "in any kind of inquiry, we begin with an inherited set of beliefs, theories, principles, policies and practices."[6] They are the antecedents that determine what we investigate in the world and how we go about those investigations. Unless and until those antecedents are shown to be inadequate, they remain the basis of our investigations. And so like Hume, Peirce attempted to ground his argument in the concrete while acknowledging the conceptual baggage we all bring to a knowledge of the world.

To argue a pragmatist point of view is not to deny the ethical, or moral. Rather, it is to insist that they ride behind and below our decisions, influencing our choices and then our judgments. The trick, then, is to see *how* we chart or map the ideas that argue their presentation. The broadly pragmatic argues a complex rather than simplistic ethic, one in which everything is contingent on the moral suppositions we espouse and the propositions we believe result necessarily from them. There is no Olympian, independent observer to say, "Yes, that's right," because there is nothing but dynamic exchanges in which beliefs dictate actions that question or enforce beliefs.

In evaluating the efficacy of a belief set, Peirce argued, in a way Plato would have embraced, the first step was to perceive its consequences. "Consider the practical effects of the objects of your conception. Then, your conception of those effects is the whole of your conception of the object."[7] In effect, he proposed an if-then proposition based on a specific goals or value. The mind-set we bring to a problem or question, and thus its formulation, Peirce wrote, has three properties. First, it is something we must be aware of; second, it permits us to face the world with some surety; third, it establishes a habit of thought and a set of procedures or actions.[8] When experience contradicts a settled belief, an ingrained habit, two things occur.

First, we have moral distress and, in extreme cases, moral injury, "that combination of emotional and cognitive consequences resulting from the commission, failure to prevent or intervene, or the observation of actions which constitute a violation of one's core values."[9] That describes the "queasy feeling" in a nutshell: believing this, how can I/we act in that way? That was the dilemma the cartographers and statisticians confronted in the Tobacco Problem. If cancer limits human life, and if life is a moral value we embrace, then how can one take on the American Tobacco Consortium assignment *without* feeling queasy? What does it say about a nation's morality when a national cancer atlas presents as complete data that are restricted to a single race? What does that say about us as citizens believing (at least in theory) in equality as a signal virtue?

The second and more general damage occurs when the ethical propositions we in theory embrace are demonstrably ignored in practice. Then "a patch of ground gives way," and our moral suppositions are challenged, their power eroded. The ethical injunctions that would otherwise follow become empty rhetoric whose power to organize our world diminishes and then disappears.[10] When moral definitions are eroded, the ethics that follow on them become inconsequential curiosities without any real-world substance.

What results is a thinly theoretical posture argued by those with little experience in the complex realities whose ethics of practice they seek to judge. For their part, professionals like the NACIS members have little knowledge of the means by which their ethical aspirations and moral sensibilities can be understood, let alone deployed in the experiential world.[11] They just know what it's like to take on a job they feel queasy about. Unlike Gorgias, they cannot take pride in the result.

When Morals Conflict

Once one is comfortable with the idea of ethics and morals as underlying determinants, the nature of resulting debates about the world we present in our choices is shifted. We see these issues not simply as acceptable differences between individuals ("everybody has an opinion") but from a shared social perspective of grounded collectively rather than eccentrically. This doesn't mean all is necessarily clear. But where differences arise, their basis becomes obvious and can be a matter of focused debate.

In April 1992, I gave a talk titled "Reporting and Research in the Electronic Age" at the Poynter Institute, a journalism think tank in St. Petersburg, Florida. In those sessions, during what is now called the First Gulf War, an editor proudly showed attendees pages of his newspaper's coverage of the "new soldier," well equipped and ferociously motivated to extend American democratic ideals in the then new Iraqi conflict. "When my country goes to war," the editor proudly told session participants, "so does my newspaper."

Did that mean he would modify or withhold news reports of civilian casualties resulting from US military activities? Did that mean he simply repeated whatever officials said? Was his newspaper a civilian *Stars and Stripes*? Of course not, he replied. Journalistic integrity required truthful reportage. But, he continued, patriotism is every citizen's ethical duty in times of war. If the United States is engaged in a moral battle for good, then those who criticize US troop activities are attacking the morally good. Patriotism became for this editor a defining social and journalistic virtue by which the truths his paper promoted were to be assessed. Not lying, of course. But where the truth was in question (and when is it not?), patriotism required that the government get the benefit of the doubt. That is how American soldiers from Kentucky, Mississippi, and Tennessee became "local" patriots in Iraq (see fig. 3.2).

When it was suggested that real patriotism and good journalism required skepticism, a critical rather than supportive voice, the editor was disconcerted. When asked if reflecting the official view didn't make his paper a mere propaganda arm of the government rather than an at least semi-independent public voice, he grew irritated. And so the issue became the nature of patriotism as much as the role of the journalist in a nation's conflicted roles.

We can map wealth as a source of pride and assume that the poor among us are of little consequence ("the business of government is business"). Alternately, we can map poverty and its consequences as a civil violation of promised equalities of opportunity ("the business of government is the health and security of its peoples"). Either way, we are mapping not simply data but an idea about what is important to us and to society. At the least, the morals underlying a map (or graph, or graphic, etc.), and its resulting ethics, may be identified and then considered on the basis of those suppositions and embedded presuppositions. Thus the first map calls on economic standards as its metric; the second calls on indices of education, health, and social franchise as its standard. The result of the latter approach is a pragmatic virtue ethic enforcing the idea of communal care over individual advance.

Practicalities

Peirce's interest in the practical and its context was grounded in his desire to improve the theoretical. He was, after all, a logician and philosopher. Here the focus is reversed. My goal has been to focus on the practical by revealing its theoretical grounding. From this perspective, the difference between definitions of moral injury—operating at very different scales of interest—come into stark relief. There is the original, early twentieth-century definition of an injury to the nation by individuals whose lives do not measure up to some official standard. The needs and realities of those persons, even their very existence, could be dismissed in favor of a vision of the nation (healthy and strong) and its progress (idiots don't help the bottom line, they breed more idiots). There is also the more modern definition in which moral injuries are visited on individuals tasked in the Hegelian sense through a conflict with the greater powers that be.

The first, today, is typically framed in economic terms. Ideas of community, mutual aid, and solidarity are quaint notions impeding the business of the nation. And so, to take one example, because the medical needs of an aging society are assumed to be expensive, some argue that those who are long-lived should be denied curative treatments.[12] Ethically, good senior citizens "too old for health care" should willingly accept diminished care standards to promote the needs of younger persons.[13] If they demur, not only is their patriotism questioned (selfish!) but their place within a society that defines its own health on the basis of economic standards (affordable versus unaffordable persons). But there is also the moral good that accrues over time to the individual in his or her need, and thus a sense of moral injury (some would say violation) when utilitarian ethical standards disastrously affect individual lives. Redlining neighborhoods may have made good banking sense, but the generations whose home prices were affected and whose mobility was restricted were injured by the practice. Funding education through local real estate taxes is efficient. That it has robbed generations of the education they require to be engaged citizens, well, so it goes.

And so from the start the conflict exists between an ethical yardstick that is broad and abstract and another that is individually focused and grounded in a morality whose suppositions advance from the start ideas of community and mutuality as central. It therefore is important to note—almost a conclusion—that with almost every example cited, allegiance to the second definition rather than the first presents consequential economic and social benefits. A communal morality ("We the people ...") is in almost all cases more efficient, less costly in any but the short term, and in the long run more beneficial to all. It is an argument and observation made time and again since the 1840s and the reformers quoted in Edwin Chadwick's *Inquiry into the Sanitary Conditions of the Labouring Population of Great Britain.*[14]

Diminishing poverty improves the health of persons and the health of society at large. It diminishes social costs of indigent care and of the even minimal care we feel obliged to provide to the unemployable frail, albeit grudgingly, as a society. Addressing systemic income inequality means a better, more engaged electorate as well as one whose members are more employable. That means more and higher taxes will be paid by working citizenry. Educational disadvantage results in poverty, and an electorate that is disengaged, devaluing democracy itself as a shared economic and social enterprise. The result is far more costly, in the end, than acting on the presupposed value of fairness and equality of opportunity for all.

In Toronto, Canada, where I live, researchers estimate that in 2016 poverty related to ill-health cost government at all levels an estimated Can $2.9 billion a year. Some put the total cost of city poverty (including diminished taxes and increased social support) at perhaps Can $5 billion annually.[15] Nationally the calculated costs are far greater.[16] And this is in Canada, with its commitment to both national healthcare and a moderately strong social safety net.

When poverty, educational failures, ill health, and unemployment are assumed to be simply objective data on a spreadsheet, the costly implications that result are usually implicit but hidden, the human suffering too easily ignored. But maps of inequality

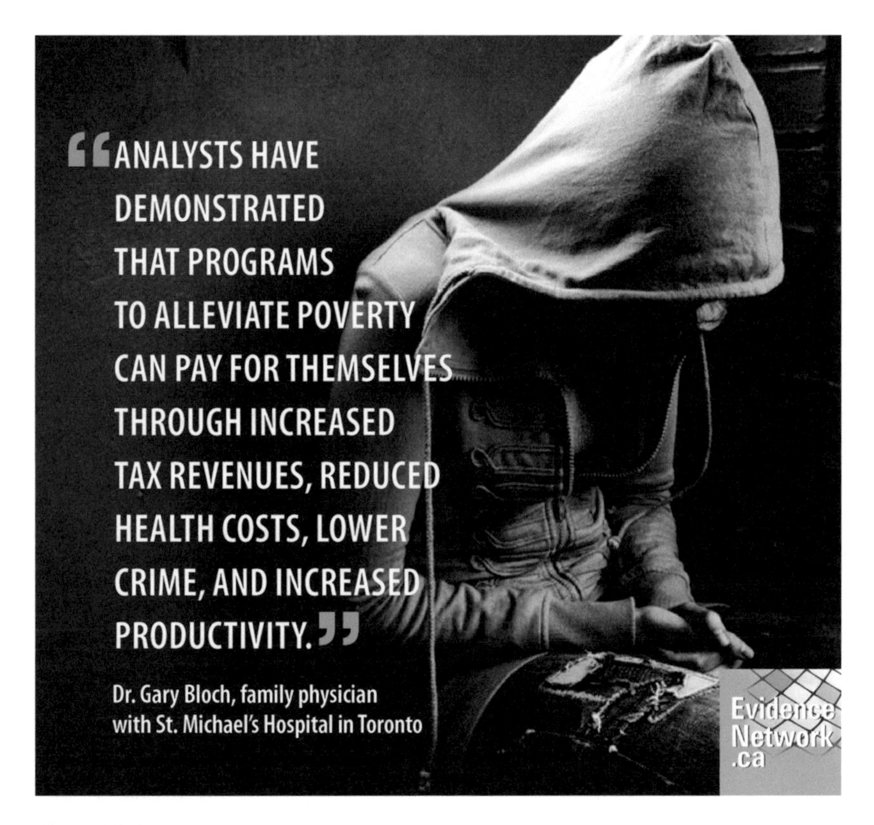

Figure 10.2
A poster in Toronto, Canada, arguing poverty is more expensive than its elimination. Courtesy Folio Designs for EvidenceNetwork.ca.

and poverty can be constructed to present opportunity surfaces for the promotion of greater communal good with positive long-term economic and social results. Rather than areas to avoid, they are sites to be engaged and improved for local and general long-term good.

We don't tend to see them this way, perhaps, because we have forgotten Plato's injunction that truth's standard is not limited but broad, not individual but shared. The true phoneme of moral debate is not the individual or economics. It is the health and welfare of the citizenry at large. At least it is supposed to be. One problem has been, as the economist Julie Nelson observes, our assumption that capitalism is a kind of automatic machine obeying "inexorable and amoral 'laws'" whose sole goal is profit, not care.[17] It would be more accurate to say that capitalism as we conceive it today is on automatic drive along a course we chose and self-consciously set. Its algorithms are typically constituted to focus on the limited and the short term, on profit rather than the social good. It doesn't have to be this way. It's just the way it is until and unless we change our perception, alter our presuppositions, change our argument and thus our focus.

Another Pragmatic

As Edmund Burke noted wryly, "It is far more easy to maintain a wrong cause, and to support paradoxical opinions to the satisfaction of a common auditory, than to establish a doubtful truth by solid and conclusive arguments."[18] It is easier for the economist to insist that he or she is simply observing the economic order rather than defining it and its costly results. It is similarly easier for the artist, cartographer, journalist, or statistician to ignore the ethical propositions of an assignment than to question them.

That, after all, is what most of us have been trained to do. We are taught that data are objective and facts are simple, observable things. We learn that the only appropriate question is whether the data we deploy are "true" and not a self-consciously fabricated, limited fiction. We are taught not to ask about the simple propositions (tobacco use encourages long life) the data were collected to argue. We are thus consequentially distanced from any deeper questioning of the research proposition's suppositions. Relative poverty is just income variation; educational performance simply a record of high school graduation rates. A map of disease is no more than a snapshot of bacterial or viral incidence. Hurricanes are simply naturally destructive events.

We are thus schooled to ignore, at least until it becomes impossible to do so, the broader implications of this or that action or analysis and its relation to the moral definitions we as citizens believe, cherish, and are pledged (at least in theory) to promote. This blinkered agnosticism is the very definition of what we mean today by "professional." The result is what Roland Barthes called a kind of "depoliticized speech" that "records facts or perceives values but refuses explanations: the order of the world can be seen as sufficient or ineffable, [but] it is never seen as significant."[19] And so we reject queasy moral concerns as *un*professional and substantive ethical concerns as irrelevancies divorced from the "real work," the work we are paid to do.

That is, we do so until it is too late. The young soldier who believes in patriotism and service to the nation is damaged when that service requires he or she perform acts that seem personally unconscionable. The resulting post-traumatic stress, an inability to live with the distance between moral definitions and professional realities, damages his or her sense of ethical personhood. The engineer who did what he was told is damaged when a train crashes, a plane drops from the sky, or a shuttle explodes because preventable errors were recognized but not addressed. Those of us who face less-violent conflicts feel a similar if lesser disjunction, and pain, in our weighing of duty and morality. Where the result diminishes the collective good, the result is moral injury in its original sense, damage to the civil public at large. From this perspective, it is that collective good, expressed in our constitutions and conventions, which must stand as the yardstick of moral supposition and ethical proposition. That it is typically more cost-efficient and thus less injurious in the long run is an added if secondary boon.

Now What?

Some may see this as a call to activism, to collectivism or socialism or some other -ism. It is instead a call to awareness, an insistence that we realize our choices matter. It asks that we see the potential effect of our work and in its preparation and presentation choose ethically and wisely. We may choose to be amoral rhetoricians free of ethical constraint, available to the highest bidder, or we may choose to acknowledge that our work is grounded in a moral framework that speaks consciously or by default to a communal good rather than simply individual advancement. We may argue that our only responsibility is to the rules others set or, alternately, to the idea of a kind of virtue ethic in which the person in society is our focus. We can choose to be like Gorgias, hired guns with allegiance only to this employer or that organization, or we can seek to be like Plato, for whom truth and its good were something more. If we choose the former path, we forfeit any ideal of substantive social responsibility; we ignore the sense of injury that occurs when our sense of personal ethics and morality is challenged by professional boundaries and commercial dictates. In so doing, we become mere mercenaries, carrying not a gun but a computer tablet.

For most of us, that is insufficient, unsatisfying to the point of moral distress. Virtue ethicists might say that's how it should be because, for our own good and that of our communities, we should want to be more. There is in law the notion of the "predicate act" that necessarily results in specific outcomes.[20] A landscape of poverty is the predicate that results in diminished educational funding, increased relative mortality, unrequited costs, and all those other things that follow on an impoverished, struggling citizenry. Because poverty is the predicate context of all these things, seeing a map of SAIPE-defined poverty, we should ask, "What is the result?" A map of disease invites questions about its causes and, if the disease is infectious, the likely pattern of its diffusion. It demands we ask about the preconditions that made a disease event inevitable and for which we as members of a society are at least in part responsible. If we let them, all or at least some charts, maps, tables, and stories open the same opportunity for

Become
Who
You Are
Practice
Philosophy!
Introductory workshop:
Monday November 16 @ 7:30pm
Tickets / info :
416-486-7198
Toronto.NewAcropolis.ca

Figure 10.3
One doesn't have to be a philosopher to "practice" philosophy. The issues it attempts to address pervade our worlds of family and work. That's the message of this sign found on a telephone pole in Toronto, Canada. Author's collection.

critical questioning. And critical questioning, here, invites consideration of the ethical suppositions and their moral presuppositions as central to who we are and what we are to do as ethical citizens.

This is not to suggest we become a nation of philosophers schooled in a literature that stretches at least from Plato through Kant to Levinas (fig. 10.3). "A nation of philosophers is as little to be expected," wrote James Madison in *The Federalist Papers* (1788), "as the philosophical race of kings." But to say we need not be philosophers by trade does not mean we can ignore the philosophies we espouse as individuals and as citizens.

We need not create the world anew, constructing from scratch a morality and consequent ethics as if such a thing had never been done before. We need only refer to the declarations, covenants, laws, and policy reports in which moral presuppositions are presented in a manner that argues a guiding and practical ethic. This would mean that, like Plato, we think of the communal rather than the limited good and, with Kant, about the lives of individuals as more than anonymous rows in a statistical spreadsheet. In this way, we assert the consequentiality of our work as social beings. We then see that the morals we assert as a nation are those we must, as citizens, enact in our lives.

Here is John Rawls's political ethic brought to the level of the practical. He argued that we need to see ourselves as if *we* are the subjects of the maps we make, the statistics we collect. We are the ones "behind the veil," members of an event class symbolized by dots on a map. We need to think as if we were *in* the maps we make and read: denizens of Skid Row, Los Angeles, or a poor citizen in Mississippi unlikely to receive a graft organ but whose organs are solicited for the good of wealthier others. We don't live in Owsley County, Kentucky (43 percent poverty), or in the poorest areas of downtown Buffalo, New York (90 percent nonwhite and poor). But we might. And thus we care about those persons as if we did because as citizens we are enjoined by the nation's moral definitions to promote the general good and the best opportunities of a more perfect union. They are us, and we, as easily, could be them. That is what the community of citizenry means, in the end.

Thinking and Acting

"It is easy to talk and write about human geographies of ethics and justice," wrote Paul Cloke, "compared to the difficulties of living out those geographies in our everyday life practices."[21] To be more than rhetoricians means that we recognize the nature of our unease and accept our responsibilities as citizens within communities where we live, where we have a chance to be effective. It would be nice to think that pointing out the distance between our best ideals and our actual programs would be all that is needed. It is rarely that easy.

It is doubtful that ATC president Thomas J. Crawford would agree to stop the publicity campaign equating long-lived smokers with healthy long lives. It is even more doubtful that the hypothetical Raleigh, North Carolina, news editor would permit a reporter to write an article ripping apart Mr. Gleason's talk as misleading piffle. It is unlikely that, as director of a small, struggling IT company, many of us would reflexively refuse the ATC contract. As Hegel knew full well, acting ethically has consequences, often unpleasant, for us as citizens trying to be virtuous and still get by in the world. The editor is beholden to bosses who are beholden to advertisers. The reporter is beholden to them all. The mapmaker has bills to pay, and to pay them, he or she must satisfy clients.

The result for the independent contractor and the salaried employee alike is the same: take the contract and feel guilty about the work; refuse it and be impoverished or, worse, unemployed. Either way, the result is "moral distress" in circumstances where "one knows the right thing to do, but institutional constraints make it nearly impossible to pursue the right course of action."[22] Those constraints result from a system of economic distribution and social governance that rarely rewards the ethical stance or the moral complaint. And so, in the Tobacco Problem, many discussants who approved the contract gave as their rationale "It's legal and that's all I need to know." Sure, the result would be one in which they could take little pride; but if it's not against the rules, as one person said charmingly, "baby needs new shoes."

The very idea of moral distress has been debated widely in medical ethics, mostly in terms of how to assuage a professional's unease rather than to address the underlying ethical dilemmas causing that distress. Some have sought to offer "conceptual and theoretical clarity."[23] The clarity typically offered parses the individual's distress and not the context that gave rise to it. And so, with that perspective, nothing changes at all.

I first encountered this in 2001 when I was hired to spend a day lecturing about bioethics to Ottawa hospital social workers. I spent the first hour reviewing the history of medical ethics and the second describing their general principles of application. In the third hour, I asked what problems the social workers saw as ethically troublesome. After all, they had hired me. It seemed the least I could do was ask what might we discuss together. All agreed the single greatest problem was that supervisors directed them to free up hospital beds by sending fragile seniors to any assisted-care facility with an open bed, even if the social workers believed the assignment was, for a particular patient, inappropriate. The problem isn't limited to their hospitals and remains exigent in many places today.

The social workers wanted to delay the transfers until more appropriate placements were available. Their responsibility, they said—personally and professionally—was to the patient's best interests and safety. An inappropriate discharge was, for them, a failure. The hospital, however, wanted these patients relocated to free beds for new and urgent cases. The hospital, after all, isn't supposed to be a long- or even mid-term care facility.[24]

Canadian hospitals are provincially funded and supervised and neither private nor "not-for-profit" institutions. Long-term care facilities are in theory regulated by provincial health ministries but are often privately owned and operated. While there is general agreement that patients needing longer-term care facilities should not remain overlong in much needed, acute care beds, the supply of affordable longer-term residence facilities is a chronic problem.

As we discussed the issue, their superior came into the room. Wearing a terrific three-piece suit below a sculpted haircut, the director for patient services (or some such title) shook my hand and warmly thanked me for sharing my knowledge with his social workers (who themselves paid my expenses and a small honorarium). He was sure they had learned a lot, and as a hospital official, he was grateful for my efforts. I told him I was learning from them, as well.

"Perhaps you can help us with something," I said. In discussing ethics as a real thing, I continued, there was this problem of the expeditious forced transfer of patients in a manner that in the professional opinion of the assembled social workers was inappropriate and potentially injurious to patients. What did he think "his" social workers should do when official directives violated their professional standards and sense of ethical responsibility?

"That doesn't happen," the supervisor assured me. A brief, short-term allocation problem had been rectified. Everything was fine. All assignments were, if not optimal, then more than acceptable. With that pronouncement and a quick final handshake, he departed. The social workers laughed, shaking their heads at my foolishness. "Well, you won't be coming back," one said to me. "So," another asked, "what do we do now?" Some talked of quitting, or at least moving to other institutions if not other professions where they would not feel queasy at the end of the day.

"Often, the underlying issue in moral distress is the gap between being responsible for delivering care and having the authority to determine what that care should be."[25] And so we talked about the problem. The social workers could point to professional ethics statements, hospital policy declarations, and, if they wished, broad political proclamations to support their views of what should be done. But while their responsibility as social workers was to the patients, as employees they were in liege to the institution and its policies. They had mortgages and car payments and kids in school. Like the Map-Off Ltd. participants, they needed their jobs.

We talked about documenting the problem. They could map the imbalance between demand and supply in assisted-care facilities and nursing homes, mapping the distance between discharge locations and family homes to show how many patients being discharged were, as a result, being isolated from their personal support communities. We discussed the possibility of union action ("Not our union," they laughed, "they don't do social"). We talked about involving local media. We talked about putting the problem before their elected members of the provincial legislature if not also their Parliamentary representatives. But any of those actions would have resulted, if not in their firing, they said, in their being condemned as whistle-blowing malcontents with a dismal work future.

It's one thing to see what is needed, I said. It's a very different thing to fight for it. That means documenting the problem in the context of the promises we make as a society or, in this case, a professional organization whose members, in theory, have a duty to care. But documentation is only the beginning. To act on it is to invite censure. Hegel knew that. It's why he called it tragedy.

It is hard to turn down work that is needed to pay the bills, to challenge a boss whose choices are inappropriate. Sometimes that is what one does because if one does not, it is hard to look in the mirror. And so I return here to where I began, with one change. Ethics is about our whole manner of being, not simply as individuals but as citizens in communities we seek to serve. We are responsible, as such, for not simply our own character but that of the community as well. Understanding what is right or wrong, what to condemn and what to promote, is not impossible. It may be uncomfortable and, in the short term, seem impractical but to ignore that understanding whatever the cost is to deny our own sense of rectitude and self. "If the tradition of the virtues was able to survive the horrors of the last dark ages," wrote Alasdair MacIntyre, "we are not entirely without grounds for hope."[26]

Across the *longue durée* of history, we have heard, time and again, a call for Aquinas's *conscientia*, a governing conscience over the immediate and pedestrian needs of the moment. It is not simply that, as Montaigne insisted, "life should be an aim to itself, a purpose unto itself," but more particularly that purpose is or should be a good life in Plato's sense, one serving the community at large rather than the particular needs of the self-serving moment. The goal here has been to insist on that possibility while mapping the effects of its failure both on us, in our distress, and on society at large.

The choice is yours. But please remember: your choice will affect us all.

Notes

Preface

1. Mary Midgley, *Evolution as a Religion: Strange Hopes and Stranger Fears*, rev. ed. (New York: Routledge, 2002), 2.

2. Mary Midgley, *Are You an Illusion?* (New York: Routledge, 2014), 19.

3. John Law, *After Method: Mess in Social Science Research* (New York: Routledge, 2004).

4. John Law and Annemarie Mol, *Complexities: Social Studies of Knowledge Practices* (Durham, NC: Duke University Press, 2002).

Chapter 1

1. Andrew Jameton, *Nursing Practice: The Ethical Issues* (Englewood Cliffs, NJ: Prentice Hall, 1984), 6.

2. Mark W. Roche, "Introduction to Hegel's Theory of Tragedy," *PhaenEx* 1, no. 2 (2006): 11–20.

3. Hallie Golden, "Rocket Engineer Who Predicted Space Shuttle *Challenger* Disaster Dies," Associated Press/*Toronto Star*, March 24, 2016, http://www.thestar.com/news/world/2016/03/24/rocket-engineer-who-predicted-space-shuttle-challenger-disaster-dies.html.

4. Ibid.

5. Renata D'Aliesio, "Failure to Safeguard," *Globe and Mail* (Toronto), May 13, 2016, http://www.theglobeandmail.com/news/national/inquiry-exposes-holes-in-canadian-forces-mental-health-caresystem/article30021281.

6. Tessy A. Thomas and Lawrence B. McCullough, "A Philosophical Taxonomy of Ethically Significant Moral Distress," *Journal of Medicine and Philosophy* 40, no. 1 (2015): 102–120.

7. David Wood, "The Grunts: Damned If They Kill, Damned If They Don't," *Huffington Post*, March 18, 2014, http://projects.huffingtonpost.com/moral-injury/the-grunts.

8. Christy A. Reentmeister, "Moral Damage to Health Care Professionals and Trainees: Legalism and Other Consequences for Patients and Colleagues," *Journal of Medicine and Philosophy* 33 (2008): 27–43.

9. Alan Cribb, "Integrity at Work: Managing Routine Moral Stress as Professional Roles," *Nursing Philosophy* 12 (2001): 119–127.

10. Stephen Pattison and Andrew Edgar, "The Problem with Integrity," *Nursing Philosophy* 12 (2011): 81.

11. Jonathan Hait and Jesse Graham, "When Morality Opposes Justice: Conservatives Have Moral Intuitions That Liberals May Not Recognize," *Social Justice Research* 20, no. 1 (2006): 98–116.

12. Alan Cribb, "Integrity at Work," 120.

13. Curt Petrovich, "Back to Zero: Curt Petrovich, Typhoon Haiyan, the Philippines, 2013," *Back Story*, CBC Radio, July 16, 2016, http://www.cbc.ca/radio/backstory/back-to-zero-curt-petrovich-typhoon-haiyan-the-philippines-2013-1.3285514.

14. Nancy Berlinger, *Are Workarounds Ethical? Managing Moral Problems in Health Care Systems* (New York: Oxford University Press, 2016), 2.

15. Bruce, Jennings, Frederick J. Wertz, and Mary Beth Morrissy, "Nudging for Health and the Predicament of Agency: The Relational Ecology of Autonomy and Care," *Journal of Theoretical and Philosophical Psychology* 36, no. 2 (2016): 81–99.

16. Daniel Kahneman, *Thinking Fast and Slow* (New York: Farrar, Straus & Giroux), 2011.

17. Peter H. Ditto, David A. Pizarro, and David Tannenbaum, "Motivated Moral Reasoning," in *Psychology of Learning and Motivation*, vol. 50, *Moral Judgments and Decision Making*, ed. B. H. Ross, D. M. Bartles, C. W. Bauman, et al. (San Diego, CA: Academic Press, 2009), 307–338.

18. Alan Cribb, "Integrity at Work," 123.

19. Peter T. Ellison, "A Review of Sarah Blaffer Hrdy, *Mothers and Others*," *Evolutionary Psychology* 7, no. 3 (2009): 442.

20. I am obliged to my friend Dr. Kenneth Hirsch for this reference and more generally for insights into issues of moral stress, distress, and post-traumatic stress.

21. W. Bullard, "The Placement of High-Grade Imbecile Girls," *Boston Medical and Surgical Journal* 160, no. 2 (June 1909): 776–777.

22. *Buck v. Bell* 274 U.S. 200, 1927.

23. Corinna Delkeskamp-Hayes, "Morality at the Expense of Others: Equality, Solidarity, Taxes, and Debts in European Public Health Care," *Journal of Medicine and Philosophy* 40, no. 2 (2015): 121–136.

24. John Meadowcroft, "Just Healthcare? The Moral Failure of Single-Tier Basic Healthcare," *Journal of Medicine and Philosophy* 40, no. 2 (2015): 152–168.

25. The bioethics literature is filled with this kind of argument. For an example see the special issue, some of whose articles have already been cited: "Handicapped by Egalitarianism: Europe's Public Health Care Systems," ed. Corinna Delkeskamp-Hayes, *Journal of Medicine and Philosophy* 40, no. 2 (2015).

26. Christopher Hamlin, *Public Health and Social Justice in the Age of Chadwick: 1800–1854* (New York: Cambridge University Press, 1998), 13.

27. The tension between these two ethics—economic and social—in the British debates over how to respond to the threat of cholera in the 1830s. Tom Koch, *Disease Maps: Epidemics on the Ground* (Chicago: University of Chicago Press, 2011), 104–108.

28. The "social progress index" is one example. For example, Leyland Cecco, "Canada Takes Second Spot Globally on Social-Progress Ranking," *Globe and Mail* (Toronto), June 29, 2016, http://www.theglobeandmail.com/news/social-progress-index-canada-isalright/article30647376.

29. Tom Koch, *Thieves of Virtue: When Bioethics Stole Medicine* (Cambridge, MA: MIT Press, 2011).

30. Robert M. Veatch, *Hippocratic, Religious, and Secular Medical Ethics: The Points of Conflict* (Washington, DC: Georgetown University Press, 2012), 68.

31. Tom Koch, "The Hippocratic Thorn in Bioethics' Hide," *Journal of Medicine and Philosophy* 39, no. 1 (2013): 75–88.

32. Brighid Kelly, "Preserving Moral Integrity: A Follow-Up Study with New Graduate Nurses," *Journal of Advanced Nursing* 28 (1998): 1134–1145, 1141.

33. Mark W. Roche, "Introduction to Hegel's Theory of Tragedy," *PhaenEx* 1, no. 2 (2006): 13–14.

34. Nancy Berlinger, *Are Workarounds Ethical?*, 14.

35. Judith Thomson, *The Realm of Rights* (Cambridge, MA: Harvard University Press, 1990), 2001.

36. Alasdair MacIntyre, *After Virtue*, 2nd ed. (Notre Dame, IN: University of Notre Dame Press, 1984), 41.

37. R. G. Collingwood, *An Essay on Metaphysics* (1939; Washington, DC: Regnery, 1972). For a discussion of Collingwood's work, see Giuseppina D'Oro and James Connelly, "Robin George Collingwood," in *The Stanford Encyclopedia of Philosophy*, ed. Edward N. Zalta, http://plato.stanford.edu/archives/sum2015/entries/collingwood.

38. J. L. Austin, *How to Do Things with Words*, 2nd ed. (Cambridge, MA: Harvard University Press, 1975), 4–7.

39. Roland Barthes, "The Imagination of the Sign," in *A Barthes Reader*, ed. Susan Sontag (New York: Hill & Wang, 1982), 211–218.

40. Roland Barthes, *The Eiffel Tower and Other Mythologies*, trans. Richard Howard (New York: Farrar, Straus & Giroux, 1979); Roland Barthes, *Mythologies*, trans. Annette Lavers (New York: Hill & Wang, 1972), 9.

41. Barthes, *Mythologies*, 9.

42. Wallace S. Snyder, *Principles and Practices for Advertising Ethics* (American Advertising Federation, 2011), https://www.aaf.org/_PDF/AAF%20Website%20Content/513_Ethics/IAE_Principles_Practices.pdf.

43. Denis Wood, "The Map as a Kind of Talk: Brian Harley and the Confabulation of the Inner and Outer Voice," *Visual Communication* 1, no. 2 (2002): 139–161.

44. Timothy Barney, *Mapping the Cold War: Cartography and the Framing of America's International Power* (Chapel Hill: University of North Carolina Press, 2015), 15.

45. Daniel Callahan, "Individual Good and Common Good: A Communitarian Approach to Bioethics," *Perspectives in Biology and Medicine* 46, no. 4 (2003): 298.

46. Denis Wood and John Fels, *The Natures of Maps: Cartographic Constructions of the Natural World* (Chicago: University of Chicago Press, 2008), xv—xvii.

47. Joseph P. Lawrence, *Socrates among Strangers* (Evanston, IL: Northwestern University, 2015), x. This is a point Lawrence returns to many times.

48. Judith Tyner, *Persuasive Cartography: An Examination of the Map as a Subjective Tool of Communication* (Ann Arbor, MI: University Microfilms, 1974); Judith Tyner, "Persuasive Cartography," *Journal of Geography* 81 (July–August, 1982): 140–144.

49. Ian Muehlenhaus, "Going Viral: The Look of Online Persuasive Maps," *Cartographica*49, no. 1 (2014): 18–34.

50. David Hume, *An Enquiry concerning Human Understanding*, ed. Tom L. Beacham (1748; New York: Oxford University Press, 1999), http://www.earlymoderntexts.com/pdfs/hume1748.pdf.

51. Plato's *Gorgias* is carefully reviewed and lovingly considered in Susan Levin, *Plato's Rivalry with Medicine: A Struggle and Its Dissolution* (New York: Oxford University Press, 2014), 8–14.

52. Clifford Gertz, *The Interpretation of Cultures: Selected Essays* (New York: Basic Books, 1973), https://chairoflogicphiloscult.files.wordpress.com/2013/02/clifford-geertz-the-interpretation-of-cultures.pdf.

53. Mary Midgley, *Are You an Illusion?* (New York: Routledge, 2014), 3.

54. John Snow, *On the Mode of Communication of Cholera*, 2nd ed. (London: Churchill, 1855), http://www.ph.ucla.edu/epi/snow/snowbook.html.

55. Edmund A. Parkes, "Review: *Mode of Communication of Cholera* by John Snow," *British and Foreign Medico-churgical Review* 15 (1855): 449–456.

56. For a more detailed discussion of these varying ideas about cholera and the alternate maps made of what is known as the Broad Street outbreak, see Koch, *Disease Maps*.

57. George Rosen, *A History of Public Health*, 2nd ed. (Baltimore, MD: The Johns Hopkins University Press, 1993), 24–26.

58. "History of the Rise, Progress, Ravages, Etc., of the Blue Cholera of India," *Lancet* 17, no 429 (1831): 241–248.

59. For a discussion of Snow's relation to cholera, see Koch, *Disease maps*, 144–162.

60. Koch, "The Hippocratic Thorn in Bioethics' Hide."

61. Hippocrates, *Airs, Waters, and Places*, trans. Francis Adams (Cambridge, MA: The Internet Classics Archive), http://classics.mit.edu/Hippocrates/airwatpl.8.8.html.

62. See Peter Vinten-Johansen, Howard Brody, Nigel Paneth, Stephen Rachman, and Michael Rip, *Cholera, Chloroform, and the Science of Medicine: A Life of John Snow* (New York: Oxford University Press, 2003). Snow's history as an apprentice is given in chapter 2, and his writings on that experience, and its relation to his work, are described in various later chapters.

Chapter 2

1. Tom Koch, *Cartographies of Disease: Maps, Mapping, and Medicine* (Redlands, CA: Esri Press, 2015).

2. Tom Koch, *Thieves of Virtue: When Bioethics Stole Medicine* (Cambridge, MA: MIT Press, 2012).

3. Anuradha Mathur and Dilip da Cunha, *Mississippi Floods: Designing a Shifting Landscape* (New Haven, CT: Yale University Press, 2001).

4. Bieke Cattoor and Chris Perkins, "Re-cartographies of Landscape: New Narratives in Architectural Atlases," *Cartographic Journal* 51, no. 2 (2014): 166–178.

5. Sheri Fink, *Five Days at Memorial* (New York: Crown, 2013), 15–23.

6. NOAA (National Oceanic and Atmospheric Administration), "Historical Hurricane Tracks," 2013, US Department of Commerce, National Oceanographic and Marine Service, http://csc.noaa.gov/hurricanes/#.

7. NOAA, "Hurricane Betsy: September 6–13, 1965," 2013, http://www.wpc.ncep.noaa.gov/tropical/rain/betsy1965.html.

8. NOAA, "Hurricane Bret," 2013, http://www.atmos.umd.edu/~stevenb/hurr/99/bret.

9. NOAA, "Hurricane Wilma," Dec. 27, 2005, http://www.nws.noaa.gov/om/data/pdfs/WilmaPSDA.pdf.

10. CDC/EPA Taskforce, *Environmental Health Needs and Habitability Assessment, Hurricane Katrina* (Washington, DC: Centers for Disease Control and Prevention and US Environmental Protection Agency, 2005).

11. Todd Litman, "Evaluating Transportation Equity," *World Transport Policy and Practice* 8, no. 2 (2002): 50–65.

12. John Renee, Tom Sanchez, Pam Jenkins, and Robert Peterson, "Challenge of Evacuating the Carless in Five Major U.S. Cities: Identifying the Key Issues," *Journal of the Transportation Research Board* (Transportation Research Board of the National Academies), no. 2119 (2009): 36–44, http://trrjournalonline.trb.org/doi/abs/10.3141/2119-05.

13. Alexandra Enders and Zachary Brandt, "Using Geographic Information System Technology to Improve Emergency Management and Disaster Response for People with Disabilities," *Journal of Disability Policy Studies* 17, no. 4 (1997): 223–229.

14. June Isaacson Kailes and Alexandra Enders, "Moving beyond 'Special Needs,'" *Journal of Disability Policy Studies* 17, no. 4 (2007): 230–237.

15. Nathaniel Rich, "The Lower Ninth Ward in New Orleans Gives New Meaning to 'Urban Growth,'" *New York Times Magazine*, March 25, 2012.

16. Mathew Ericson, "When Maps Shouldn't Be Maps," *New York Times*, October 11, 2011.

17. Mary Midgley, *Wickedness: A Philosophical Essay* (New York: Routledge Classics, 1984), 72–73.

18. Jonathan Haidt, "The Emotional Dog and Its Rational Tail: A Social Intuitionist Approach to Moral Judgment," *Psychological Review* 108 (2001): 814–834.

19. James Fieser, "Ethics," *Internet Encyclopedia of Philosophy*, http://www.iep.utm.edu/ethics/#H2.

20. Alasdair MacIntyre, *A Short History of Ethics* (New York: Collier Books, 1966).

21. Alasdair MacIntyre, *After Virtue*, 2nd ed. (Notre Dame, IN: University of Notre Dame Press, 1984), 61.

22. Per Nortvedt, "The Normativity of Clinical Health Care: Perspectives on Moral Realism," *Journal of Medicine and Philosophy* 37, no. 3 (2012): 296–309.

23. Judith Tyner, "Persuasive Cartography," *Journal of Geography* 81 (July–August 1982): 140–144. The article was a condensation of her dissertation, "Persuasive Cartography: An Examination of the Map as a Subjective Tool of Communication" (Ann Arbor, MI: University Microfilms, 1974).

24. Brian J. Harley, "Can There Be a Cartographic Ethics?" *Cartographic Perspectives* 10 (1991): 9–17.

25. Ian Muehlenhaus, "Going Viral: The Look of Online Persuasive Maps," *Cartographica* 49, no. 1 (2014): 18–34; also see his "The Design and Composition of Persuasive Maps," *Cartography and Geographic Information Science* 39, no. 2 (2013): 401–414.

26. This was the point that Denis Wood made in his discussion of Tom Van Sant and Lloyd Van Warren's famous satellite composite image of the world: "This is less a dividing up than a grinding or pulverizing of reality, done in this case with multispectral scanners." Denis Wood, *The Power of Maps* (New York: Guilford Press, 1992), 51–53.

27. Mark Monmonier, "Ethics and Map Design: Six Strategies for Confronting the Traditional One-Map Solution," *Cartographic Perspectives* 10 (1991): 3–9.

28. Cattoor and Perkins, "Re-cartographies of Landscape."

29. W. E. Morris, "David Hume," in *Stanford Encyclopedia of Philosophy*, ed. Edward N. Zalta, http://plato.stanford.edu/archives/spr2013/entries/hume.

30. Jacques Bertin, *Semiology of Graphics: Diagrams, Networks, Maps*, trans. William J. Berg (Redlands, CA: Esri Press, 1983).

31. Tom Koch, *The News as Myth: Fact and Context in Journalism* (Westport, CT: Greenwood Press, 1990), 59.

32. Investigative reportage may attempt to assess the statements of officials through a deeper, more independent examination of an event and its context. But even here, the work is often about finding an expert who contradicts the official statement, the witness whose narrative may differ from the official.

33. Annemarie Mol and John Law, "Complexities: An Introduction," in *Social Studies of Knowledge Practices*, ed. John Law and Annemarie Mol (Durham, NC: Duke University Press, 2006), 3–5.

34. Stewart Elden and Eduardo Mendieta, eds., *Reading Kant's Geography* (Albany: State University of New York Press, 2011).

35. John Macmurray, *The Self as Agent* (London: Faber & Faber, 1957), 39.

36. David Harvey, *Social Justice and the City* (Cambridge: Blackwell, 1973).

37. Morris, "David Hume."

38. Patrick McHaffie, Michael Dobson, Sona K. Andrews, et al., "Ethical Problems in Cartography: A Roundtable Commentary," *Cartographic Perspectives* 7 (1991): 6.

39. Andrew Pickering, *The Mangle of Practice: Time, Agency, and Science* (Chicago: University of Chicago Press, 1997).

40. Tom Koch, "False Truths: Ethics and Mapping as a Profession," *Cartographic Perspectives* 54 (2006): 4–15.

41. Richard A. Shweder, "Ethnographic Methods in Contemporary Perspective," in *Ethnography and Human Development*, ed. Richard Jessor, Anne Colby, and Richard A. Shweder (Chicago: University of Chicago Press, 1996), 17.

Chapter 3

1. Nicholas Schiller, "Finding a Socratic Method for Information Literacy Instruction," in *Critical Thinking within the Library Program*, ed. John Spencer and Christopher Millson-Martula (New York: Routledge, 2009), 52.

2. Peter Singer, *Practical Ethics*, 2nd ed. (New York: Cambridge University Press, 2003), 12.

3. Tom Koch, "Bioethics as Ideology: Conditional and Unconditional Values," *Journal of Medicine and Philosophy* 31, no. 3 (2006): 251–268.

4. See, e.g., Richard C. Lewontin, *Biology as Ideology: The Doctrine of DNA* (New York: Harper Perennial, 1993). And, of course, there is the Darwinian ideology of individuality and competition as natural, criticized early on by Kropotkin and more recently by evolutionary biologists. For a brief review, see my "Prince Kropotkin: Public Health's Patron Saint," *International Journal of Epidemiology* 43, no. 6 (2014): 1681–1685, http://ije.oxfordjournals.org/content/early/2014/10/21/ije.dyu206.

5. Koch, "Bioethics as Ideology."

6. Denis Wood, "The Map as a Kind of Talk: Brian Harley and the Confabulation of the Inner and Outer Voice," *Visual Communication* 1, no. 2 (2002): 139–161.

7. Talcott Parsons, *The Social System* (London: Routledge & Kegan Paul, 1951).

8. Harold Perkin, *The Rise of Professional Society: England since 1880* (London: Routledge, 1989).

9. Brian J. Harley, "Can There Be a Cartographic Ethics?" *Cartographic Perspectives* 10 (1991): 10.

10. Roland Barthes, "The Imagination of the Sign," in *A Barthes Reader*, ed. Susan Sontag (New York: Hill & Wang, 1982), 211–218.

11. Farid M. Shamji and Ronald MacCormick, "How Many Deaths Can Be Directly Attributed to Cigarette Smoking Every Year?" *Canadian Journal of Diagnosis* 31, no. 6 (June 16, 2014): 29.

12. Tom Koch, *The News as Myth: Fact and Context in Journalism* (Westport, CT: Greenwood Press, 1990), 9–10.

13. Arthur H. Robinson, Joel L. Morrison, P. C. Muehrcke, et al., *Elements of Cartography*, 6th ed. (Hoboken, NJ: John Wiley & Sons, 1995).

14. Karen S. Cook, "A Lifelong Curiosity about Maps," *Cartographic Perspectives* 51 (2005): 43–54.

15. Nicholas Lemann, "Atlas Shrugs: The New Geography Argues That Maps Have Shaped the World," *New Yorker*, April 9, 2001, 131–134, http://www.newyorker.com/magazine/2001/04/09/atlas-shrugs.

16. Harley, "Can There Be a Cartographic Ethics?"

17. Denis Wood and John Fels, *The Natures of Maps: Cartographic Constructions of the Natural World* (Chicago: University of Chicago Press, 2008).

18. Konrad Yakabuski, "Attacks on Joseph Boyden's Identity Should Set Off Alarm Bells," *Globe and Mail* (Toronto), December 29, 2016.

19. Stephen J. Ward, *The Invention of Journalism Ethics: The Path to Objectivity and Beyond* (Montreal: McGill University Press, 2005). On news and facticity, see Koch, *The News as Myth*.

20. Kathy English, "The Shades of Grey of Journalism Ethics: Public Editor," *Toronto Star*, October 2, 2015.

21. David Herzog, *Mapping the News: Case Studies in GIS and Journalism* (Redlands, CA: ESRI Press, 2003).

22. Mark Monmonier, *Maps with the News: The Development of American Journalistic Cartography* (Chicago: University of Chicago Press, 1999).

23. Solomon Moore, "Slaying of Defense Lawyer in Saddam Trial Raises Concerns," *Reno Gazette-Journal*, November 9, 2005, 1C, 25. The map was also discussed in my "'False Truths': Ethics and Mapping as a Profession," *Cartographic Perspectives* 54 (spring 2006): 8, http://www.cartographicperspectives.org/index.php/journal/article/viewFile/cp54-koch/403.

24. AP/Washington Post, "Agency Shows Way for Gulf Forces," *Washington Post*, January 2, 1991.

25. For a noncommercial presentation of the map, see Koch, "False Truths," 8.

26. James Risen, *State of War* (New York: Free Press, 2006), 136.

27. For a brief popular discussion of the documentary, see Gerald Kaplan, "Why the NDP Shouldn't Be Pacifists," *Globe and Mail* (Toronto), September 20, 2016.

28. Fred Peabody, dir., *All Governments Lie: Truth, Deception and the Spirit of I. F. Stone* (White Pine Pictures, August 3, 2016), http://www.whitepinepictures.com/9212-2/?v=3e8d115eb4b3.

29. Timothy Barney, *Mapping the Cold War* (Raleigh: University of North Carolina Press, 2015).

30. Denis Cosgrove, "Epistemology, Geography and Cartography: Thoughts on the Reaction of Brian Harley's Cartographic Theories," paper presented at the Association of American Geographers annual meeting, Chicago, IL, March 10, 2006.

31. Joseph P. Lawrence, *Socrates among Strangers* (Evanston, IL: Northwestern University Press, 2015), 12.

32. Nadine Schuurman, "Critical GIS: Theorizing an Emerging Science," *Cartographica* 36, no. 4 (1999).

33. Committee on Organ Procurement and Transplantation Policy, Institute of Medicine, Committee on Organ Transplantation, *Organ Procurement and Transplantation: Assessing Current Policies and the Potential Impact of the DHHS Final Rule* (Washington, DC: National Academy Press, 1999), 58a.

34. Donna Shalala, *Final Rule: Organ Procurement and Transplantation Network*, Fed. Reg. 63, 16288 (1998).

35. *National Organ Transplant Act*, Pub. L. No. 98–507; 98 Stat 2339 (1984).

36. Susan. S. Shudd, "The Impact of Travel on Transplantation Outcomes" (PhD diss., Yale University, 1997).

37. Ronald J. Ozminkowski, Allan J. White, Andrea Hassol, and Michael Murphy, "What If Socioeconomics Made No Difference? Access to a Cadaver Kidney Transplantation as an Example," *Medical Care* 38, no. 9 (1998): 1396–1406.

38. Robert Steinbrook, "Allocating Livers—Devising a Fair System," *New England Journal of Medicine* 336, no. 6 (February 6, 1997): 436–438.

39. Ozminkowski et al., "What If Socioeconomics Made No Difference?"

40. Tom Koch, "Thcy Might as Well Be in Bolivia: Race, Ethnicity and the Problem of Solid Organ Donation," *Theoretical Medicine and Bioethics* 20, no. 6 (1999): 563–574.

41. Robert D. Gibbons, David Meltzer, and Naihua Duan, "Waiting for Organ Transplantation," *Science* 287, no. 5451 (January 14, 2000): 237–238.

42. Ozminkowski et al., "What If Socioeconomics Made No Difference?"

43. Tom Koch, *Scarce Goods: Justice, Fairness, and Organ Transplantation* (London: Praeger, 2001), 148.

44. J. P. Vistnes and A. C. Monheit, "Health Insurance Status of the Civilian Noninstitutionalized Population," AHCPR Pub. No. 97–0030 (Rockville, MD: Agency for Health Care Policy and Research, 1997), http://meps.ahrq.gov/mepsweb/data_files/publications/rf1/rf1.pdf.

45. Tom Koch and Ken Denike, "Geography, the Problem of Scale, and Processes of Allocation: The U.S. National Organ Transplant Act of 1986, Amended 1990," in *Law and Geography*, ed. Jane Holder and Carolyn Harrison (London: Oxford University Press, 2003), 109–137.

46. Erving Goffman, *The Presentation of Self in Everyday Life* (New York: Doubleday, 1979).

Chapter 4

1. LaDale Winling, "HOLC Maps," UrbanOasis.org, 2012, http://www.urbanoasis.org/?s=HOLC+Maps. The maps have also been collected and made publicly available at the University of Richmond's Digital Scholarship Lab: https://dsl.richmond.edu/panorama/redlining/#loc=12/40.8586/-73.8568&opacity=0.8&city=bronx-ny.

2. The original reports are archived federally at "Owners' Loan Corporation and Federal Savings and Loan Corporation Annual Reports, 1933–1952" (Washington, DC: Federal Reserve Archive), http://fraser.stlouisfed.org/publication/?pid=70.

3. Sarah Bond, "Five GIS Projects That Are Changing the Way We Understand Racism," *Forbes*, October 25, 2016, http://www.forbes.com/sites/drsarahbond/2016/10/25/5-gis-projects-that-are-changing-the-way-we-understand-racism/#30c4439f2a44.

4. "Prize Announcement," Nobelprize.org, October 13, 2006, http://www.nobelprize.org/nobel_prizes/peace/laureates/2006/announcement.html.

5. More recently the redlined areas have been called "red-circled" amid calls for favorable state or federal policies that might "incentivize" banks to invest. Jennifer Wells, "Michael Bloomberg Could Be the One to Stop Trump," *Toronto Star*, February 16, 2016.

6. Lauren La Rose, "Bangladesh Factory Collapse Prompts Reforms, but Long-Term Impact Uncertain," *Global News*, December 17, 2013, http://globalnews.ca/news/1035856/bangladesh-factory-collapse-prompts-reforms-but-long-term-impact-uncertain.

7. Ludwig Wittgenstein, *Tractatus Logico-Philosophicus,* rev. ed., trans. C. K. Ogden (New York: Routledge, 1974).

8. Denis Wood and John Fels, *The Natures of Maps: Cartographic Constructions of the Natural World* (Chicago: University of Chicago Press, 2008), 6–7.

9. Anthony Kenny, *Wittgenstein*, rev. ed. (Malden, MA: Blackwell, 2005), 48.

10. Denis Wood, "The Map as a Kind of Talk: Brian Harley and the Confabulation of the Inner and Outer Voice," *Visual Communication* 1, no. 2 (2002): 139–161.

11. Denis Wood, "The Map's Power," paper presented at Deutscher Geographentag: Kongress für Wissenschaft, Schule, und Praxis, Passau, Germany, October 10, 2013.

12. Thomas J. Mason, Frank W. McKay, Robert Hoover, William J. Blot, and Joseph F. Fraumeni Jr., *Atlas of Cancer Mortality for U.S. Counties, 1950–1969* (Washington, DC: US Department of Health, Education, and Welfare/National Institutes of Health, 1979).

13. Ibid.

14. I discuss the history of cancer mapping and studies in Tom Koch, *Disease Maps* (Chicago: Chicago University Press, 2011), 246–248.

15. Percy Stocks, "On the Evidence for a Regional Distribution of Cancer Prevalence in England and Wales," in *Report of the International Conference on Cancer* (London, July 17–20, 1928).

16. Linda Gundersen, "Mapping It Out: Using Atlases to Detect Patterns in Health Care, Disease, and Mortality," *Annals of International Medicine* 133, no. 2(2000): 134.

17. Susan S. Devesa, Dan J. Grauman, William J. Blot, Gene A. Penello, Robert N. Hoover, and Joseph Fraumeni Jr., *Atlas of Cancer Mortality in the United States, 1950–94,* National Institutes of Health Publication No. 99–4583 (Rockland, MD: National Institutes of Health,1999), http://ratecalc.cancer.gov/archivedatlas/pdfs/text.pdf.

18. Mark Monmonier, *How to Lie with Maps*, 2nd ed. (Chicago: University of Chicago Press, 1996).

19. Tom Koch, *The News as Myth: Fact and Context in Journalism* (Westport, CT: Greenwood Press, 1990).

20. Darrell Huff, *How to Lie with Statistics* (New York: W. W. Norton, 1954).

21. J. Michael Steele, "Darrell Huff and Fifty Years of *How to Lie with Statistics*," *Statistical Science* 20, no. 3 (2005): 205–209, http://www-stat.wharton.upenn.edu/~steele/Publications/PDF/TN148.pdf.

22. Joel Best, *Damned Lies and Statistics*, updated ed. (Berkeley: University of California Press, 2012).

Chapter 5

1. See, e.g., Rebecca Vallas and Shawn Fremstead, "Disability Is a Cause and Consequence of Poverty," Talkpoverty.org, September 19, 2014, https://talkpoverty.org/2014/09/18/scholars -activists-poverty-data.

2. Americans with Disabilities Act of 1990, 42 U.S. Code, Chapter 126. Many saw this act, when passed, as a natural expansion of the Civil Rights Act of 1964 and its promise of equality—and equal opportunity—for all citizens irrespective of race. The government maintains a website regarding the ADA and its implementation at http://www.ada.gov.

3. See, e.g., Tom Beauchamp and James F. Childress, *Principles of Biomedical Ethics*, 5th ed. (New York: Oxford University Press, 2001). Beneficence is one of the basic principles the authors advance as a universal underpinning of an ethics principally applicable to medicine.

4. "Small Area Income and Poverty Estimates: About SAIPE," US Census Bureau, http://www.census.gov//did/www/saipe/about/index.html.

5. "Small Area Income and Poverty Estimates: Video Tutorials," http://www.census.gov/did/www/saipe/methods/tutorial.

6. Carmen DeNavas-Walt, Bernadette D. Proctor, and Jessica C. Smith, "Income, Poverty, and Health Insurance Coverage in the United States: 2009" (Washington, DC: US Department of Commerce, Economics and Statistics Administration, US Census Bureau, issued September 2010), https://www.census.gov/prod/2010pubs/p60-238.pdf.

7. To make your own map using more current statistics, visit http://www.census.gov/did/www/saipe/data/index.html.

8. See, e.g., William Watson, *The Inequality Trap: Fighting Capitalism Instead of Poverty* (Toronto: University of Toronto Press, 2015).

9. Suzanne Macartney, Alemayehu Bishaw, and Kayla Fontenot, "Poverty Rates for Selected Detailed Race and Hispanic Groups by State and Place: 2007–2011" (Washington, DC: US Department of Commerce, Economics and Statistics Administration, US Census Bureau, issued February 2013), 10, http://www.census.gov/prod/2013pubs/acsbr11-17.pdf.

10. Ibid., 1.

11. A. Buchanan, "Report of the Diseases Which Prevailed among the Poor of Glasgow, during the Summer of 1830," *Glasgow Medical Journal* 3 (1830): 440.

12. Gary Bloch, "Poverty: A Clinical Tool for Primary Care in Ontario," handout of the Ontario College of Family Physicians, rev. February 2013, http://ocfp.on.ca/docs/default-source/cme/poverty-and-medicine-march-2013.pdf.

13. G. L. McLaren and M. R. S. Baine, *Deprivation and Health in Scotland: Insights from NHS Data* (Edinburgh: ISD Scotland Publications, 1998), http://www.scotpho.org.uk/downloads/deprivation/isd-deprivationreport-1998.pdf.

14. "Premature Mortality—from All Causes, Aged under 75 Years," in *Long-Term Monitoring of Health Inequalities* (Edinburgh: St. Andrew's House, 2011), part 3, http://www.gov.scot/Publications/2011/10/21133633/3.

15. Francis P. Boscoe, Kevin A. Henry, Recinda L. Sherman, and Christopher J. Johnson, "The Relationship between Cancer Incidence, Stage and Poverty in the United States," *International Journal of Cancer*139 (2016): 607–612.

16. James Agee and Walker Evans, *Cotton Tenants: Three Families*, ed. John Summers (Brooklyn, NY: Melville House, 2013), 191–204. This was a reissue of a 1930s piece, originally written for *Fortune* magazine, before their writing *Let Us Now Praise Famous Men* (New York: Houghton Mifflin, 1939).

17. Edward R. Murrow, "Harvest of Shame," *CBS Reports*, November 26, 1960, http://www.youtube.com/watch?v=yJTVF_dya7E.

18. Trymaine Lee and Matt Black, "Geography of Poverty: A Journey through Forgotten America," produced by Amy Pereira, Mina Liu, and Sam Petulla, *MSNBC*, 2015, http://www.msnbc.com/interactives/geography-of-poverty/index.html.

19. Adam Haslett, "A Poet's Brief," in *Cotton Tenants: Three Families*, by James Agee and Walker Evans, ed. John Summers (Brooklyn, NY: Melville House, 2013), 14.

20. Agee and Evans, *Cotton Tenants*, 36.

21. Linda McQuaid, "The Upside of Kevin O'Leary's Political Ambitions," *Toronto Star*, January 22, 2016, http://www.thestar.com/opinion/commentary/2016/01/22/the-upside-of-kevin-olearys-political-ambitions.html. The Brandeis quote is usually sourced to Raymond Lonegran, *Mr. Justice Brandeis, Great American* (St. Louis, MO: Modern View Press, 1941), 41.

22. Richard Wilkinson and Michael Marmot, eds., *Social Determinants of Health: The Solid Facts*, 2nd ed. (Copenhagen, Denmark: World Health Organization, European Office, 2003), 23.

23. Jonathan Kozol, *Savage Inequalities: Children in America's Schools* (New York: Harper Perennial, 1991).

24. Jonathan Kozol, *Fire in the Ashes: Twenty-five Years among the Poorest Children in America* (New York: Crown, 2012).

25. Jonathan Kozol, *Amazing Grace: The Lives of Children and the Conscience of a Nation* (New York: Harper Perennial, 1995).

26. For a popular review of the recent technical literature, see Erika Hayasaki, "How Poverty Affects the Brain," *Newsweek*, August 25, 2016, http://www.newsweek.com/2016/09/02/how-poverty-affects-brains-493239.html.

27. Dylan Matthews, "Child Poverty in the US Is a Disgrace: Experts Are Embracing This Simple Plan to Fix It," *Vox*, April 27, 2017, https://www.vox.com/policy-and-politics/2017/4/27/15388696/child-benefit-universal-cash-tax-credit-allowance.

28. Christopher Hamlin, *Public Health and Social Justice in the Age of Chadwick: Britain, 1800–1854* (New York: Cambridge University Press, 1998).

29. Ibid., 70.

30. John F. Pickstone, "Ferriar's Fever to Kay's Cholera: Disease and Social Structure in Cottonopolis," *History of Science* 22 (1984): 404, http://articles.adsabs.harvard.edu/full/1984HisSc..22..401P.

31. Buchanan, "Report of the Diseases Which Prevailed among the Poor of Glasgow," 440.

32. "The fear that Manchester fever would prove so virulent, and would extend its reach from poor to rich, was an obvious component of the [positive social] response." Pickstone, "Ferriar's Fever to Kay's Cholera," 404.

33. John Lynch, George Davey Smith, Sam Harper, Marianne Hillemeier, et al., "Is Income Inequality a Determinant of Population Health? Part 2: A Systematic Review," *Milbank Quarterly* 82, no. 2 (2004): 359.

34. "Editorial: The Big Idea," *British Medical Journal* 312 (April 20, 1996): 985.

35. Juha Mikkonen and Dennis Raphael, *Social Determinants of Health: The Canadian Facts* (Toronto: York University School of Health Policy and Management, 2010), http://www.thecanadianfacts.org/the_canadian_facts.pdf.

36. Rodrick Wallace, Yi-Shan Huang, Peter Gould, and Deborah Wallace, "The Hierarchical Diffusion of AIDS," *Social Science and Medicine* 44, no. 7 (1997): 940.

37. Peter J. Hotez, "Tropical Diseases: The New Plague of Poverty," *New York Times*, August 9, 2012, SR4.

38. Jennifer Yang, "L.A.'s Skid Row: Ground Zero for the City's Largest Tuberculosis Outbreak in a Decade," *Toronto Star*, February 25, 2013, http://thestar.blogs.com/worlddaily/2013/02/street-scenes-from-skid-row-in-downtown-los-angeles-the-last-refuge-for-people-with-nowhere-else-to-go.html.

39. "Scientists Believe Thousands of People Have Been Exposed to a Deadly Outbreak of Tuberculosis in Downtown Los Angeles," (UK) *Daily Mail*, February 22, 2013, http://www.dailymail.co.uk/news/article-2283043/Thousands-exposed-deadly-TB-outbreak-Los-Angeles.html.

40. Hayley Fox, "Skid Row TB Epidemic Is 'Alarming,' but the Community Is Well-Versed in Disease," *Southern California Public Radio: Blog Downtown*, February 22, 2013, http://blogdowntown.com/2013/02/7146-skid-row-tb-epidemic-is-alarming-but-the.

41. Richard G. Wilkinson, *Unhealthy Societies: The Afflictions of Inequality* (New York: Routledge, 1996), 226.

42. Ibid., 27.

43. Kao-Ping Chua, "The Case for Universal Health Care" (Reston, VA: American Medical Student Association, 2008), https://www.amsa.org/wp-content/uploads/2015/03/CaseForUHC.pdf.

44. John Lynch, George Davey Smith, Sam Harper, Marianne Hillemeier, et al., "Is Income Inequality a Determinant of Population Health? Part 1: A Systematic Review," *Milbank Quarterly* 82, no. 1 (2004): 18.

45. Ching-Chi Hsieh and M.D. Pugh, "Poverty, Income Inequality, and Violent Crime: A Meta-analysis of Recent Aggregate Data Studies," *Criminal Justice Review* 18, no. 2 (1993): 182–202.

46. Kate E. Pickett and Richard G. Wilkinson, "Adolescent Birth Rates, Total Homicides, and Income Inequality in Rich Countries," *American Journal of Public Health* 95, no. 7 (2005): 1181–1183.

47. Lynch, Davey Smith, Harper, Hillemeier, et al., "Is Income Inequality a Determinant of Population Health? Part 2."

48. Carmen DeNavas-Walt, Bernadette D. Proctor, and Jessica C. Smith, "Income, Poverty, and Health Insurance Coverage in the United States: 2008" (Washington, DC: US Department of Commerce, Economics and Statistics Administration, US Census Bureau, issued September 2009), http://www.census.gov/prod/2009pubs/p60-236.pdf.

49. Harry Bradford, "Bangladesh to Raise Minimum Wage for Garment Workers," *Huffington Post*, May 12, 2013, http://www.huffingtonpost.com/2013/05/12/bangladesh-minimum-wage-garment-workers_n_3263347.html.

50. "Measuring Poverty," *Wikipedia*, last modified March 21, 2017, http://en.wikipedia.org/wiki/Measuring_poverty.

51. Tracy Hunter, "The Gini Coefficient, a Measure of Income Inequality," illustration in "Measuring Poverty," *Wikipedia*, https://en.wikipedia.org/wiki/Measuring_poverty#/media/File:2014_Gini_Index_World_Map,_income_inequality_distribution_by_country_per_World_Bank.svg.

52. Tom Koch, "Plague to Ebola: 1690–2015," *Cartographies of Disease: Maps, Mapping, and Medicine*, new ed. (Redlands, CA: Esri Press, 2017), 331–348.

Chapter 6

1. Education Law Center (ELC), Campaign for Fiscal Equity, "History" (New York: Education Law Center, 2013), http://www.edlawcenter.org/.

2. *Campaign for Fiscal Equity, Inc. et al. v. State of New York et al.*, 86 N.Y. 2d 307, 655 N.E. 2d 661, 631 N.Y.S. 2d 565 (June 15, 1995), http://www.edlawcenter.org/assets/files/pdfs/cfe/CFE%201995%20Decision.pdf.

3. *Campaign for Fiscal Equity (CFE), Inc. v. State of New York*, 86 N.Y. 2d 307 (June 13, 1996).

4. *Campaign for Fiscal Equity (CFE), Inc. et al. v. State of New York et al.*, 100 N.Y. 2d 908 (2003), http://www.edlawcenter.org/assets/files/pdfs/cfe/CFE%202006%20Decision.pdf.

5. Bess Keller, "N.Y. System of State Aid Thrown Out," *Education Week*, January 17, 2001, http://www.edweek.org/ew/articles/2001/01/17/18newyork.h20.html.

6. Saskia Sassen, *The Global City: New York, London, Tokyo* (Princeton, NJ: Princeton University Press, 1991), 261.

7. William J. Wilson, ed., *The Ghetto Underclass: Social Science Perspectives*, Annals of the American Academy of Political and Social Science, vol. 501 (Newbury Park, CA: Sage, 1989).

8. John D. Kasarda, "Urban Industrial Transition and the Underclass," in *The Ghetto Underclass: Social Science Perspectives*, ed. William J. Wilson, Annals of the American Academy of Political and Social Science, vol. 501 (Newbury Park, CA: Sage, 1989), 26–47.

9. Tom Koch and Ken Denike, "Geography, Justice, and Inequality: The New York City School Funding Controversy," *Journal of Geography* 102, no. 5 (2003): 193–201.

10. Jonathan Kozol, *Savage Inequalities: Children in America's Schools* (New York: Harper Perennial, 1991), 237.

11. Frederick P. Shaffer, "Memorandum of Law of the Association of the Bar of the City of New York, Amicus Curiae. Kruger et al. v. Bloomberg et al. For order and judgment pursuant to Article 78 of CPLR, *Superior Court of the State of New York*, Index No. 102510/03, May 28, 2003: 6, http://www.nycbar.org/pdf/report/AMICUS%20BRIEF.pdf.

12. Jason DeParle, "For Poor, Leap to College Often Ends in a Hard Fall," *New York Times*, December 22, 2012, http://www.nytimes.com/2012/12/23/education/poor-students-struggle-as-class-plays-a-greater-role-in-success.html.

13. Community Service Society, *Mapping Poverty in New York City: Pinpointing the Impact of Poverty, Community by Community* (New York: United Way of New York City, 2006), 13, http://b.3cdn.net/nycss/cc0e2b7c121eba2938_20m6ifgc8.pdf.

14. *Campaign for Fiscal Equity (CFE), Inc. et al. v. State of New York et al.*, 100 N.Y. 2d 908 (2003).

15. Patricia Cohen, "Prosperity Caught in Gap, Study Finds," *New York Times/Honolulu Star-Advertiser*, February 4, 2015, 9, http://www.pressreader.com/usa/honolulu-star-advertiser/20150204/textview.

16. Kristen Lewis and Sarah Burd-Sharps, "High School Graduation in New York City: Is Neighborhood Still Destiny?" Social Research Council: Measure of America (New York: Data2.Go), May 2016. https://www.measureofamerica.org/project/.

17. Eleanor Barkhorn, "Why Are American Schools Still Segregated?" *Atlantic.com*, November 13, 2013, http://www.theatlantic.com/education/archive/2013/11/why-are-american-schools-still-segregated/281126.

18. Jeremy E. Fiel, "Decomposing School Resegregation: Social Closure, Racial Imbalance, and Racial Isolation," *American Sociological Review*78, no. 5 (October 2013): 828–848, http://asr.sagepub.com/content/78/5/828.full.pdf+html.

19. Laura Bliss, "How School Districts Seal Their Students into Poverty," *CityLab* (from the *Atlantic*), July 22, 2015, http://www.citylab.com/politics/2015/07/how-school-districts-seal-their-students-into-poverty/399116/?utm_source=SFTwitter.

20. Sandra Tan, "Stacking the Deck against Buffalo's Six 'Failing Schools,'" *Buffalo News*, July 23, 2013, A1.

21. New York State Education Department, *Public School Total Cohort Graduation Rate and Enrollment Outcome Summary, 2011–12 School Year*, 2013, http://www.p12.nysed.gov/irs/pressRelease/20130617/School-enroll-outcomes-and-diplomas-June172013.pdf.

22. "Education: Best High Schools," *U.S. News and World Report*, http://www.usnews.com/education/best-high-schools.

23. Cory Turner, ed., "Why America's Schools Have a Money Problem," *Morning Edition*, NPR, April 18, 2016, http://www.npr.org/2016/04/18/474256366/why-americas-schools-have-a-money-problem?sc=tw.

24. Joseph Popiolkowski, "New Census Report Finds Majority of Buffalo's Children Live in Poverty: Statistics Show Rate Has Jumped from 45% to 50.6%," *Buffalo News*, September 18, 2014, http://www.buffalonews.com/city-region/new-census-report-finds-majority-of-buffalos-children-live-in-poverty-20140918.

25. Dan Telvock, "Asthma Plagues Peace Bridge Neighborhood," *Investigative Post*, May 25, 2014, http://www.investigativepost.org/2013/05/25/asthma-epidemic-near-peace-bridge.

26. Dan Telvock, "Rochester Leads on Lead While Buffalo Dallies," *Investigative Post*, November 12, 2014, https://www.investigativepost.org/2014/11/12/buffalo-lacks-leadership-lead-poisoning-problem.

27. Kathy Georgiades, Michael H. Boyle, and Eric Duku, "Contextual Influences on Children's Mental Health and School Performance: The Moderating Effects of Family Immigrant Status," *Child Development* 78, no. 5 (2007): 1572–1591.

28. Doug Sanders, "Where to Find School Bullies? Not Where You Might Expect," *Globe and Mail* (Toronto), September 17, 2016, http://www.theglobeandmail.com/opinion/where-to-find-school-bullies-not-where-you-might-expect/article31930773.

29. Economic Innovation Group (EIG), *The 2016 Distressed Communities Index: An Analysis of Community Well-Being across the United States* (Washington, DC: Economic Innovation Group, 2016), http://eig.org/wp-content/uploads/2016/02/2016-Distressed-Communities-Index-Report.pdf. See also http://eig.org/dci.

30. Nelson D. Schwartz, "Poorest Areas Have Missed Out on Boons of Recovery, Study Finds," *New York Times*, February 24, 2016, http://www.nytimes.com/2016/02/25/business/economy/poorest-areas-have-missed-out-on-boons-of-recovery-study-finds.html?ref=topics&_r=0.

31. *Texas Department of Housing and Community Affairs et al. v. Inclusive Communities Project, Inc. et al.*, 576 USC, Docket No. 13-1371 (June 25, 2015).

32. Kriston Capps, "What the Supreme Court's 'Disparate Impact' Decision Means for the Future of Fair Housing," *CityLab* (from the *Atlantic*), June 25, 2015, http://www.citylab.com/housing/2015/06/what-the-supreme-courts-disparate-impact-decision-means-for-the-future-of-fair-housing/396704.

33. Joseph P. Lawrence, *Socrates among Strangers* (Evanston, IL: Northwestern University Press, 2015), x.

Chapter 7

1. *Browder v. Gayle*, 142 F. Supp. 707 (1956); *Browder v. Gayle*, 352 U.S. 903 (1956).

2. "An Act to authorize the President to award a gold medal on behalf of the Congress to Rosa Parks in recognition of her contributions to the Nation," 106th Congress Public Law 26, May 4, 1999 (S. 531), http://www.gpo.gov/fdsys/pkg/PLAW-106publ26/html/PLAW-106publ26.htm.

3. *Brown v. Board of Education of Topeka*, Kansas 347 U.S. 483 (1954), 349 U.S. 294 (1955).

4. *Plessy v. Ferguson*, 163 U.S. 537 (1896).

5. John Rawls, *A Theory of Justice*, rev. ed. (1971; Oxford: Oxford University Press, 1999), 3.

6. Bryan C. Pilkington, "Dignity, Health, and Membership: Who Counts as One of Us?" *Journal of Medicine and Philosophy* 41, no. 1 (2016): 119.

7. Klaus Schaffer and Elliott Sclar, *Access for All: Transportation and Urban Growth* (New York: Columbia University Press, 1980), 3.

8. Harvey J. Miller, "Measuring Space-Time Accessibility Benefits within Transportation Networks: Basic Theory and Computational Procedures," *Geographical Analysis* 31, no. 2 (1999): 187–212.

9. United Nations, Convention on the Rights of Persons with Disabilities, Preamble (a), 2007, http://www.un.org/disabilities/documents/convention/convoptprot-e.pdf.

10. Richard L. Church and James R. Marston, "Measuring Accessibility for People with Disability," *Geographical Analysis* 35, no. 1 (2003): 84.

11. Janin Hadlaw, "The London Underground Map: Imagining Modern Time and Space," *Design Issues* 19, no. 1 (2003): 25–35.

12. Ken Garland, *Mr. Beck's Underground Map* (Weald, Middlesex: Capital Transport Publishing, 2003), 25.

13. Ibid., 7.

14. Jennifer Quinn, "Bob Crow Was Champion of London Transport Workers," *Toronto Star*, March 12, 2014, http://www.thestar.com/news/world/2014/03/11/bob_crow_was_champion_of_london_transport_workers.html.

15. Tom Koch, "Spaced Out in the City: The Wrinkled World of Transit for Those with Limited Mobility," *Disability Studies Quarterly* 26, no. 2 (2008), http://dsq-sds.org/article/view/94/94.

16. Elizabeth Czupta, "Broken CTA Facilities, Slow Repairs Create Problems for Disabled Customers," *ChicagoTalks*, May 12, 2009, http://www.chicagotalks.org. This was one of a series of reports

on the failure of the Chicago Transit Authority to accommodate mobility-limited users. Sued in 2000 by disability rights groups, CTA officials agreed to maintain a database of all complaints filed under the Americans with Disabilities Act. For more, see Kirsten Steinbeck, "Injury and Equipment Breakdowns Continue to Trouble Some Disabled CTA Riders," *ChicagoTalks*, May 12, 2009, http://www.chicagotalks.org/?p=2208.

17. Sasha Blair-Goldensohn, "New York Has a Great Subway, if You're Not in a Wheelchair," *New York Times*, March 27, 2017, https://www.nytimes.com/2017/03/29/opinion/new-york-has-a-great-subway-if-youre-not-in-a-wheelchair.html.

18. Anna I. Torres-Davis, "The Need for Improved Transportation Options for the Elderly and the Elder Advocate's Role," *Journal of Poverty Law and Policy* 42, nos. 5–6 (2008): 281–291.

19. Melanie A. Rapino and Thomas J. Cooke, "Commuting, Gender Roles, and Entrapment: A National Study Utilizing Spatial Fixed Effects and Control Groups," *Professional Geographer* 63, no. 2 (2011): 277–278.

20. Carole Thomas, *Female Forms: Experiencing and Understanding Disability* (Buckingham: Open University Press, 2002), 43–44. Also see her "Disability Theory: Key Ideas, Issues, and Thinkers," in *Disability Studies Today*, ed. Colin Barnes, Len Barton, and Mike Oliver (Malden, MA: Routledge, 2002), 38–57; Imrie Rob and Claire Edwards, "The Geographies of Disability: Reflections on the Development of a Sub-Discipline," *Geography Compass* 1, no. 3 (2007): 623–649, http://onlinelibrary.wiley.com/doi/10.1111/j.1749-8198.2007.00032.x/pdf.

21. Alison Porter, "Compromise and Constraint: Examining the Nature of Transport Disability in the Context of Local Travel," *World Transport Policy and Practice* 8, no. 2 (2002): 9–16.

22. Inger Marie Lid and Per Koren Solvang, "(Dis)ability and the Experience of Accessibility in the Urban Environment," *European Journal of Disability Research* 10, no. 2 (2016): 181–194.

23. Union of the Physically Impaired against Segregation (UPIAS), *Fundamental Principles of Disability* (London: UPIAS, 1976), 3. "Disability is a situation caused by social conditions. ... It is society which disables physically impaired people."

24. United Nations, Convention on the Rights of Persons with Disabilities, 2008, https://www.un.org/development/desa/disabilities/convention-on-the-rights-of-persons-with-disabilities.html.

25. For a discussion of disability theory and justice, see Jonas-Sébastion Beaudry, "Beyond (Models of) Disability?" *Journal of Medicine and Philosophy* 41, no. 1 (2016): 215.

26. John Pickles, *A History of Spaces: Cartographic Reason, Mapping and the Geo-coded World* (London: Routledge, 2004).

27. Bieke Cattoor and Chris Perkins, "Re-cartographies of Landscape: New Narratives in Architectural Atlases," *Cartographic Journal* 51, no. 2 (2014): 167.

28. Todd Litman, "Evaluating Transportation Equity," *World Transport Policy and Practice* 8, no. 2 (2002): 50–65.

29. The British Equality Act 2010 is reproduced online at http://www.legislation.gov.uk/ukpga/2010/15/pdfs/ukpga_20100015_en.pdf.

30. Details on the 2010 legislation are accessible in the British archives online at http://www.legislation.gov.uk/ukpga/2010/15.

31. Alice Maynard, "Can Measuring the Benefits of Accessible Transport Enable a 'Seamless' Journey?" *Journal of Transport and Land Use* 2 (2009): 21–30.

32. By 2015 the system had been changed again, although the basic program remained unchanged. See https://tfl.gov.uk/plan-a-journey.

33. Mei-Po Kwan, Alan T. Murray, Morton E. O'Kelly, and Michael Tiefelsdorf, "Recent Advances in Accessibility Research: Presentation, Methodology, and Applications," *Journal of Geographical Systems* 5 (2003): 129–138, http://meipokwan.org/Paper/JGS_2003_Conclude.pdf.

34. Harvey J. Miller, "Place-Based versus People-Based Geographic Information Science," *Geography Compass* 1, no. 3 (2007): 503–535.

35. Mei-Po Kwan, "Gender and Individual Access to Urban Opportunities: A Study Using Space-Time Measures," *Professional Geographer* 51, no. 2 (1999): 211–227.

36. Miller, "Measuring Space-Time Accessibility Benefits."

37. James R. Marston, Reginald G. Golledge, and C. Michael Costanzo, "Investigating Travel Behavior of Non-driving Blind and Vision Impaired People: The Role of Public Transit," *Professional Geographer* 49, no. 2 (1997): 235–345.

38. See, e.g., Richard L. Church and James R. Marston, "Measuring Accessibility for People with Disability," *Geographical Analysis* 35, no. 1 (2003): 83–96.

39. Barbara Starfield, "The Hidden Inequality in Health Care," *International Journal of Equity in Health* 10, no. 15 (2011), http://www.equityhealthj.com/content/10/1/15.

40. Wenwu Tang and David A. Bennett, "The Explicit Representation of Context in Agent-Based Models of Complex Adaptive Spatial Systems," *Annals of the Association of American Geographers* 100, no. 5 (2010): 1128–1155.

41. Mark Ovenden, *Transit Maps of the World* (London: Penguin, 2003).

Chapter 8

1. See, e.g., Editorial, "Hospitals Must Embrace Donor Organ Programs to Save Lives," *Toronto Star*, April 28, 2014, http://www.thestar.com/opinion/editorials/2014/04/28/hospitals_must_embrace_donor_organ_programs_to_save_lives_editorial.html.

2. Richard Titmuss, *The Gift Relationship: From Human Blood to Social Policy* (New York: Pantheon Books, 1971).

3. Nancy Scheper-Hughes, "Rotten Trade, Millennial Capitalism, Human Values and Global Justice in Organs Trafficking," *Journal of Human Rights* 2, no. 2 (2003): 197–226.

4. Joseph J. Fins, "Severe Brain Injury and Organ Donation: A Call for Temperance," *Virtual Mentor* 14, no. 3 (2012): 221–226.

5. Joseph J. Fins, *Rights Come to Mind: Brain Injury, Ethics, and the Struggle for Consciousness* (New York: Cambridge University Press, 2015), 54–58.

6. Franklin G. Miller and Robert D. Truog, "Rethinking the Ethics of Vital Organ Donations," *Hastings Center Report* 38, no. 6 (2008): 38–46.

7. Robert D. Truog and Franklin G. Miller, "The Dead Donor Rule and Organ Transplantation," *New England Journal of Medicine* 359, no. 7 (2008): 674, http://www.nejm.org/doi/full/10.1056/NEJMp0804474#t=article. For a discussion of these issues, see Tom Koch, *Thieves of Virtue: When Bioethics Stole Medicine* (Cambridge, MA: MIT Press, 2012), 60–64.

8. National Organ Transplant Act, Pub. L. No. 98-507, 98 Stat. 2339 (1984).

9. Titmuss, *The Gift Relationship.*

10. James F. Blumstein, "Government's Role in Organ Transplantation Policy," *Journal of Health Politics, Policy and Law* 14, no. 1 (1989): 5–40.

11. Task Force on Organ Transplantation, Department of Health and Human Services, *Organ Transplantation: Issues and Recommendations* (Washington, DC: Government Printing Office, 1986), xix.

12. Ibid., xxi.

13. Martin Benjamin, Carl Cohen, and Eugene Grochowski, "What Transplantation Can Teach Us about Health Care Reform," *New England Journal of Medicine* 330, no. 12 (1994): 858–860, http://www.nejm.org/doi/full/10.1056/NEJM199403243301211.

14. Nancy Scheper-Hughes, "The Global Traffic in Human Organs," *Current Anthropology* 41, no. 2 (2000): 197.

15. Steven A. Finkler, "Cost-Effectiveness of Regionalization: The Heart Surgery Example," *Inquiry* 16, no. 3 (1979): 266, http://www.ncbi.nlm.nih.gov/pmc/articles/PMC1072250/pdf/hsresearch00532-0070.pdf.

16. The map (fig. 8.1) was published on the UNOS website in 2014. By 2016, the map had been changed to include a brighter color spectrum of reds and oranges and a different projection. See https://www.unos.org/transplantation/matching-organs/regions.

17. Dario Del Rizzo et al., "The Role of Donor Age and Ischemic Time on Survival following Orthotropic Heart Transplantation," *Journal of Heart and Lung Transplant* 18, no. 4 (1999): 310–319, http://www.ncbi.nlm.nih.gov/m/pubmed/10226895/?i=2&from=/14666043/related.

18. Richard Morrill, "Efficiency and Equity of Optimum Location Networks," *Antipode* 6, no. 1 (1974): 43.

19. Donna Shalala, "Final Rule: Organ Procurement and Transplantation Network," *Federal Register* 63, no. 16288 (1998). Also see Tom Koch, "The Organ Transplant Dilemma," *OR/MS Today* 26, no. 1 (1999): 22–28, http://www.orms-today.org/orms-2-99/kochmain.html.

20. For a discussion of the "Final Rule," see Tom Koch, *Scarce Goods: Justice, Fairness, and Organ Transplantation* (Westport, CT: Praeger Books, 2001), 57–58, 73–74.

21. Koch, "The Organ Transplant Dilemma."

22. David M. Smith, "Geography and Ethics: A Moral Turn?" *Progress in Human Geography* 21, no. 4 (1997): 583–590.

23. Alan B. Pritsker, "Organ Transplantation Allocation Policy Analysis," *OR/MS Today* 25, no. 4 (1998), http://www.orms-today.org/orms-8-98/transplant.html.

24. Tom Koch, *The Limits of Principle: Deciding Who Lives and What Dies* (Westport, CT: Praeger Books, 1998).

25. Tom Koch, "Transplantation: Fairness vs. Efficiency," *OR/MS Today* 25, no. 3 (October 1998): 8.

26. Robert Steinbrook, "Allocating Livers: Devising a Fair System," *New England Journal of Medicine* 336, no. 6 (February 1997): 436–438.

27. This was the subject of a fine dissertation by Susan Shudd, "The Impact of Travel on Transplantation Outcomes" (PhD diss., Yale University, 1997).

28. Koch, *Scarce Goods*.

29. In 2015 UNOS listed the total cost of a heart transplant from the first admission to the six-month evaluation, and drugs, at $997,000. See UNOS, "Transplant Living," http://www.transplantliving.org/before-the-transplant/financing-a-transplant/the-costs.

30. Nick Cassavetes, dir., *John Q.* (New Line Cinema, February 2002).

31. Institute of Medicine Committee on Organ Procurement and Transplantation Policy, *Organ Procurement and Transplantation: Assessing Current Policies and the Potential Impact of the DHHS Final Rule* (Washington, DC: Institute of Medicine, 1999), 68.

32. Ibid., 35–36.

33. David R. Williams, "Race, Socioeconomic Status, and Health: The Added Effects of Racism and Discrimination," *Annals of the New York Academy of Sciences* 896 (1999): 173, https://deepblue.lib.umich.edu/bitstream/handle/2027.42/71908/j.1749-6632.1999.tb08114.x.pdf?sequence=1.

34. Vanessa Grubbs, "Good for Harvesting, Bad for Planting," *Health Affairs* 25, no. 1 (2007): 232–237, http://content.healthaffairs.org/content/26/1/232.full.

35. Centers for Disease Control (CDC), "U.S. Public Health Service Syphilis Study at Tuskegee," "The Tuskegee Timeline," page last updated December 8, 2016, http://www.cdc.gov/tuskegee/timeline.htm.

36. Rebecca Skloot, *The Immortal Life of Henrietta Lacks* (New York: Broadway Books, 2010).

37. Organ Procurement and Transplantation Network (OPTN), "National Data," (Washington, DC: Health Resources and Services Administration, US Department of Health and Human Services), http://optn.transplant.hrsa.gov/latestData/rptData.asp.

38. US Census Bureau, "State and County Quick Facts," accessed June 7, 2014, https://www.census.gov/quickfacts/table/PST045216/00.

39. Population data were recovered from a US Census Bureau data site, accessed June 9, 2014, https://www.census.gov/quickfacts/table/PST045216/00.

40. Mark Schweda and Silke Schicktanz, "Why Public Moralities Matter: The Relevance of Socio-empirical Premises for the Ethical Debate on Organ Markets," *Journal of Medicine and Philosophy* 39, no. 3 (2014): 218.

41. Nancy Scheper-Hughes, "The Global Traffic in Human Organs," *Current Anthropology* 41, no. 2 (2000): 197.

Chapter 9

1. Peter Singer, *A Darwinian Left: Politics, Evolution, and Cooperation* (New Haven, CT: Yale University Press, 1999), 37.

2. Adam Haslett, "A Poet's Brief," in *Cotton Tenants: Three Families*, by James Agee and Walker Evans, ed. John Summers (Brooklyn, NY: Melville House, 2013), 13.

3. Jeff McMahan, *The Ethics of Killing: Problems at the Margins of Life* (New York: Oxford University Press, 2002), 218.

4. Chris Kaposy, "A Disability Critique of the New Prenatal Test for Down Syndrome," *Kennedy Institute of Ethics Journal* 23, no. 4 (2013): 311.

5. Waldo Tobler, "A Computer Movie Simulating Urban Growth in the Detroit Region," *Economic Geography* 46, no. 2 (1970): 234–240.

6. United Nations, *The Universal Declaration of Human Rights* (1948; New York: United Nations Department of Public Information, 2007), http://www.un.org/en/documents/udhr.

7. Robert Coles, *Children of Crisis: Selections from the Pulitzer Prize—Winning Five-Volume Children of Crisis Series* (Boston: Little, Brown, 2003).

8. Andrea Elliott and Ruth Fremson, "Invisible Child," *New York Times Magazine*, December 9, 2013.

9. Peter J. Hotez, "Tropical Diseases: The New Plague of Poverty," *New York Times*, August 9, 2012, SR4.

10. Dan Smith, *The State of the World Atlas*, 9th ed. (New York: Penguin Books, 2012).

11. Michael Kidron and Dan Smith, *The War Atlas: Armed Conflict, Armed Peace* (Portsmouth, NH: Heinemann Educational Publishers, 1983).

12. On this point, see my "Fighting Disease, like Fighting Fires: The Lessons Ebola Teaches," *Canadian Geographer* 60, no. 2 (2016), doi:10.1111/cag.12258.

13. Lauren La Rose, "Bangladesh Factory Collapse Prompts Reforms, but Long-Term Impact Uncertain," *Global News*, December 13, 2013, http://globalnews.ca/news/1035856/bangladesh-factory-collapse-prompts-reforms-but-long-term-impact-uncertain.

14. Jennifer Wells, "Little Changed on Anniversary of Bangladesh Factory Collapse: Wells," *Toronto Star*, April 22, 2016, http://www.thestar.com/business/2016/04/22/little-changed-on-anniversary-of-bangladesh-factory-collapse-wells.html.

15. James A. Tyner, *War, Violence, and Population: Making the Body Count* (New York: Guilford Press, 2009), 196.

16. Robert J. Bellah, Richard Madesen, William M. Sullivan, Ann Swidler, and Steven M. Tripton, *Habits of the Heart: Individualism and Commitment in American Life* (New York: Harper & Row, 1985), 6.

17. Ibid., 37. These quotes are the core of Bellah et al.'s analysis of contemporary American life and its reflection of Tocqueville's conclusions.

18. Alexis de Tocqueville, *Journey to America*, ed. J. P. Mayer, trans. George Lawrence (London: Faber & Faber, 1959), 15. These are Tocqueville's edited notebooks. There are a variety of print editions by various translators, as well as various online versions. One from Penn State, for example, can be found at http://seas3.elte.hu/coursematerial/LojkoMiklos/Alexis-de-Tocqueville-Democracy-in-America.pdf.

19. Marshall Berman, *All That Is Solid Melts into Air* (New York: Penguin Books, 1988), 15.

20. Jonathan Schlefer, "Today's Most Mischievous Misquotation," *Atlantic Monthly* 281, no. 3 (1998): 16–19, http://www.mindspring.com/~mfpatton/smithmisquoted.pdf.

Chapter 10

1. Susan Levin, *Plato's Rivalry with Medicine: A Struggle and Its Dissolution* (New York: Oxford University Press, 2014), 19.

2. This view of the fourth estate as the broadcaster for prior, official estates is long-standing. It ignores, however, the move to investigative journalism, editorial arguments, and the broad political perspective of many journals and journalists. For a more detailed discussion of the limits of the reportorial form, and potentials for others, see my *The News as Myth: Fact and Context in Journalism* (Westport, CT: Greenwood Press, 1990).

3. Ulf Strohmayer and Matthew Hannah, "Domesticating Postmodernism," *Antipode* 24, no. 1 (1992): 36.

4. John Rawls, *A Theory of Justice*, rev. ed. (1971; Oxford: Oxford University Press, 1999), 121; and for a commentary, see Brian Barry, *The Liberal Theory of Justice: A Critical Examination of the Principal Doctrines in "A Theory of Justice" by John Rawls* (New York: Oxford University Press, 1973), 11.

5. Max Tholl, "A Line Can Turn into a Horrifyingly Rigid Reality," *The Idea List*, April 4, 2016, http://idealistmag.com/borders/a-line-can-turn-into-a-horrifyingly-rigid-reality.

6. Cheryl J. Misak, Douglas B. White, and Robert D. Truog, "Medically Inappropriate or Futile Treatment: Deliberation and Justification," *Journal of Medicine and Philosophy* 41, no. 1 (2016): 96.

7. Charles S. Peirce, "How to Make Our Ideas Clear," *Popular Science Monthly* 12 (January 1878): 294, https://en.wikisource.org/wiki/Popular_Science_Monthly/Volume_12/January_1878/Illustrations_of_the_Logic_of_Science_II.

8. Ibid., 292.

9. Kenneth Hirsch, personal communication, October 2015. Ken Hirsch is a psychiatrist whose interest in moral stress and injury stems from his treatment of US veterans with post-traumatic stress. In those cases, he seeks to help patients to perceive a way to reconcile their moral values with the realities of war and their actions in war as soldiers under the direction of military superiors.

10. Misak et al., "Medically Inappropriate or Futile Treatment," 96.

11. Nicky Priaulx, Martin Weinel, and Anthony Wrigley, "Rethinking Moral Expertise," *Health Care Analysis*, August 8, 2014, https://www.academia.edu/7943443/Rethinking_Moral_Expertise_Health_Care_Analysis_2014_with_N_Priaulx_and_M_Weinel.

12. Famously, this argument gained currency among bioethicists in the late 1980s and into the 1990s. See Daniel Callahan, *Setting Limits: Medical Goals in an Aging Society* (New York: Simon & Schuster, 1987).

13. Robert H. Binstock and Stephen G. Post, eds., *Too Old for Health Care? Controversies in Medicine, Law, Economics, and Ethics* (Baltimore, MD: The Johns Hopkins University Press, 1991).

14. Christopher Hamlin's detailed study of both Chadwick's report and the social context in which it was created remains a critical text in this area. See Hamlin, *Public Health and Social Justice in the Age of Chadwick: Britain, 1800–1854* (Cambridge: Cambridge University Press, 1998).

15. Gary Bloch, "The Cost of Poverty Affects Us All," *Toronto Star*, December 6, 2016, A13, https://www.thestar.com/opinion/commentary/2016/12/06/the-cost-of-poverty-affects-us-all.html. For detailed figures, see Nate Laurie, *The Cost of Poverty: An Analysis of the Economic Cost of Poverty in Ontario* (Toronto: Ontario Association of Food Banks, 2008).

16. Canada without Poverty, "Basic Statistics," http://www.cwp-csp.ca/poverty/just-the-facts.

17. Julie A. Nelson, *Economics for Humans* (Chicago: University of Chicago Press, 2006), 12.

18. Edmund Burke, "Maxims and Opinions, Moral, Political and Economical …," in *Burke's Writing and Speeches*, vol. 1 (London: John C. Nimmo, 1887), 35.

19. Susan Sontag, ed., *A Barthes Reader* (New York: Hill & Wang, 1982), 130.

20. The idea of the predicate act is usually framed in terms of criminal actions whose predicate is an earlier and greater violation. Its best-known use in the United States has been in the Racketeer Influenced and Corrupt Organizations Act (RICO). Here I apply the idea in a broader and more general context.

21. Paul Cloke, "Deliver Us from Evil? Prospects for Living Ethically and Acting Politically in Human Geography," *Progress in Human Geography* 26, no. 5 (2002): 588.

22. Andrew Jameton, *Nursing Practice: The Ethical Issues* (Englewood Cliffs, NJ: Prentice Hall, 1984), 6.

23. Tessy A. Thomas and Lawrence B. McCullough, "A Philosophical Taxonomy of Ethically Significant Moral Distress," *Journal of Medicine and Philosophy* 400, no.1 (2015): 103.

24. Kelly Grant, "'Discharge Him at All Costs': A Case Study in Overcrowding at Ontario's Hospitals," *Globe and Mail* (Toronto), May 9, 2017, https://beta.theglobeandmail.com/news/national/ontario-hospital-overcrowding/article34918036/?ref=http://www.theglobeandmail.com&; Kelly Grant, "Bad Hospital Discharges among Top Complaints, Ontario Watchdog Finds," *Globe and Mail* (Toronto), May 12, 2017, https://beta.theglobeandmail.com/news/national/bad-hospital-discharges-among-top-complaints-ontario-watchdog-finds/article34963271/?ref=http://www.theglobeandmail.com&.

25. Bonnie Chan, "Moral Distress," *Qmentum Quarterly: Quality in Health Care* 7, no. 2 (summer 2014): 13, http://www.accreditation.ca/sites/default/files/qq-2014-summer-en.pdf.

26. Alasdair MacIntyre, *Whose Justice? Which Rationality?* (Notre Dame, IN: University of Notre Dame Press, 1988), 263.

References

Agee, James, and Walker Evans. 1939. *Let Us Now Praise Famous Men*. New York: Houghton Mifflin.

Agee, James, and Walker Evans. 2013. *Cotton Tenants: Three Families*. Ed. John Summers. Brooklyn, NY: Melville House.

AP/Washington Post. 1991. Agency shows way for Gulf forces. *Washington Post*, January 2, A13. http://www.highbeam.com/doc/1P2-1042125.html.

Austin, J. L. 1975. *How to Do Things with Words*. 2nd ed. Cambridge, MA: Harvard University Press.

Barkhorn, Eleanor. 2013. Why are American schools still segregated? *Atlantic.com*, November 13. http://www.theatlantic.com/education/archive/2013/11/why-are-american-schools-still-segregated/281126.

Barney, Timothy. 2015. *Mapping the Cold War: Cartography and the Framing of America's International Power*. Chapel Hill: University of North Carolina Press.

Barry, Brian. 1973. *The Liberal Theory of Justice: A Critical Examination of the Principal Doctrines in "A Theory of Justice" by John Rawls*. New York: Oxford University Press.

Barthes, Roland. 1972. *Mythologies*. Trans. Annette Lavers. New York: Hill & Wang.

Barthes, Roland. 1979. *The Eiffel Tower and Other Mythologies*. Trans. Richard Howard. New York: Farrar, Straus & Giroux.

Barthes, Roland. 1982. The imagination of the sign. In *A Barthes Reader*, ed. Susan Sontag, 211–218. New York: Hill & Wang.

Beauchamp, Tom, and James F. Childress. 2001. *Principles of Biomedical Ethics*. 5th ed. New York: Oxford University Press.

Beaudry, Jonas-Sébastion. 2016. Beyond (models of) disability? *Journal of Medicine and Philosophy* 41 (1): 210–228.

Bellah, Robert J., Richard Madesen, William M. Sullivan, Ann Swidler, and Steven M. Tripton. 1985. *Habits of the Heart: Individualism and Commitment in American Life*. New York: Harper & Row.

Benjamin, Martin, Carl Cohen, and Eugene Grochowski. 1994. What transplantation can teach us about health care reform. *New England Journal of Medicine* 330 (12): 858–860. http://www.nejm.org/doi/full/10.1056/NEJM199403243301211.

Berlinger, Nancy. 2016. *Are Workarounds Ethical? Managing Moral Problems in Health Care Systems*. New York: Oxford University Press.

Berman, Marshall. 1988. *All That Is Solid Melts into Air*. New York: Penguin Books.

Bertin, Jacques. 2011. *Semiology of Graphics: Diagrams, Networks, Maps*. Trans. W. J. Berg. Redlands, CA: Esri Press.

Best, Joel. 2012. *Damned Lies and Statistics*. Updated ed. Berkeley: University of California Press.

Binstock, Robert H., and Stephen G. Post, eds. 1991. *Too Old for Health Care? Controversies in Medicine, Law, Economics, and Ethics*. Baltimore, MD: The Johns Hopkins University Press.

Blair-Goldensohn, Sasha. 2017. New York has a great subway, if you're not in a wheelchair. *New York Times*, March 27. https://www.nytimes.com/2017/03/29/opinion/new-york-has-a-great-subway-if-youre-not-in-a-wheelchair.html.

Bliss, Laura. 2015. How school districts seal their students into poverty. *CityLab* (from the *Atlantic*), July 22. http://www.citylab.com/politics/2015/07/how-school-districts-seal-their-students-into-poverty/399116/?utm_source=SFTwitter.

Bloch, Gary. 2013. Poverty: A clinical tool for primary care in Ontario. Handout of the Ontario College of Family Physicians, rev. February 2013. http://ocfp.on.ca/docs/default-source/cme/poverty-and-medicine-march-2013.pdf.

Blumstein, James F. 1989. "Government's role in organ transplantation policy." *Journal of Health Politics, Policy and Law* 14 (1): 5–39.

Boscoe, Frank. 2014. The relationship between poverty and cancer incidence in the United States. Paper presented at the American Association of Geographers Annual Meeting, Tampa, FL, April 10.

Boscoe, Francis P., Kevin A. Henry, Recinda L. Sherman, and Christopher J. Johnson. 2016. The relationship between cancer incidence, stage and poverty in the United States. *International Journal of Cancer* 139:607–612.

Bradford, Harry. 2013. Bangladesh to raise minimum wage for garment workers. *Huffington Post*, May 12. http://www.huffingtonpost.com/2013/05/12/bangladesh-minimum-wage-garment-workers_n_3263347.html.

Buchanan, A. 1830. Report of the diseases which prevailed among the poor of Glasgow, during the summer of 1830. *Glasgow Medical Journal* 3:440.

Bullard, W. 1909. The placement of high-grade imbecile girls. *Boston Medical and Surgical Journal* 160 (2): 776–777.

Burke, Edmund. 1887. Maxims and opinions, moral, political and economical. ... In *Burke's Writing and Speeches*, vol. 1, John C. Nimmo, ed. London: The Strand.

Callahan, Daniel. 1987. *Setting Limits: Medical Goals in an Aging Society*. New York: Simon & Schuster.

Callahan, Daniel. 2003. Individual good and common good: A communitarian approach to bioethics. *Perspectives in Biology and Medicine* 46 (4): 496–507.

Capps, Kriston. 2015. What the Supreme Court's "disparate impact" decision means for the future of fair housing. *CityLab* (from the *Atlantic*), June 25. http://www.citylab.com/housing/2015/06/what-the-supreme-courts-disparate-impact-decision-means-for-the-future-of-fair-housing/396704.

Cassavetes, N., dir. 2002. *John Q.* New Line Cinema, February.

Cattoor, Bieke, and Chris Perkins. 2014. Re-cartographies of landscape: New narratives in architectural atlases. *Cartographic Journal* 51 (2): 166–178.

CDC/EPA Taskforce. 2005. *Environmental Health Needs and Habitability Assessment, Hurricane Katrina*. Washington, DC: Centers for Disease Control and Prevention and US Environmental Protection Agency.

Cecco, Leyland. 2016. Canada takes second spot globally on social-progress ranking. *Globe and Mail* (Toronto), June 29. http://www.theglobeandmail.com/news/social-progress-index-canada-isalright/article30647376/.

Centers for Disease Control (CDC). 2013. U.S. Public Health Service Syphilis Study at Tuskegee. The Tuskegee timeline. Page last updated December 8, 2016. http://www.cdc.gov/tuskegee/timeline.htm.

Chan, Bonnie. 2014. Moral distress. *Qmentum Quarterly: Quality in Health Care* 7 (2): 12–18. http://www.accreditation.ca/sites/default/files/qq-2014-summer-en.pdf.

Chua, Kao-Ping. 2008. The case for universal health care. Reston, VA: American Medical Student Association. https://www.amsa.org/wp-content/uploads/2015/03/CaseForUHC.pdf.

Church, Richard L., and James R. Marston. 2003. Measuring accessibility for people with disability. *Geographical Analysis* 35 (1): 83–96.

Cloke, Paul. 2002. Deliver us from evil? Prospects for living ethically and acting politically in human geography. *Progress in Human Geography* 26 (5): 587–604.

Cohen, Patricia. 2015. Prosperity caught in gap, study finds. *New York Times/Honolulu Star-Advertiser*, February 4. http://www.pressreader.com/usa/honolulu-star-advertiser/20150204/textview.

Coles, Robert. 2003. *Children of Crisis: Selections from the Pulitzer Prize–Winning Five-Volume Children of Crisis Series*. Boston: Little, Brown.

Collingwood, Robin G. 1939/1972. *An Essay on Metaphysics*. Washington, DC: Regnery.

Community Service Society. 2006. *Mapping Poverty in New York City: Pinpointing the Impact of Poverty, Community by Community*. New York: United Way of New York City. http://b.3cdn.net/nycss/cc0e2b7c121eba2938_20m6ifgc8.pdf.

Cook, Karen S. 2005. A lifelong curiosity about maps. *Cartographic Perspectives* 51:43–54.

Cooper, Edmund. 1854. *Report on an enquiry and examination in the state of the drainage of the homes situate in that part of the Parish of St. James, Westminster*. London: Metropolitan Commission of Sewers.

Cosgrove, Denis. 2006. Epistemology, geography and cartography: Thoughts on the reaction of Brian Harley's cartographic theories. Paper presented at the Association of American Geographers Annual Meeting, Chicago, IL, March 10.

Cribb, Alan. 2001. Integrity at work: Managing routine moral stress as professional roles. *Nursing Philosophy* 12:119–127.

Czupta, Elizabeth. 2009. Broken CTA facilities, slow repairs create problems for disabled customers. *ChicagoTalks*, May 12. http://www.chicagotalks.org.

D'Aliesio, Renata. 2016. Failure to safeguard. *Globe and Mail* (Toronto), May 13. http://www.theglobeandmail.com/news/national/inquiry-exposes-holes-in-canadian-forces-mental-health-caresystem/article30021281.

Delkeskamp-Hayes, Corinna, ed. 2015a. Handicapped by egalitarianism: Europe's public health care systems. Special issue, *Journal of Medicine and Philosophy* 40:2.

Delkeskamp-Hayes, Corinna. 2015b. Morality at the expense of others: Equality, solidarity, taxes, and debts in European public health care. *Journal of Medicine and Philosophy* 40 (2): 121–136.

Del Rizzo, Dario, Alan H. Menkis, Peter W. Pflugfelder, Richard J. Novick, F. Neil MCKenzie, Walter Boyd, and William J. Kostuk. 1999. The role of donor age and ischemic time on survival following orthotropic heart transplantation. *Journal of Heart and Lung Transplantation* 18 (4): 310–319. http://www.ncbi.nlm.nih.gov/m/pubmed/10226895/?i=2&from=/14666043/related.

DeNavas-Walt, Carmen, Bernadette D. Proctor, and Jessica C. Smith. 2009. Income, poverty, and health insurance coverage in the United States: 2008. Washington, DC: US Department of Commerce, Economics and Statistics Administration, US Census Bureau. http://www.census.gov/prod/2009pubs/p60-236.pdf.

DeNavas-Walt, Carmen, Bernadette D. Proctor, and Jessica C. Smith. 2010. Income, poverty, and health insurance coverage in the United States: 2009. Washington, DC: US Department of Commerce, Economics and Statistics Administration, US Census Bureau. https://www.census.gov/prod/2010pubs/p60-238.pdf.

DeParle, Jason. 2012. For poor, leap to college often ends in a hard fall. *New York Times*, December 22. http://www.nytimes.com/2012/12/23/education/poor-students-struggle-as-class-plays-a-greater-role-in-success.html.

Devesa, Susan S., Dan J. Grauman, William J. Blot, Gene A. Pennello, Robert N. Hoover, and Joseph F. Fraumeni Jr. 1999. *Atlas of Cancer Mortality in the United States: 1950–1994*. Washington, DC: US Government Printing Office (NIH Publ. No. [NIH] 99-4564). https://archive.org/stream/atlasofcancermor00nati/atlasofcancermor00nati_djvu.txt.

Ditto, Peter H., David A. Pizarro, and David Tannenbaum. 2009. Motivated moral reasoning. In *Psychology of Learning and Motivation*, vol. 50, ed. B. H. Ross, 307–338. http://www.sciencedirect.com/science/journal/00797421/50?sdc=1.

D'Oro, Giusepina, and James Connelly. 2015. Robin George Collingwood. In *The Stanford Encyclopedia of Philosophy*, ed. Edward N. Zalta. http://plato.stanford.edu/archives/sum2015/entries/collingwood.

Economic Innovation Group (EIG). 2016. *The 2016 Distressed Communities Index: An Analysis of Community Well-Being across the United States*. Washington, DC: Economic Innovation Group. http://eig.org/wp-content/uploads/2016/02/2016-Distressed-Communities-Index-Report.pdf.

Editorial: The big idea. 1996. *British Medical Journal* 312:985.

Editorial: Hospitals must embrace donor organ programs to save lives. 2014. *Toronto Star*, April 28. http://www.thestar.com/opinion/editorials/2014/04/28/hospitals_must_embrace_donor_organ_programs_to_save_lives_editorial.html.

Elden, Stewart, and Eduardo Mendieta, eds. 2011. *Reading Kant's Geography*. Albany: SUNY Press.

Elliott, Andrea, and Ruth Fremson. 2013. Invisible child. *New York Times Magazine*, December 9. http://www.nytimes.com/projects/2013/invisible-child/#/?chapt=0.

Ellison, Peter T. 2009. A review of Sarah Blaffer Hrdy, *Mothers and Others*. *Evolutionary Psychology* 7 (3): 442–448.

Enders, Alexandra, and Zachary Brandt. 1997. Using geographic information system technology to improve emergency management and disaster response for people with disabilities. *Journal of Disability Policy Studies* 17 (4): 223–229.

English, Kathy. 2015. The shades of grey of journalism ethics: Public editor. *Toronto Star*, October 2. http://www.thestar.com/opinion/public_editor/2015/10/02/the-shades-of-grey-of-journalism-ethics-public-editor.html.

Ericson, Mathew. 2011. When maps shouldn't be maps. *New York Times*, October 11. http://www.ericson.net/content/2011/10/when-maps-shouldnt-be-maps.

Fieser, James. 2001. Ethics. *Internet Encyclopedia of Philosophy*. http://www.iep.utm.edu/ethics/#H2.

Fiel, Jeremy A. 2013. Decomposing school resegregation: Social closure, racial imbalance, and racial isolation. *American Sociological Review* 78 (5): 828–848. http://asr.sagepub.com/content/78/5/828.full.pdf+html.

Fink, Sheri. 2013. *Five Days at Memorial*. New York: Crown Publishers.

Finkler, Steven A. 1979. Cost-effectiveness of regionalization: The heart surgery example. *Inquiry* 16 (3): 266. http://www.ncbi.nlm.nih.gov/pmc/articles/PMC1072250/pdf/hsresearch00532-0070.pdf.

Fins, Joseph J. 2012. Severe brain injury and organ donation: A call for temperance. *Virtual Mentor* 14 (3): 221–226.

Fins, Joseph J. 2015. *Rights Come to Mind: Brain Injury, Ethics, and the Struggle for Consciousness*. New York: Cambridge University Press.

Fox, Hayley. 2013. Skid Row TB epidemic is "alarming," but the community is well-versed in disease. *Blogdowntown*, Southern California Public Radio, February 22. http://blogdowntown.com/2013/02/7146-skid-row-tb-epidemic-is-alarming-but-the.

Garland, Ken. 2003. *Mr. Beck's Underground Map*. Weald, Middlesex: Capital Transport Publishing.

Georgiades, Kathy, Michael H. Boyle, and Eric Duku. 2007. Contextual influences on children's mental health and school performance: The moderating effects of family immigrant status. *Child Development* 78 (5): 1572–1591.

Gertz, Clifford. 1973. *The Interpretation of Cultures: Selected Essays*. New York: Basic Books.

Gibbons, Robert D., David Meltzer, and Nai-hua Duan. 2000. Waiting for organ transplantation. *Science* 287 (5451): 237–238.

Goffman, Erving. 1979. *The Presentation of Self in Everyday Life*. New York: Doubleday.

Golden, Hallie. 2016. Rocket engineer who predicted space shuttle *Challenger* disaster dies. Associated Press/*Toronto Star*, March 24. http://www.thestar.com/news/world/2016/03/24/rocket-engineer-who-predicted-space-shuttle-challenger-disaster-dies.html.

Grant, Kelly. 2017a. "Discharge him at all costs": A case study in overcrowding at Ontario hospitals. *Globe and Mail* (Toronto), May 9. https://beta.theglobeandmail.com/news/national/ontario-hospital-overcrowding/article34918036/.

Grant, Kelly. 2017b. Bad hospital discharges among top complaints, Ontario watchdog finds. *Globe and Mail* (Toronto), May 12. https://beta.theglobeandmail.com/news/national/bad-hospital-discharges-among-top-complaints-ontario-watchdog-finds/article34963271/.

Grubbs, Vanessa. 2007. Good for harvesting, bad for planting. *Health Affairs* 25 (1): 232–237. http://content.healthaffairs.org/content/26/1/232.full.

Gundersen, Linda. 2000. Mapping it out: Using atlases to detect patterns in health care, disease, and mortality. *Annals of Internal Medicine* 133 (2): 161–164.

Hadlaw, Janin. 2003. The London Underground map: Imagining modern time and space. *Design Issues* 19 (1): 25–35.

Haidt, Jonathan, and Jesse Graham. 2006. When morality opposes justice: Conservatives have moral intuitions that liberals may not recognize. *Social Justice Research* 20 (1): 98–116.

Hamlin, Christopher. 1998. *Public Health and Social Justice in the Age of Chadwick: 1800–1854*. New York: Cambridge University Press.

Harley, Brian J. 1991. Can there be a cartographic ethics? *Cartographic Perspectives* 10:9–17. http://www.nacis.org/documents_upload/cp10summer1991.pdf.

Harvey, David. 1973. *Social Justice and the City*. Oxford: Blackwell.

Haslett, Adam. 2013. A poet's brief. In *Cotton Tenants: Three Families*, by James Agee and Walker Evans. Ed. John Summers. Brooklyn, NY: Melville House.

Hayasaki, Erika. 2016. How poverty affects the brain. *Newsweek*, August 25. http://www.newsweek.com/2016/09/02/how-poverty-affects-brains-493239.html.

Herzog, David. 2003. *Mapping the News: Case Studies in GIS and Journalism*. Redlands, CA: Esri Press.

Hippocrates. 2003. *Airs, Waters, and Places*. Trans. Francis Adams. Cambridge, MA: The Internet Classics Archive. http://classics.mit.edu/Hippocrates/airwatpl.8.8.html.

Hotez, Peter. J. 2012. Tropical diseases: The new plague of poverty. *New York Times*, August 9, SR4.

Hsieh, Ching-Chi, and M. D. Pugh. 1993. Poverty, income inequality, and violent crime: A meta-analysis of recent aggregate data studies. *Criminal Justice Review* 18 (2): 182–202.

Huff, Darrell. 1954. *How to Lie with Statistics*. New York: W. W. Norton.

Hume, David. 1748/1999. *An Enquiry concerning Human Understanding*. Ed. Tom L. Beacham. Oxford: Oxford University Press. http://www.earlymoderntexts.com/pdfs/hume1748.pdf.

Hunter, Tracy. 2014. The Gini coefficient, a measure of income inequality. Illustration in "Measuring Poverty." *Wikipedia*. https://en.wikipedia.org/wiki/Measuring_poverty#/media/File:2014_Gini_Index_World_Map,_income_inequality_distribution_by_country_per_World_Bank.svg.

Imrie, Rob, and Claire Edwards. 2007. The geographies of disability: Reflections on the development of a sub-discipline. *Geography Compass* (3): 623–649.

Institute of Medicine Committee on Organ Procurement and Transplantation Policy. 1999. *Organ Procurement and Transplantation: Assessing Current Policies and the Potential Impact of the DHHS Final Rule*. Washington, DC: Institute of Medicine.

Jameton, Andrew. 1984. *Nursing Practice: The Ethical Issues*. Englewood Cliffs, NJ: Prentice Hall.

Jennings, Bruce, Frederick J. Wertz, and Mary Beth Morrissey. 2016. Nudging for health and the predicament of agency: The relational ecology of autonomy and care. *Journal of Theoretical and Philosophical Psychology* 36 (2): 81–99.

Kahneman, Daniel. 2011. *Thinking Fast and Slow*. New York: Farrar, Straus & Giroux.

Kailes, June I., and A. Enders. 2007. Moving beyond "special needs." *Journal of Disability Policy Studies* 17 (4): 230–237.

Kaplan, Gerald. 2016. Why the NDP shouldn't be pacifists. *Globe and Mail* (Toronto), September 20. http://www.theglobeandmail.com/news/politics/why-the-ndp-shouldnt-be-pacifists/article31969227/.

Kaposy, Chris. 2013. A disability critique of the new prenatal test for Down syndrome. *Kennedy Institute of Ethics Journal* 23 (4): 299–324.

Kasarda, John D. 1989. Urban industrial transition and the underclass. In *The Ghetto Underclass: Social Science Perspectives*, ed. William J. Wilson, 26–47. Annals of the American Academy of Political and Social Science, vol. 501. Newbury Park, CA: Sage.

Keller, Bess. 2001. N.Y. system of state aid thrown out. *Education Week*, January 17. http://www.edweek.org/ew/articles/2001/01/17/18newyork.h20.html.

Kelly, B. 1998. Preserving moral integrity: A follow-up study with new graduate nurses. *Journal of Advanced Nursing* 28 (5): 1134–1145.

Kenny, Anthony. 2005. *Wittgenstein*. Rev. ed. Malden, MA: Blackwell.

Kidron, Michael, and Dan Smith. 1983. *The War Atlas: Armed Conflict, Armed Peace*. Portsmouth, NH: Heinemann Educational Publishers.

Koch, Tom. 1990. *The News as Myth: Fact and Context in Journalism*. Westport, CT: Greenwood Press.

Koch, Tom. 1998. *The Limits of Principle: Deciding Who Lives and What Dies*. Westport, CT: Praeger Books.

Koch, Tom. 1998. Transplantation: Fairness vs. efficiency. *OR/MS Today* 25 (3): 8.

Koch, Tom. 1999a. The organ transplant dilemma. *OR/MS Today* 26 (1): 22–28. http://www.orms-today.org/orms-2-99/kochmain.html.

Koch, Tom. 1999b. They might as well be in Bolivia: Race, ethnicity and the problem of solid organ donation. *Theoretical Medicine and Bioethics* 20 (6): 563–575.

Koch, Tom. 2002. *Scarce Goods: Justice, Fairness, and Organ Transplantation*. Westport, CT: Praeger Books.

Koch, Tom. 2005. *Cartographies of Disease: Maps, Mapping, and Medicine*. Redlands, CA: Esri Press.

Koch, Tom. 2006. False truths: Ethics and mapping as a profession. *Cartographic Perspectives* 54:4–15.

Koch, Tom. 2006. Bioethics as ideology: Conditional and unconditional values. *Journal of Medicine and Philosophy* 31 (3): 251–268.

Koch, Tom. 2008. Spaced out in the city: The wrinkled world of transit for those with limited mobility. *Disability Studies Quarterly* 26 (2). http://dsq-sds.org/article/view/94/94.

Koch, Tom. 2011a. *Disease Maps: Epidemics on the Ground*. Chicago: University of Chicago Press.

Koch, Tom. 2011b. *Thieves of Virtue: When Bioethics Stole Medicine*. Cambridge, MA: MIT Press.

Koch, Tom. 2014. The Hippocratic thorn in bioethics' hide: Cults, sects, and strangeness. *Journal of Medicine and Philosophy* 39 (1): 75–88.

Koch, Tom. 2014. Prince Kropotkin: Public health's patron saint. *International Journal of Epidemiology* 43 (6): 1681–1685. http://ije.oxfordjournals.org/content/early/2014/10/21/ije.dyu206.

Koch, Tom. 2016. Fighting disease, like fighting fires: The lessons Ebola teaches. *Canadian Geographer* 60:2. doi:10.1111/cag.12258.

Koch, Tom, and Ken Denike. 2003a. Geography, justice, and inequality: The New York City school funding controversy. *Journal of Geography* 102 (5): 193–201.

Koch, Tom, and Ken Denike. 2003b. Geography, the problem of scale, and processes of allocation: The US National Organ Transplant Act of 1986, amended 1990. In *Law and Geography*, ed. Jane Holder and Carolyn Harrison, 109–137. London: Oxford University Press.

Koch, Tom, and Kenneth Denike. 2009. Crediting his critics' concerns: Remaking John Snow's map of Broad Street cholera, 1854. *Social Science and Medicine* 69 (8): 1246–1251.

Koch, Tom, Ken Denike, Warren Gill, and Raymond Torchinsky. 2010. Accessibility and access: A new approach to transportation barriers. Paper presented at American Association of Geographers Annual Meeting, Washington, DC, April 16.

Kozol, Jonathan. 1991. *Savage Inequalities: Children in America's Schools*. New York: Harper Perennial.

Kozol, Jonathan. 1995. *Amazing Grace: The Lives of Children and the Conscience of a Nation*. New York: Harper Perennial.

Kozol, Jonathan. 2005. *The Shame of the Nation: The Restoration of Apartheid Schooling in America*. New York: Three Rivers Press.

Kozol, Jonathan. 2012. *Fire in the Ashes: Twenty-five Years among the Poorest Children in America*. New York: Crown Publishers.

Kwan, Mei-Po. 1999. Gender and individual access to urban opportunities: A study using space-time measures. *Professional Geographer* 51 (2): 211–227.

Kwan, Mei-Po, Alan T. Murray, Morton E. O'Kelly, and Michael Tiefelsdorf. 2003. Recent advances in accessibility research: Presentation, methodology, and applications. *Journal of Geographical Systems* 5:129–138. http://meipokwan.org/Paper/JGS_2003_Conclude.pdf.

La Rose, Lauren. 2013. Bangladesh factory collapse prompts reforms, but long-term impact uncertain. *Global News*, December 17. http://globalnews.ca/news/1035856/bangladesh-factory-collapse-prompts-reforms-but-long-term-impact-uncertain.

Law, John. 2004. *After Method: Mess in Social Science Research*. New York: Routledge.

Law, John, and Annemarie Mol. 2002. *Complexities: Social Studies of Knowledge Practices*. Durham, NC: Duke University Press.

Lawrence, Joseph P. 2015. *Socrates among Strangers*. Evanston, IL: Northwestern University Press.

Lee, Trymaine, and Black Matt. 2015. Geography of poverty: A journey through forgotten America. *MSNBC*. Produced by Amy Pereira, Mina Liu, and Sam Petulla. http://www.msnbc.com/interactives/geography-of-poverty/index.html.

Lemann, Nicholas. 2000. Atlas shrugs: The new geography argues that maps have shaped the world. *New Yorker*, April 9, 131–134.

Levin, Susan. 2014. *Plato's Rivalry with Medicine: A Struggle and Its Dissolution*. New York: Oxford University Press.

Lewis, Kristen, and Sarah Burd-Sharps. 2016. High school graduation in New York City: Is neighborhood still destiny? Social Research Council: Measure of America (New York: Data2.Go), May 2016. http://www.measureofamerica.org/d2gnyc/high-school-graduation-in-new-york-city.

Lewontin, Richard C. 1993. *Biology as Ideology: The Doctrine of DNA*. New York: Harper Perennial.

Liao, Matthew S. 2016. Review of *What We Owe Each Other*, by T. M. Scanlon. http://www.smatthewliao.com/wp-content/uploads/2008/06/scanlon.pdf.

Lid, Inger Marie, and Per Koren Solvang. 2015. (Dis)ability and the experience of accessibility in the urban environment. *European Journal of Disability Research* (December). doi:10.1016/j.alter.2015.11.003.

Litman, Todd. 2002. Evaluating transportation equity. *World Transport Policy and Practice* 8:2.

Lonegran, Raymond. 1941. *Mr. Justice Brandeis, Great American*. St. Louis, MO: Modern View Press.

Lynch, John, George Davey Smith, Sam Harper, and Marianne Hillemeier. 2004. Is income inequality a determinant of population health? Part 2: A systematic review. *Milbank Quarterly* 82 (2): 355–400.

Lynch, John, George Davey Smith, Sam Harper, Marianne Hillemeier, Nancy Ross, George A. Kaplan, and Michael Wolfson. 2004. Is income inequality a determinant of population health? Part 1: A systematic review. *Milbank Quarterly* 82 (1): 5–99.

Macartney, Suzanne, Alemayehu Bishaw, and Kayla Fontenot. 2013. *Poverty Rates for Selected Detailed Race and Hispanic Groups by State and Place: 2007–2011*. Washington, DC: US Department of Commerce, Economics and Statistics Administration, US Census Bureau. http://www.census.gov/prod/2013pubs/acsbr11-17.pdf.

MacCormick, Ronald. 2014. How many deaths can be directly attributed to cigarette smoking every year? *Canadian Journal of Diagnosis* 31 (6): 29.

MacIntyre, Alasdair. 1966. *A Short History of Ethics*. New York: Collier Books.

MacIntyre, Alasdair. 1984. *After Virtue*. 2nd ed. Notre Dame, IN: University of Notre Dame Press.

Macmurray, John. 1957. *The Self as Agent*. London: Faber & Faber.

Marston, James R., Reginald G. Golledge, and C. Michael Costanzo. 1997. Investigating travel behavior of non-driving blind and vision impaired people: The role of public transit. *Professional Geographer* 49 (2): 235–345.

Mason, Thomas J., Frank W. McKay, Robert Hoover, William J. Blot, and Joseph F. Fraumeni Jr. 1979. *Atlas of Cancer Mortality for U.S. Counties: 1950–1969*. DHEW Pub. No. (NIH) 75-780). Washington, DC: US Department of Health, Education, and Welfare/National Institutes of Health.

Mathur, Anuradha, and Dilip da Cunha. 2001. *Mississippi Floods: Designing a Shifting Landscape*. New Haven, CT: Yale University Press.

Matthews, Dylan. 2017. Child poverty in the US is a disgrace: Experts are embracing this simple plan to fix it. *Vox*, April 27. https://www.vox.com/policy-and-politics/2017/4/27/15388696/child-benefit-universal-cash-tax-credit-allowance.

Maynard, Alice. 2009. Can measuring the benefits of accessible transport enable a "seamless" journey? *Journal of Transport and Land Use* 2:21–30.

McHaffie, Patrick, Sona Karentz Andrews, Michael Dobson, and Anon. 1991. Ethical problems in cartography: A roundtable commentary. *Cartographic Perspectives* 7:3–13.

McLaren, G. L., and M. R. S. Baine. 1998. *Deprivation and Health in Scotland: Insights from NHS Data*. Edinburgh: ISD Scotland Publications. http://www.scotpho.org.uk/downloads/deprivation/isd-deprivationreport-1998.pdf.

McMahan, Jeff. 2002. *The Ethics of Killing: Problems at the Margins of Life*. New York: Oxford University Press.

McQuaid, Linda. 2016. The upside of Kevin O'Leary's political ambitions. *Toronto Star*, January 22. http://www.thestar.com/opinion/commentary/2016/01/22/the-upside-of-kevin-olearys-political-ambitions.html.

Meadowcroft, John. 2015. Just healthcare? The moral failure of single-tier basic healthcare. *Journal of Medicine and Philosophy* 40 (2): 152–168.

Midgley, Mary. 1984. *Wickedness: A Philosophical Essay*. New York: Routledge Classics.

Midgley, Mary. 2002. *Evolution as a Religion: Strange Hopes and Stranger Fears*. Rev. ed. New York: Routledge.

Midgley, Mary. 2014. *Are You an Illusion?* New York: Routledge.

Mikkonen, Juha, and Dennis Raphael. 2010. *Social Determinants of Health: The Canadian Facts*. Toronto: York University School of Health Policy and Management. http://www.thecanadianfacts.org.

Miller, Franklin G., and Robert D. Truog. 2008. Rethinking the ethics of vital organ donations. *Hastings Center Report* 38 (6): 38–46.

Miller, Harvey J. 1999. Measuring space-time accessibility benefits within transportation networks: Basic theory and computational procedures. *Geographical Analysis* 31 (2): 187–212.

Miller, Harvey J. 2007. Place-based versus people-based geographic information science. *Geography Compass* 1 (3): 503–535.

Misak, Cheryl J., Douglas B. White, and Robert D. Truog. 2016. Medically inappropriate or futile treatment: Deliberation and justification. *Journal of Medicine and Philosophy* 41 (1): 90–114.

Mol, Annemarie, and John Law. 2006. Complexities: An introduction. In *Social Studies of Knowledge Practices*, ed. John Law and Annemarie Mol, 1–23. Durham, NC: Duke University Press.

Monmonier, Mark. 1991. Ethics and map design: Six strategies for confronting the traditional one-map solution. *Cartographic Perspectives* 10:3–9.

Monmonier, Mark. 1996. *How to Lie with Maps*. 2nd ed. Chicago: University of Chicago Press.

Monmonier, Mark. 1999. *Maps with the News: The Development of American Journalistic Cartography*. Chicago: University of Chicago Press.

Morrill, Richard. 1974. Efficiency and equity of optimum location networks. *Antipode* 6 (1): 41–46.

Morris, W. E. 2013. David Hume. In *Stanford Encyclopedia of Philosophy*, ed. Edward N. Zalta. http://plato.stanford.edu/archives/spr2013/entries/hume.

Muehlenhaus, Ian. 2013. The design and composition of persuasive maps. *Cartography and Geographic Information Science* 39 (2): 401–414.

Muehlenhaus, Ian. 2014. Going viral: The look of online persuasive maps. *Cartographica* 49 (1): 18–34.

Murrow, Edward R. 1960. Harvest of shame. *CBS Reports*, November 26. http://www.youtube.com/watch?v=yJTVF_dya7E.

Institute of Medicine (NIM), Committee on Organ Transplantation. n.d. *Organ Procurement and Transplantation: Assessing Current Policies and the Potential Impact of the DHHS Final Rule*. Washington, DC: National Academy Press.

National Oceanic and Atmospheric Administration (NOAA). 2013. Historical hurricane tracks. US Department of Commerce, National Oceanographic and Marine Service. http://csc.noaa.gov/hurricanes.

Nortvedt, Per. 2012. The normativity of clinical health care: Perspectives on moral realism. *Journal of Medicine and Philosophy* 37 (3): 296–309.

New York State Department of Education. 2013. *Public School Total Cohort Graduation Rate and Enrollment Outcome Summary, 2011–12 School Year*. http://www.p12.nysed.gov/irs/pressRelease/20130617/School-enroll-outcomes-and-diplomas-June172013.pdf.

Organ Procurement and Transplantation Network (OPTN). 2014. National data. Washington, DC: Health Resources and Services Administration, US Department of Health and Human Services. http://optn.transplant.hrsa.gov/latestData/rptData.asp.

Ovenden, Mark. 2003. *Transit Maps of the World*. London: Penguin.

Owners' Loan Corporation, and Federal Savings and Loan Corporation Annual Reports, 1933–1952. Washington, DC: Federal Reserve Archive. http://fraser.stlouisfed.org/publication/?pid=70.

Ozminkowski, Ronald J., Allan J. White, Andrea Hassol, and Michael Murphy. 1998. What if socioeconomics made no difference? Access to a cadaver kidney transplantation as an example. *Medical Care* 38 (9): 1396–1406.

Ozminkowski, Ronald J., Allan J. White, Andrea Hassol, and Michael Murphy. 1997. Minimizing racial disparity regarding receipt of a cadaver kidney transplant. *American Journal of Kidney Diseases* 30 (6): 749–759.

Parkes, Edmund A. 1855. Review: *Mode of Communication of Cholera* by John Snow. *British and Foreign Medico-Chirurgical Review* 15:449–456.

Parsons, Talcott. 1951. *The Social System*. London: Routledge & Kegan Paul.

Perkin, Harold. 1989. *The Rise of Professional Society: England since 1880*. London: Routledge.

Pattison, Stephen, and Andrew Edgar. 2011. The problem with integrity. *Nursing Philosophy* 12:81–82.

Peabody, Fred, dir. 2016. *All Governments Lie: Truth, Deception and the Spirit of I. F. Stone*. White Pine Pictures, August 3. http://www.whitepinepictures.com/9212-2/?v=3e8d115eb4b3.

Peirce, Charles S. 1878. How to make our ideas clear. *Popular Science Monthly* 12:286–302. https://en.wikisource.org/wiki/Popular_Science_Monthly/Volume_12/January_1878/Illustrations_of_the_Logic_of_Science_II.

Petrovich, Curt. 2016. Back to zero: Curt Petrovich, Typhoon Haiyan, the Philippines, 2013. *Back Story*. CBC Radio, July 16. http://www.cbc.ca/radio/backstory/back-to-zero-curt-petrovich-typhoon-haiyan-the-philippines-2013-1.3285514.

Pickering, Andrew. 1997. *The Mangle of Practice: Time, Agency, and Science*. Chicago: University of Chicago Press.

Pickett, Kate E., and Richard G. Wilkinson. 2005. Adolescent birth rates, total homicides, and income inequality in rich countries. *American Journal of Public Health* 95 (7): 1181–1183.

Pickles, John. 2004. *A History of Spaces: Cartographic Reason, Mapping and the Geo-coded World*. London: Routledge.

Pickstone, John F. 1984. Ferriar's fever to Kay's cholera: Disease and social structure in Cottonopolis. *History of Science* 22:401–419. http://articles.adsabs.harvard.edu/full/1984HisSc.22.401P.

Pilkington, Bryan C. 2016. Dignity, health, and membership: Who counts as one of us? *Journal of Medicine and Philosophy* 41 (1): 115–129.

Popiolkowski, Joseph. 2014. New census report finds majority of Buffalo's children live in poverty: Statistics show rate has jumped from 45% to 50.6%. *Buffalo News*, September 18. http://www.buffalonews.com/city-region/new-census-report-finds-majority-of-buffalos-children-live-in-poverty-20140918.

Porter, Allison. 2002. Compromise and constraint: Examining the nature of transport disability in the context of local travel. *World Transport Policy and Practice* 8 (2): 9–16.

Priaulx, Nicky, Martin Weinel, and Anthony Wrigley. 2014. Rethinking moral expertise. *Health Care Analysis*, August 8. http://www.academia.edu/7943443/Rethinking_Moral_Expertise_Health_Care_Analysis_2014_.

Pritsker, Alan B. 1998. Organ transplantation allocation policy analysis. *OR/MS Today* 25 (4). http://www.orms-today.org/orms-8-98/transplant.html.

Quinn, Jennifer. 2014. Bob Crow was champion of London transport workers. *Toronto Star*, March 12. http://www.thestar.com/news/world/2014/03/11/bob_crow_was_champion_of_london_transport_workers.html.

Raphael, Denis L., and Toba Bryant. 2014. Income inequality is killing thousands of Canadians a year. *Toronto Star*, November 23. http://www.thestar.com/opinion/commentary/2014/11/23/income_inequality_is_killing_thousands_of_canadians_every_year.html.

Rapino, Melanie A., and Thomas J. Cooke. 2011. Commuting, gender roles, and entrapment: A national study utilizing spatial fixed effects and control groups. *Professional Geographer* 63 (2): 277–294.

Rawls, John. 1971/1993. *A Theory of Justice*. Rev. ed. Oxford: Oxford University Press.

Reentmeister, Christy A. 2008. Moral damage to health care professionals and trainees: Legalism and other consequences for patients and colleagues. *Journal of Medicine and Philosophy* 33:27–43.

Renee, John, Tom Sanchez, Pam Jenkins, and Robert Peterson. 2009. Challenge of evacuating the carless in five major U.S. cities: Identifying the key issues. *Transportation Research Record: Journal of the Transportation Research Board* 2119:36–44. http://trrjournalonline.trb.org/doi/abs/10.3141/2119-05.

Rich, Nathaniel. 2012. The Lower Ninth Ward in New Orleans gives new meaning to "urban growth." *New York Times Magazine*, March 25. http://www.nytimes.com/2012/03/25/magazine/the-lower-ninth-ward-new-orleans.html?hpw&_r=0.

Risen, James. 2006. *State of War*. New York: Free Press.

Robinson, Arthur H., Joel L. Morrison, P. C. Muehrcke, A. John Kimerling, and Stephen G. Guptill. 1995. *Elements of Cartography*. 6th ed. Hoboken, NJ: John Wiley & Sons.

Roche, Mark W. 2006. Introduction to Hegel's theory of tragedy. *PhaenEx* 1 (2): 11–20.

Rosen, George. 1993. *A History of Public Health*. 2nd ed. Baltimore, MD: The Johns Hopkins University Press.

Sanders, Doug. 2016. Where to find school bullies? Not where you might expect. *Globe and Mail* (Toronto), September 17. http://www.theglobeandmail.com/opinion/where-to-find-school-bullies-not-where-you-might-expect/article31930773

Sassen, Saskia. 1991. *The Global City: New York, London, Tokyo*. Princeton, NJ: Princeton University Press.

Scanlon, Thomas. 1998. *What We Owe to Each Other*. Cambridge, MA: Harvard University Press.

Schaeffer, Klaus, and Elliott Sclar. 1980. *Access for All: Transportation and Urban Growth*. New York: Columbia University Press.

Scientists believe thousands of people have been exposed to a deadly outbreak of tuberculosis in downtown Los Angeles. 2013. *Daily Mail*, February 22. http://www.dailymail.co.uk/news/article-2283043/Thousands-exposed-deadly-TB-outbreak-Los-Angeles.html.

Schlefer, Jonathan. 1998. Today's most mischievous misquotation. *Atlantic Monthly* 281 (3): 16–19. http://www.mindspring.com/~mfpatton/smithmisquoted.pdf.

Schuurman, Nadine. 1999. Critical GIS: Theorizing an emerging science. *Cartographica* (Monograph 53) 36:4.

Schwartz, Nelson D. 2016. Poorest areas have missed out on boons of recovery, study finds. *New York Times*, February 24.

Schweda, Mark, and Silke Schicktanz. 2014. Why public moralities matter: The relevance of socio-empirical premises for the ethical debate on organ markets. *Journal of Medicine and Philosophy* 39 (3): 217–222.

Scottish Government. 2011. Premature mortality—from all causes, aged under 75 years. In *Long-Term Monitoring of Health Inequalities*. Edinburgh: St. Andrew's House. http://www.gov.scot/Publications/2011/10/21133633/3.

Shafran, David, Martin L. Smith, Barbara J. Daly, and David Goldfarb. 2016. Transplant ethics: Let's begin the conversation anew. *HEC Forum* 28 (2): 141–152. doi:10.1007/s10730-015-9285-5.

Shalala, Donna. 1998. Final rule: Organ procurement and transplantation network. *Federal Register* 63:16288.

Scheper-Hughes, Nancy. 2000. The global traffic in human organs. *Current Anthropology* 41 (2): 191–224.

Scheper-Hughes, Nancy. 2003. Rotten trade, millennial capitalism, human values and global justice in organs trafficking. *Journal of Human Rights* 2 (2): 197–226.

Shudd, Susan S. 1997. The impact of travel on transplantation outcomes. PhD diss., Yale University.

Shweder, Richard A. 1996. Ethnographic methods in contemporary perspective. In *Ethnography and Human Development*, ed. Richard Jessor, Anne Colby, and Richard A. Shweder, 3–52. Chicago: University of Chicago Press.

Singer, Peter. 1999. *A Darwinian Left: Politics, Evolution, and Cooperation*. New Haven, CT: Yale University Press.

Singer, Peter. 2003. *Practical Ethics*. 2nd ed. New York: Cambridge University Press.

Skloot, Rebecca. 2010. *The Immortal Life of Henrietta Lacks*. New York: Broadway Books.

Smith, Dan. 2012. *The State of the World Atlas*. 9th ed. New York: Penguin Books.

Smith, David M. 1997. Geography and ethics: A moral turn? *Progress in Human Geography* 21 (4): 583–590.

Snow, John. 1855. *On the Mode of Communication of Cholera*. 2nd ed. London: Churchill.

Snyder, Wallace S. 2011. *Principles and Practices for Advertising Ethics*. American Advertising Federation. https://www.aaf.org/_PDF/AAF%20Website%20Content/513_Ethics/IAE_Principles_Practices.pdf.

Starfield, Barbara. 2011. The hidden inequality in health care. *International Journal of Equity in Health* 10 (15). http://www.equityhealthj.com/content/10/1/15.

Steele, J. Michael. 2005. Darrell Huff and fifty years of *How to Lie with Statistics*. *Statistical Science* 20 (3): 205–209. http://www-stat.wharton.upenn.edu/~steele/Publications/PDF/TN148.pdf.

Steinbeck, Kirsten. 2009. Injury and equipment breakdowns continue to trouble some disabled CTA riders. *ChicagoTalks*, May 12. http://www.chicagotalks.org/?p=2208.

Steinbrook, Robert. 1997. Allocating livers—devising a fair system. *New England Journal of Medicine* 336 (6): 436–438.

Stocks, Percy. 1928. On the evidence for a regional distribution of cancer prevalence in England and Wales. *Report of the International Conference on Cancer* (London, UK), July 17–20, July 28.

Strohmayer, Ulf, and Matthew Hannah. 1992. Domesticating postmodernism. *Antipode* 24 (1): 29–55.

Tan, Sandra. 2013. Stacking the deck against Buffalo's six "failing schools." *Buffalo News*, July 23, A1.

Tang, Wenwu, and David A. Bennett. 2010. The explicit representation of context in agent-based models of complex adaptive spatial systems. *Annals of the Association of American Geographers* 100 (5): 1128–1155.

Task Force on Organ Transplantation. 1986. *Organ Transplantation: Issues and Recommendations*. Washington, DC: Government Printing Office.

Telvock, Dan. 2014. Asthma plagues Peace Bridge neighborhood. *Investigative Post*, May 25. http://www.investigativepost.org/2013/05/25/asthma-epidemic-near-peace-bridge.

Telvock, Dan. 2014. Rochester leads on lead while Buffalo dallies. *Investigative Post*, November 12. https://www.investigativepost.org/2014/11/12/buffalo-lacks-leadership-lead-poisoning-problem.

Tholl, Max. 2016. A line can turn into a horrifyingly rigid reality. *Idea List*. http://idealistmag.com/borders/a-line-can-turn-into-a-horrifyingly-rigid-reality.

Thomas, Carole. 1999. *Female Forms: Experiencing and Understanding Disability*. Buckingham: Open University Press.

Thomas, Carole. 2002. Disability theory: Key ideas, issues, and thinkers. In *Disability Studies Today*, ed. Colin Barnes, Len Barton, and Mike Oliver, 38–57. Malden, MA: Routledge.

Thomas, Tessy A., and Lawrence B. McCullough. 2015. A philosophical taxonomy of ethically significant moral distress. *Journal of Medicine and Philosophy* 40 (1): 102–120.

Thomson, Judith. 1990/2001. *The Realm of Rights*. Cambridge, MA: Harvard University Press.

Titmuss, Richard. 1971. *The Gift Relationship: From Human Blood to Social Policy*. New York: Pantheon Books.

Toble, Waldo. 1970. A computer movie simulating urban growth in the Detroit region. *Economic Geography* 46 (2): 234–240.

de Tocqueville, Alexis. 1959. *Journey to America*. Ed. J. P. Mayer. Trans. G. Lawrence. London: Faber & Faber.

Torres-Davis, Anna I. 2008. The need for improved transportation options for the elderly and the elder advocate's role. *Journal of Poverty Law and Policy* 42 (5–6): 281–291.

Truog, Robert D., and Franklin G. Miller. 2008. The dead donor rule and organ transplantation. *New England Journal of Medicine* 359 (7): 674. http://www.nejm.org/doi/full/10.1056/NEJMp0804474#t=article.

Turner, Cory. 2016. Why America's schools have a money problem. *Morning Edition*, NPR, April 18. http://www.npr.org/2016/04/18/474256366/why-americas-schools-have-a-money-problem?sc=tw.

Tyner, James A. 2009. *War, Violence, and Population: Making the Body Count*. New York: Guilford Press.

Tyner, Judith. 1974. Persuasive cartography: An examination of the map as a subjective tool of communication. PhD diss., University of California, Los Angeles.

Tyner, Judith. 1982. Persuasive cartography. *Journal of Geography* 81:140–144.

Union of Physically Impaired against Segregation (UPIAS). 1976. *Fundamental Principles of Disability*. London: UPIAS.

United Nations. 1948/2007. *Universal Declaration of Human Rights*. New York: United Nations Department of Public Information. http://www.un.org/en/documents/udhr.

United Nations. 2007. *Convention on the Rights of Persons with Disabilities*. http://www.un.org/disabilities/documents/convention/convoptprot-e.pdf.

UNOS. 2015. Transplant living. http://www.transplantliving.org/before-the-transplant/financing-a-transplant/the-costs

US Census Bureau. 2015. State and county quick facts. https://www.census.gov/quickfacts/table/PST045216/00.

Vallas, Rebecca, and Shawn Fremstead. 2014. Disability is a cause and consequence of poverty. *TalkPoverty.org*, September 18. https://talkpoverty.org/2014/09/19/disability-cause-consequence-poverty/.

Veatch, Robert M. 2012. *Hippocratic, Religious, and Secular Medical Ethics: The Points of Conflict*. Washington, DC: Georgetown University Press.

Vinten-Johansen, Peter, Howard Brody, Nigel Paneth, Steven Rachman, and Michael Russell Rip. 2003. *Cholera, Chloroform, and the Science of Medicine: A Life of John Snow*. New York: Oxford University Press.

Vistnes, J. P., and A. C. Monheit. 1997. *Health Insurance Status of the Civilian Noninstitutionalized Population: 1996*. AHCPR Pub. No. 97-0030. Rockville, MD: Agency for Health Care Policy and Research. http://meps.ahrq.gov/mepsweb/data_files/publications/rf1/rf1.pdf.

Wallace, Rodrick, Yi-Shan Huang, Peter Gould, and Deborah Wallace. 1997. The hierarchical diffusion of AIDS. *Social Science and Medicine* 44 (7): 935–947.

Ward, Stephen J. 2005. *The Invention of Journalism Ethics: The Path to Objectivity and Beyond*. Montreal, PQ: McGill University Press.

Watson, William. 2015. *The Inequality Trap: Fighting Capitalism instead of Poverty*. Toronto: University of Toronto Press.

Wells, Jennifer. 2016a. Little changed on anniversary of Bangladesh factory collapse: Wells. *Toronto Star*, April 22. http://www.thestar.com/business/2016/04/22/little-changed-on-anniversary-of-bangladesh-factory-collapse-wells.html.

Wells, Jennifer. 2016b. Michael Bloomberg could be the one to stop Trump. *Toronto Star*, February 16. http://www.thestar.com/business/2016/02/16/michael-bloomberg-could-be-the-one-to-stop-trump-wells.html.

Whitehead, Henry. 1855. Mr. Whitehead's report. In *Report of the Cholera Outbreak in the Parish of St. James, Westminster, during the Autumn of 1854*, 120–167. London: J. Churchill.

Wiggins, Osborne P., and Michael A. Schwartz. 2005. Richard Zaner's phenomenology of the clinical encounter. *Theoretical Medicine and Bioethics* 26 (1): 73–84.

Wilkinson, Richard G. 1996. *Unhealthy Societies: The Afflictions of Inequality*. New York: Routledge.

Wilkinson, Richard, and Michael Marmot, eds. 2003. *Social Determinants of Health: The Solid Facts*. 2nd ed. Copenhagen, Denmark: World Health Organization (European Office).

Williams, David R. 1999. Race, socioeconomic status, and health: The added effects of racism and discrimination. *Annals of the New York Academy of Sciences* 896:220–243. https://deepblue.lib.umich.edu/bitstream/handle/2027.42/71908/j.1749-6632.1999.tb08114.x.pdf?sequence=1.

Wilson, William J. ed. 1989. *The Ghetto Underclass: Social Science Perspectives*. Annals of the American Academy of Political and Social Science, vol. 501. Newbury Park, CA: Sage.

Wittgenstein, Ludwig. 1974. *Tractatus Logico-Philosophicus*. Rev. ed. Trans. C. K. Ogden. New York: Routledge.

Wood, David. 2014. The grunts: Damned if they kill, damned if they don't. *Huffington Post*, March 18. http://projects.huffingtonpost.com/moral-injury/the-grunts.

Wood, Denis. 1992. *The Power of Maps*. New York: Guilford Press.

Wood, Denis. 2002. The map as a kind of talk: Brian Harley and the confabulation of the inner and outer voice. *Visual Communication* 1 (2): 139–161.

Wood, Denis. 2013. The map's power. Paper presented at Deutscher Geographentag: Kongress für Wissenschaft, Schule, und Praxis, Passau, Germany, October 10.

Wood, Denis, and John Fels. 2008. *The Natures of Maps: Cartographic Constructions of the Natural World*. Chicago: University of Chicago Press.

Yakabuski, Konrad. 2016. Attacks on Joseph Boyden's identity should set off alarm bells. *Globe and Mail* (Toronto), December 29. http://www.theglobeandmail.com/opinion/attacks-on-joseph-boydens-identity-should-set-off-alarm-bells/article33444228.

Yang, Jennifer. 2013. L.A.'s Skid Row: Ground zero for the city's largest tuberculosis outbreak in a decade. *Toronto Star*, February 25. http://thestar.blogs.com/worlddaily/2013/02/street-scenes-from-skid-row-in-downtown-los-angeles-the-last-refuge-for-people-with-nowhere-else-to-go.html.

Legal Citations

Americans with Disabilities Act of 1990. (ADA) 42 U.S. Code. Chapter 126. http://www.ada.gov.

An Act to authorize the President to award a gold medal on behalf of the Congress to Rosa Parks in recognition of her contributions to the Nation. 106th Congress Public Law 26, May 4, 1999 [S. 531]. http://www.gpo.gov/fdsys/pkg/PLAW-106publ26/html/PLAW-106publ26.htm.

Browder v. Gayle, 142 F. Supp. 707 (1956).

Browder v. Gayle, 352 U.S. 903 (1956).

Brown v. Board of Education of Topeka, Kansas 347 U.S. 483 (1954) 349 U.S. 294 (1955).

Campaign for Fiscal Equity, Inc. et al. v. State of New York et al., 86 N.Y. 2d 307, 655 N.E.2d 661, 631 N.Y.S.2d 565 (June 15, 1995). http://www.edlawcenter.org/assets/files/pdfs/cfe/CFE%201995%20Decision.pdf.

Campaign for Fiscal Equity (CFE), Inc. v. State of New York, 86 N.Y. 2d 307 (June 13, 1996).

Campaign for Fiscal Equity (CFE), Inc. et al. v. State of New York et al., 100 N.Y. 2d 908 (2003). http://www.edlawcenter.org/assets/files/pdfs/cfe/CFE%202006%20Decision.pdf (accessed January 14, 2014).

Legal Information Institute. 2006. *Campaign for Fiscal Equality, Inc. v. State*, 85 N.Y. 2d 307 (June 13, 1995). Cornell University Law School. https://www.law.cornell.edu/nyctap/comments/i95_0156.htm#issue.

National Organ Transplant Act, Pub. L. No. 98-507; 98 Stat 2339 (1984).

Plessy v. Ferguson, 163 U.S. 537 (1896).

Racketeer Influenced and Corrupt Organizations Act (RICO). 18 U.S. C. Crimes and Criminal Procedures § 1961–1968 (84 Stat. 933-923).

Shaffer, Frederick P. 2003. Memorandum of law of the Association of the Bar of the City of New York, Amicus Curiae. *Kruger et al. v. Bloomberg et al.* For order and judgment pursuant to Article 78 of CPLR. *Superior Court of the State of New York*. Index No. 102510/03. May 28, 2003. http://www.nycbar.org/pdf/report/AMICUS%20BRIEF.pdf.

US Supreme Court. 2015. *Texas Department of Housing and Community Affairs, et al. v. Inclusive Communities Project Inc. et al.* U.S.C. 576 Docket No. 13-1371 (June 25). http://www.supremecourt.gov/opinions/14pdf/13-1371_m64o.pdf.

Index

Basic Bioethics

Arthur Caplan, editor

Books Acquired under the Editorship of Glenn McGee and Arthur Caplan

Peter A. Ubel, *Pricing Life: Why It's Time for Health Care Rationing*

Mark G. Kuczewski and Ronald Polansky, eds., *Bioethics: Ancient Themes in Contemporary Issues*

Suzanne Holland, Karen Lebacqz, and Laurie Zoloth, eds., *The Human Embryonic Stem Cell Debate: Science, Ethics, and Public Policy*

Gita Sen, Asha George, and Piroska Östlin, eds., *Engendering International Health: The Challenge of Equity*

Carolyn McLeod, *Self-Trust and Reproductive Autonomy*

Lenny Moss, *What Genes Can't Do*

Jonathan D. Moreno, ed., *In the Wake of Terror: Medicine and Morality in a Time of Crisis*

Glenn McGee, ed., *Pragmatic Bioethics*, 2nd edition

Timothy F. Murphy, *Case Studies in Biomedical Research Ethics*

Mark A. Rothstein, ed., *Genetics and Life Insurance: Medical Underwriting and Social Policy*

Kenneth A. Richman, *Ethics and the Metaphysics of Medicine: Reflections on Health and Beneficence*

David Lazer, ed., *DNA and the Criminal Justice System: The Technology of Justice*

Harold W. Baillie and Timothy K. Casey, eds., *Is Human Nature Obsolete? Genetics, Bioengineering, and the Future of the Human Condition*

Robert H. Blank and Janna C. Merrick, eds., *End-of-Life Decision Making: A Cross-National Study*

Norman L. Cantor, *Making Medical Decisions for the Profoundly Mentally Disabled*

Margrit Shildrick and Roxanne Mykitiuk, eds., *Ethics of the Body: Post-Conventional Challenges*

Alfred I. Tauber, *Patient Autonomy and the Ethics of Responsibility*

David H. Brendel, *Healing Psychiatry: Bridging the Science/Humanism Divide*

Jonathan Baron, *Against Bioethics*

Michael L. Gross, *Bioethics and Armed Conflict: Moral Dilemmas of Medicine and War*

Karen F. Greif and Jon F. Merz, *Current Controversies in the Biological Sciences: Case Studies of Policy Challenges from New Technologies*

Deborah Blizzard, *Looking Within: A Sociocultural Examination of Fetoscopy*

Ronald Cole-Turner, ed., *Design and Destiny: Jewish and Christian Perspectives on Human Germline Modification*

Holly Fernandez Lynch, *Conflicts of Conscience in Health Care: An Institutional Compromise*

Mark A. Bedau and Emily C. Parke, eds., *The Ethics of Protocells: Moral and Social Implications of Creating Life in the Laboratory*

Jonathan D. Moreno and Sam Berger, eds., *Progress in Bioethics: Science, Policy, and Politics*

Eric Racine, *Pragmatic Neuroethics: Improving Understanding and Treatment of the Mind-Brain*

Martha J. Farah, ed., *Neuroethics: An Introduction with Readings*

Jeremy R. Garrett, ed., *The Ethics of Animal Research: Exploring the Controversy*

Books Acquired under the Editorship of Arthur Caplan

Sheila Jasanoff, ed., *Reframing Rights: Bioconstitutionalism in the Genetic Age*

Christine Overall, *Why Have Children? The Ethical Debate*

Yechiel Michael Barilan, *Human Dignity, Human Rights, and Responsibility: The New Language of Global Bioethics and Bio-Law*

Tom Koch, *Thieves of Virtue: When Bioethics Stole Medicine*

Timothy F. Murphy, *Ethics, Sexual Orientation, and Choices about Children*

Daniel Callahan, *In Search of the Good: A Life in Bioethics*

Robert Blank, *Intervention in the Brain: Politics, Policy, and Ethics*

Gregory E. Kaebnick and Thomas H. Murray, eds., *Synthetic Biology and Morality: Artificial Life and the Bounds of Nature*

Dominic A. Sisti, Arthur L. Caplan, and Hila Rimon-Greenspan, eds., *Applied Ethics in Mental Healthcare: An Interdisciplinary Reader*

Barbara K. Redman, *Research Misconduct Policy in Biomedicine: Beyond the Bad-Apple Approach*

Russell Blackford, *Humanity Enhanced: Genetic Choice and the Challenge for Liberal Democracies*

Nicholas Agar, *Truly Human Enhancement: A Philosophical Defense of Limits*

Bruno Perreau, *The Politics of Adoption: Gender and the Making of French Citizenship*

Carl Schneider, *The Censor's Hand: The Misregulation of Human-Subject Research*

Lydia S. Dugdale, ed., *Dying in the Twenty-First Century: Towards a New Ethical Framework for the Art of Dying Well*

John D. Lantos and Diane S. Lauderdale, *Preterm Babies, Fetal Patients, and Childbearing Choices*

Harris Wiseman, *The Myth of the Moral Brain: The Limits of Moral Enhancement*

Nicholas G. Evans, Tara C. Smith, and Maimuna S. Majumder, eds., *Ebola's Message: Public Health and Medicine in the Twenty-First Century*

Jason L. Schwartz and Arthur L. Caplan, eds., *Vaccination Ethics and Policy: An Introduction with Readings*

Tom Koch, *Ethics in Everyday Places: Mapping Moral Stress, Distress, and Injury*

Printed in the United States
by Baker & Taylor Publisher Services